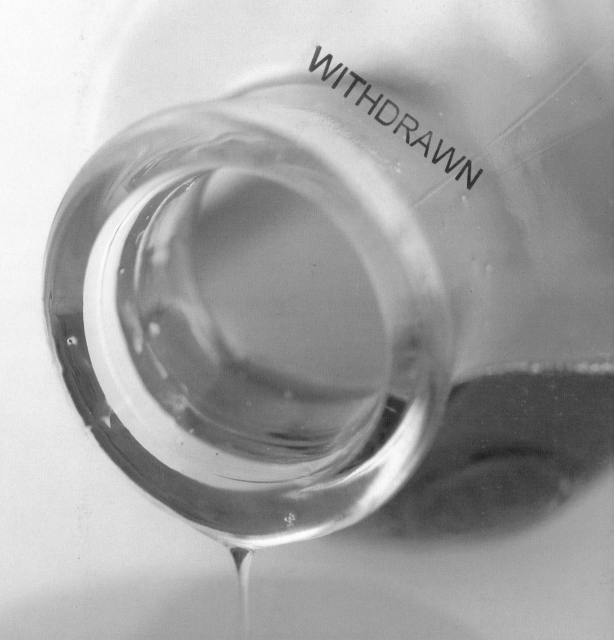

the complete book of
massage

THIS IS A CARLTON BOOK

Design © 2004 Carlton Books

Text copyright © 2004 Carlton pages 1–121 and pages 316–320
Text copyright © 2001 Mary Atkinson pages 122–315

This edition published by
Carlton Books Limited 2011
20 Mortimer Street
London W1T 3JW

10 9 8 7 6 5 4 3

Material for this book has previously appeared under the titles *Body Massage* (Carlton, 2004),
The Art of Indian Head Massage (Carlton, 2000) and *Hand & Foot Massage* (Carlton, 2001).
The views and advice given by the authors of the individual titles are not necessarily the
views or advice of the other author.

A CIP catalogue record for this book is available from the British Library.

ISBN 978 1 84732 946 2

Printed and bound in Dubai

Senior Executive Editor: Lisa Dyer
Cover design: Lucy Coley
Design: Barbara Zuñiga, Simon Mercer and Michael Spender
Art Direction: Trevor Newman and Diane Spender
Editors: Claire Richardson and Camilla MacWhannell
Picture Research: Alex Pepper
Photography: John Davis
Production Manager: Dawn Cameron

The author and publisher have made every effort to ensure that all information is correct and up to date
at the time of publication. Neither the author nor the publisher can accept responsibility for any accident, injury or damage that results from using the ideas, information and advice offered in this book.

It is important to consult your doctor before commencing any massage programme. This is particularly
the case if you have any existing medical condition, have had recent surgery or are pregnant. All
instructions should be read carefully. This book is not intended to replace personal instruction or
professional medical advice. The contraindications/cautions listed are guidelines only.

MARY ATKINSON with ESME FLOYD

the complete book of
massage

CARLTON
BOOKS

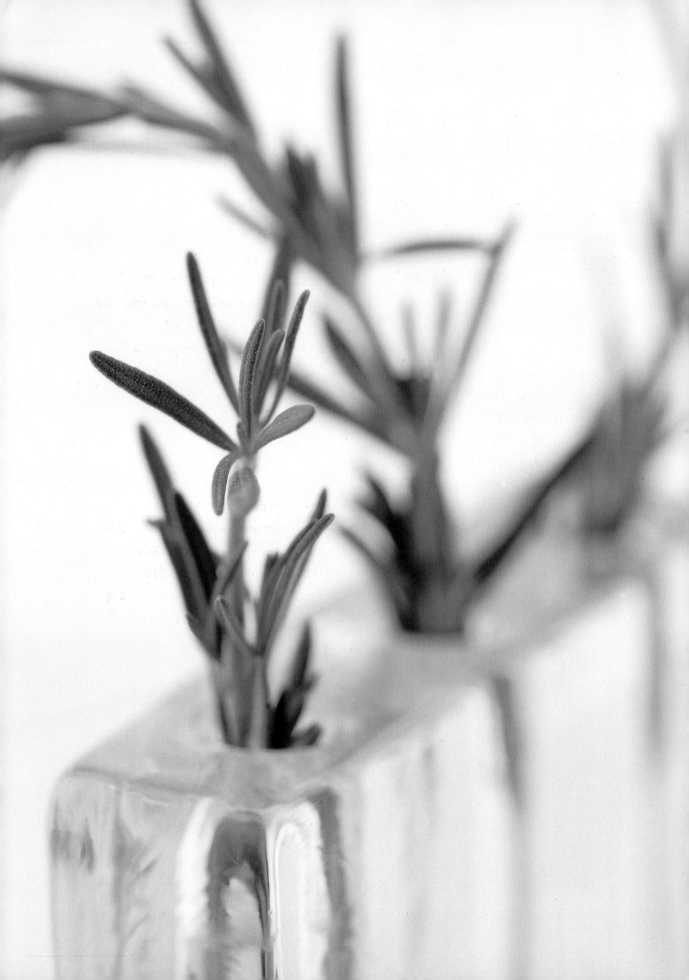

Contents

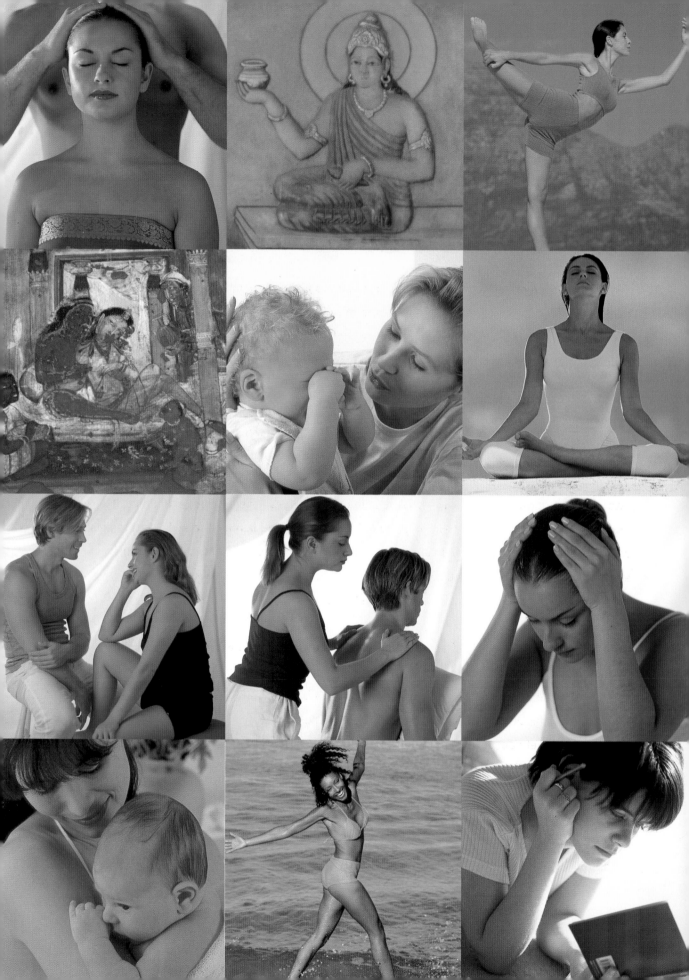

Introduction

The healing touch of massage is one of the best gifts you can give your body. It has been used in human societies for thousands of years as one of the principle therapies for both mind and body healing. Massage is not only an aid for relaxing away stress and tension and stimulating healing, it also boosts circulation and helps tired bodies to rejuvenate themselves, ready for the rigours of everyday life.

All too often we take our bodies for granted, expecting them to work all day with little or no reward. Learning to use massage can give your body the special treat it needs and the practice benefits the giver as well as the receiver. It encourages closeness and caring, boosts body awareness by the power of touch and teaches the hands to 'hear' the body beneath them. It gives you emotional 'time out', allowing you to focus entirely on the massage and how it makes you feel, boosting self-awareness and revitalizing the mind-body connection. The soothing strokes and deep breathing techniques discourage worry and stress and give the giver and receiver the chance to get in touch with their real feelings.

Designed to show you how to share the caring and healing touch of massage, the book will also help you develop your own unique massage style. Divided into three main sections – whole-body, hands and feet, and Indian head – the book is a complete guide, covering techniques for the head, back, neck and shoulders, arms and legs, hands and feet, and the abdomen. Whether you want to target specific areas of the body or learn how to perform a top-to-toe massage, this book will show you how to give your friends and family all the benefits of a professional massage in the privacy of your own home and how to use your own healing touch to solve body problems and ease stress, once and for all.

Understanding
massage

Massage has been used for centuries to heal, invigorate and relax the mind and body, reaching all the major organs as well as helping the muscles, bones and soft tissue stay healthy.

The massage principle is simple: touch means stimulation. This means that wherever touch is used, the body reacts. Because of the changing landscape of the skin and the body parts it protects, differing levels of touch on the body elicit a range of responses; a soft stroke of the forearm may induce relaxation, but a deeper touch might help the blood vessels in the lower arm take blood back to the heart or stimulate and deepen blood flow to painful muscles.

It is important that anyone using massage, even if it is just at home, has a basic understanding of how it works on different areas of the body. This chapter will help you understand some of the fundamental principles, techniques and benefits of massage.

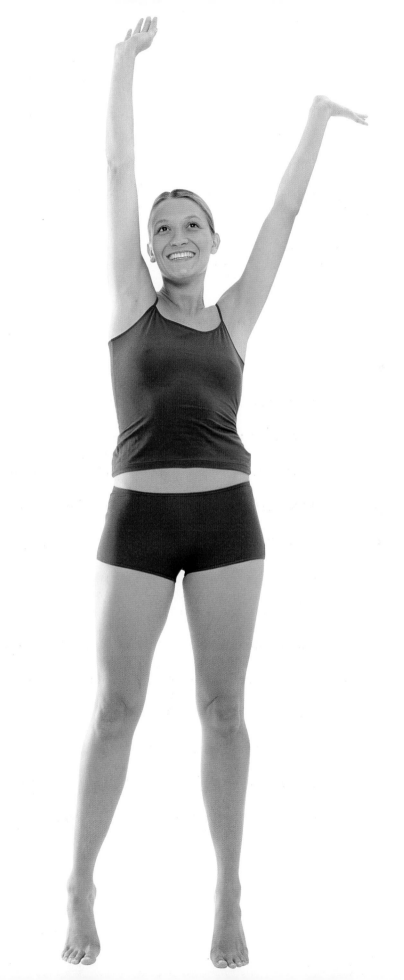

Helping your body

In order for our bodies to work efficiently, the many complex systems that exist under our skin have to work together in a coordinated way. Bones, muscles and soft tissues help us to move. A circulatory system consisting of heart, lungs arteries and blood allows oxygen to be transported around the body to keep cells alive. The nervous system keeps the brain informed of what's going on and allows us to think, act and feel. Our digestive system helps us absorb energy from food and keeps us hydrated with water. An immune system prevents attack from viruses, bacteria and other micro-organisms that could cause us harm or spread disease.

Massage can help each of these systems work optimally, boosting general health and well-being and encouraging healing and growth, right down to a microscopic level.

Bones, muscles and soft tissues

Thanks to our skeletal system, the network of bones and of soft tissues that surround them, our bodies are capable of an amazing range of movements. The effects of massage on the skeletal system are long term – they continue to work long after the actual massage ends, stimulating healing and repair of soft tissue adhesions for up to a month afterwards.

Muscles are made up of bundles of fibres that glide over each other and contract to generate movement. Muscles are attached to bones by tendons and bones are attached to each other by ligaments. Muscle fibres only work in one direction – that is, they contract to shorten themselves but cannot extend. This is why, all around the body, muscles are arranged in opposing pairs so that as one contracts the other expands to allow movement in all directions. Muscles, tendons and ligaments can all be affected by adhesions and small scars or tears that create sore spots. These can stop the tissues from working properly, and can also become severe if left untreated. Massage helps to break down these adhesions.

Circulation

Massage not only stimulates the general circulation system of the body, but it also boosts circulation at a very localized level. Our bodies are made up of thousands of cells and every one of them needs a regular supply of blood. Blood brings all the ingredients the cells need for growth, nutrition and repair; it also takes away waste products and toxins. Massage stimulates the flow of blood and boosts the supply of nutrients – such as minerals and vitamins for health and sugar for energy – and the removal of toxins.

Lymphatic drainage

The body has another, separate, circulatory system that transports a fluid called lymph around the body via a series of glands and vessels. Impurities and toxins are filtered through the glands (called lymph nodes) and the clean fluid drains back into the bloodstream. This helps the immune system by removing bacteria, viruses and other foreign matter, thus fighting infection and draining away excess fluid. Damaged or stiff tissues can become thick and fibrous, causing blockage of the pores and affecting lymph drainage. Massage helps fluids to travel towards the heart and also stimulates muscle contractions that remove fluid blockages. Lymphatic drainage is one of the reasons that all the techniques in this book – and all good massage therapists – work from the outside of the body in towards the heart.

Nervous system

There are two nervous systems that run throughout the body. The first, the sympathetic nervous system, responds to pressure, touch, temperature and so on, passing messages to the brain and responding to sensory stimulation. The second, the parasympathetic nervous system, is the unconscious system that controls body functions, such as heart rate, liver function, digestion and metabolism – the 'behind the scenes' mechanisms that work constantly to keep you alive. Massage stimulates both of the nervous systems, working on the sympathetic system's nerve endings and receptors in the skin and muscles to reduce tension and overactivity and also the parasympathetic nervous system, having a positive effect on conditions such as abnormal blood pressure, digestive disorders, migraine and insomnia.

Skin

The skin is the body's largest organ, providing a flexible protective covering to all body parts, giving us shape and holding us together, containing body fluids and acting as the first line of defence against injury and invasion by bacteria, viruses and microbes. There are three main layers – the upper, epidermis; the middle, dermis; and the lower, subcutaneous.

The epidermis, which is the visible, outer layer of skin, is constantly regenerating itself, producing new cells in the lower layers that rise to the surface and are eventually shed. The dermis lies directly underneath the epidermis and is filled with a rich supply of blood vessels, lymph, nerve endings, sweat and oil glands and hair follicles. The subcutaneous layer lies beneath the dermis and provides a storage facility for fat, which acts as a heat insulator and also provides a protective layer. Massage boosts circulation in all three layers of skin, encouraging renewal, growth and repair, preventing build-up of dead skin cells and stimulating sweat glands to remove waste products and clear out the pores. It gives the skin a healthy glow and promotes cellular healing at every level.

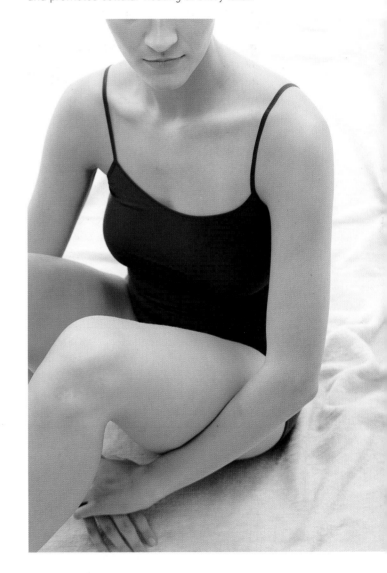

RIGHT **By stimulating circulation, massage boosts the health of the skin.**

Cautions and contraindications

Qualified massage therapists use a range of techniques to treat different problems. The purpose of this book is to give you a general understanding of the therapeutic effects of massage and how you can use it to help yourself, your family and friends to relax and unwind. If you have health problems, always consult a professional before massage.

Massage is generally considered to be an extremely safe form of therapy, but even so there are a few situations in which it might do more harm than good. Several conditions – known as contraindications – are adversely affected by massage. Check before you start that your massage partner is not suffering from any of these and if you have any doubts about safety DO NOT MASSAGE. If you're worried, you'll be tense and won't give a good massage – it's better to wait and seek professional advice, and then you may be able to go ahead with no worries at a later date.

Never give a massage if the person to be massaged has any of the following:

Inflammation

Never massage over inflamed or sore soft tissues because it could make them worse. Look for bruising, swelling, tender or sore muscles or areas of skin, heat and redness in the skin, or pain and dysfunction in the affected area. Swollen or sore lymph nodes (in the neck, underarms and groin) are to be avoided. If you are in doubt, try the ten-second test – apply enough pressure to the area to cause mild discomfort and maintain it for ten seconds. If discomfort decreases it's probably safe to treat, but if it increases you should wait until the inflammation has died down.

Bone and joint injuries

Avoid conditions affecting the bones and joints after injury (like whiplash, fractures, sprains and strains) because massage could aggravate the condition and cause pain.

Open wounds

You should never massage over an open wound because of the risk of infection.

Fever

People develop a high temperature when their bodies are working hard to deal with some sort of infection. Massage is not recommended for people with a temperature over 37.5°C (99.4°F) because it could jeopardize the body's defence systems by raising their temperature further.

Thrombosis

People with a history of thrombosis should not be massaged because it could encourage a clot to come loose and enter the blood. Great care should be taken with conditions known to increase thrombosis risk such as recent major surgery, varicose veins, heart disease, impact trauma, some contraceptive pills and long periods of immobility or bed rest, which reduces circulation. If you are at all concerned or worried, seek medical advice before starting a massage.

Varicose veins

A breakdown in the one-way valves of the veins in the legs causes blood to collect in the veins and gives them a blue, slightly lumpy appearance, known as varicose veins. In many cases, a light stroking over the vein will not do any harm, but deep techniques should be avoided in the leg area as they could exert pressure on already weakened vein walls, causing further problems.

Skin disorders

Disorders like psoriasis, eczema and acne can be aggravated by massage, which should also be avoided in cases of bacterial, fungal or viral infections. You should also avoid other skin problems like cold sores, blisters, sunburn, cuts and grazes, bites, stings and unexplained lumps.

Cancer

Although a trained therapist can sometimes lessen pain and tension caused by cancer, there is a risk that tumours may be spread through the body or that it might be painful. Stick to gentle stroking or consult a doctor.

Drugs and alcohol

Never give a massage to anyone who is under the influence of drugs or alcohol. These are mind- and body-altering substances that can cause people to react in an unpredictable way.

Long-term medical conditions

Although not necessarily contraindications, you should seek medical advice before massaging someone with a long-term condition like epilepsy, severe asthma, oedema, heart disease, chronic back pain, and those on long-term medication.

Other concerns

In addition, there are several other conditions that can have a bearing on the massage you choose to give. Look out for:

Diabetes

The condition can affect circulation in the feet and lower legs, and create fragile tissues that may be damaged by deep massage techniques. Sometimes massage appears to have the same effect on blood sugar levels as exercise, so diet and medication might need altering.

High or low blood pressure

Massage can cause fluctuations in blood pressure levels so be careful around people with high or low blood pressure. If you are at all concerned, seek medical advice first.

Osteoporosis

This disease is a brittle bone condition in which the bones (particularly in the back, neck and shoulders) become thin and easily broken. Deep massage techniques could cause fractures in people with severe osteoporosis, so seek medical advice.

Pregnancy

The aches and pains of pregnancy can be soothed away with the correct massage techniques, reducing swelling and pain and boosting well-being. However, massage should be avoided during the first 12 weeks – particularly around the stomach – when the risk of miscarriage and foetal disorders are greatest. Occasionally pregnant women go on to develop conditions like diabetes and high blood pressure, which could contraindicate massage (see above), or they might suffer severe nausea as a result of massage so they should be made aware of this before a session. Essential oils should not be used during pregnancy.

Children and the elderly

Both children and the elderly can benefit greatly from massage, but should not be massaged using deep techniques because they have less lean tissue and could therefore suffer pain or discomfort, and may be less likely to tell you how they feel. Being aware of how much pressure you are exerting and making sure you have a continued dialogue can help to make the massage a beneficial experience for both of you.

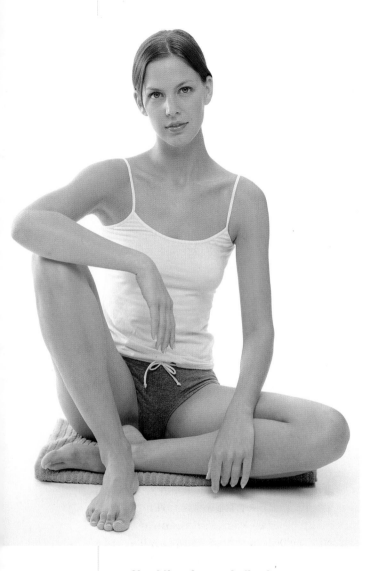

LEFT **Along with promoting the healthy function of the body, massage is an excellent way to de-stress and unwind.**

Areas to avoid

There are several places on the body where massage should not be performed under any circumstances. These are:

Eyes – The eyes are delicate and can be damaged by pressure, so avoid pressing or massaging in or around the eyes.

Sides of the neck – The side of the neck holds the carotid artery, which takes oxygen and nutrients to the brain. Pressure here can interrupt blood flow, causing faintness or dizziness and even unconsciousness. Avoid pressing hard on the sides of the neck and be careful around the backs of the ears.

Back of the knees – Behind the knee and slightly above it, there is a soft triangle of tissue that sits between the muscles of the hamstrings as they meet the knee where arteries and veins travel very close to the surface. Leg massages always concentrate on working around this area and never actually on it.

Babies' heads – The plates of a baby's skull are not fully formed for the first two or three years of life and extreme care should be taken when touching these soft areas, called the fontanelles, as well as any part of the neck and face.

Stomach in pregnancy – The stomach and abdomen of pregnant women should be avoided and extreme caution taken with massage in the lower back.

Checklist of contraindications to massage:
- Swelling or inflammation
- Fever
- Open wounds
- Bone and joint injuries
- Bleeding disorders
- Melanoma (skin cancer)
- High blood pressure
- Cancer
- Varicose veins
- Deep vein thrombosis
- Skin infections

The benefits of massage for body and mind

One of the most profound benefits of massage is deep relaxation, reducing the stress and tension that is believed to be, directly or indirectly, the cause of nearly three-quarters of all illness. Every single nerve in our bodies, including thousands in the skin, send messages to the brain, which is the control room of the nervous system. It monitors everything that goes on in our bodies as well as our moods and feelings. In this way, touch is linked to emotions, and that's why massage can help beat stress.

Coping with stress

When you are faced with a stressful situation – whether it's an immediate problem like an emergency or a long-term build-up of stress like trouble at work or tiredness – your body responds by secreting the stress hormones adrenaline and cortisol into the bloodstream. These hormones give us the famous 'fight or flight' response that is designed to allow our bodies to react to dangerous situations. When they are released, our muscles tense, ready to spring into action, and the heart and lungs work harder to pump oxygen to the arms and legs. Blood pressure, breathing and pulse rate rise, and oxygenated blood is diverted away from the stomach (halting digestion and causing the 'nervous' sensation of butterflies), the skin (causing it to turn pale), the immune system and organs like the liver and kidneys.

Our bodies are designed to respond to stress – it is only when stressful situations become prolonged that the body starts to suffer damage. Being in a constant state of alertness raises blood pressure and heart rate, and can cause problems with skin, digestion, migraine, back pain and heart

disease. Massage helps to combat the harmful effects of long-term stress because it allows the body to slow down and reduces the effects of the stress hormones. It slows breathing and relaxes muscles, which prevent more adrenaline and cortisol from being released into the bloodstream, and simultaneously stimulate the skin and major organs to boost circulation and lymphatic drainage around the whole body.

Time out and general well-being

One of the primary benefits of massage is that it gives you time to unwind and be with your thoughts, away from the strains of everyday life. Peaceful surroundings and a calming atmosphere allow the mind time out to relax and recharge. The soothing touch of massage, alongside the space to concentrate, helps to reconnect the mind-body links that can be lost through busy lifestyles. This enables your physical and emotional sides to work together to combat future stress.

The feeling of physical contact stimulates the release of endorphins – also known as feel-good chemicals – in the brain. These lift the mood, help fight pain, boost self-esteem and dissolve the effects of stress, which allow the immune system and major organs to return to functioning normally. Massage reminds your body of the pleasure of taking time out and helps to reduce blood pressure, breathing rate and stress.

The nervous system controls tension in the entire body, which is why nonphysical pressures, such as stress, can lead to physical symptoms like digestive problems and headaches. Massage helps by affecting the nerves to reduce tension and thus increase positive input to the body's systems.

Getting ready
for massage

Massage is a totally natural therapy that you can do anywhere, at any time and without any specialized equipment. However, because massage is about the mind as well as the body, and because we are affected by everything around us all the time, it is important to create the best possible environment before you start.

This chapter will take you through a few important technical points, such as which massage mediums to use, how to choose aromatherapy oils for their essential oil properties and the best way to use towels to warm, cover and comfort the person you are massaging. It also explains how to create an atmosphere for your massage that gives you a total sensory experience.

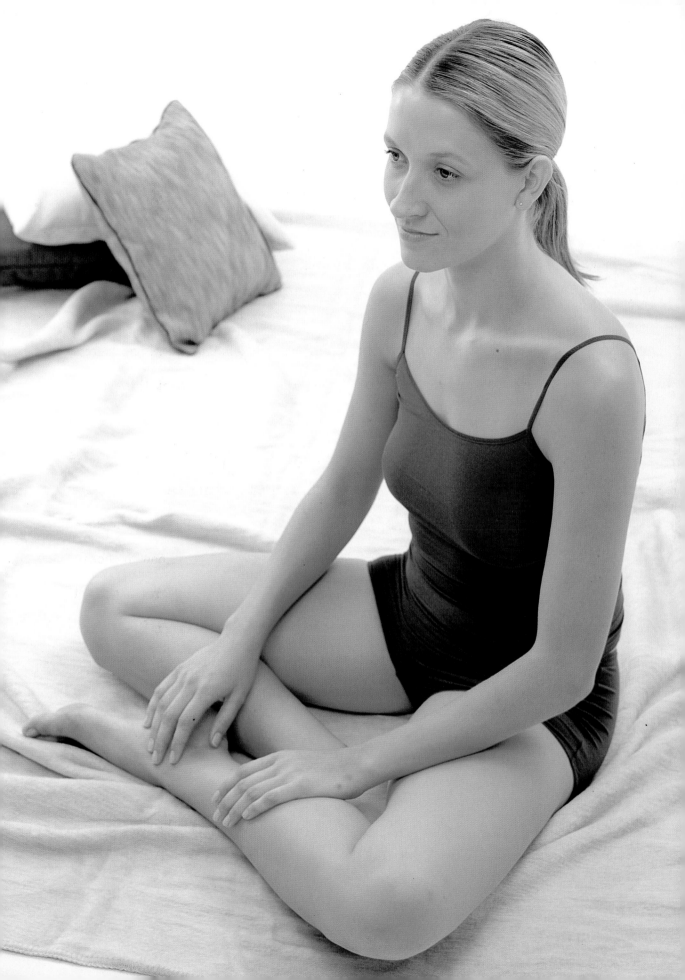

Massage mediums

In order to massage correctly, you need to make sure that your hands can glide over the skin, exerting just the right amount of pressure. To do this, you will need to use a massage medium to reduce frictional drag and to lubricate the surface of the skin. The massage medium you use depends on the skin type of the person being massaged. Skins differ greatly in the amount of oils, lotions and other mediums they absorb, so it's wise to have a few different types ready to use. It is about personal choice, so try a few before you decide which one works best for you and the person you are massaging – trust yourself and choose the one that feels right.

Lotions

Body massage lotions are a combination of oil and cream, which is good for massage because it doesn't absorb too quickly into the skin and can therefore be used sparsely. Lotions are also kind to the therapist's hands, keeping them well moisturized. Massage lotions differ from normal body lotions, which do not contain oil, so they last longer on the skin and are therefore better for massage. Some body massage lotions contain lanolin, which some people are allergic to, so most massage therapists opt for hypoallergenic lotions. Lotions are often the first choice for therapeutic massage, which requires a combination of light and deep strokes.

Creams

Excellent for massaging small areas with light contact, creams moisturize but have high levels of base oil, which means they can become slippery on larger areas. Hand and foot cream and moisturizers containing urea, which doesn't absorb as quickly as other constituents, are particularly good.

Talcum powder

Talc allows a large range of contact with minimal movement and retains a high degree of the natural friction between skin surfaces. It allows for some movement, but also means that the masseur can achieve deeper contact for correctional and friction work. It is a great alternative for people who are allergic to oils, creams and lotions and is more likely to be chosen by a professional for deep work on specific areas than for general massage.

Oils

These do not absorb into the skin very well, which means they are good for light contact, especially if you are working with children, the elderly or people with whom you want to avoid deep contact. The less oil you use, the deeper the contact; the lighter contact you require, the more oil you need, but remember the skin surface should never be so slippery that you are not in control of your strokes. Oils differ in absorption but most commonly available massage oils will be light oils, which are good for a soft, relaxing massage.

Aromatherapy oils

Essential oils can be combined with a base carrier oil, such as almond, to further the therapeutic benefits of the massage.

Caution: Essential oils are potent and can be harmful if misused, so always follow the manufacturer's instructions. Obtain oils from a reputable source and dilute in the right proportions. With the exception of lavender and tea tree, no undiluted essential oils should be applied directly onto the skin, and oils should never be eaten, drunk or applied to lips and eyes. Essential oils should be avoided in pregnancy – especially in the first 12 weeks – and help should be sought from a qualified practitioner before using them on children and the elderly. Many stores now sell ready-mixed massage oils, but the following essential oils are commonly used:

Lavender – Sleep-inducing, calming and antidepressant. May help: headaches, skin complaints, stretchmarks, high and low blood pressure, muscular pains, rheumatism and arthritis. An excellent carrier oil because of its beneficial effects.

Black pepper – Warming, stimulating and invigorating. May help: stiff and tired muscles and joints, sluggish circulation, decreased mobility. May irritate some skins.

Camomile – Sedative, antidepressant and sleep-inducing. May help: high blood pressure, general aches and pains, dry skin and eczema. Approved as safe for use with children because of its mildness, it is also good for using on the elderly.

Marjoram – Sedative, circulation-boosting and warming. May help: sore and tired muscles, joint pains, headaches and arthritis. Marjoram should not be used in combination with clary sage, as the mixture could be potentially intoxicating.

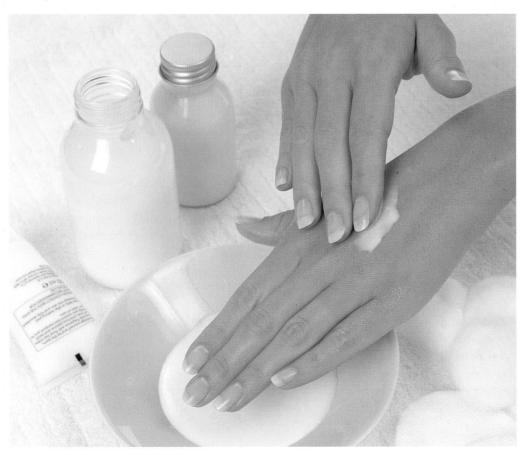

BELOW **Oils, creams and lotions have different textures and absorbabilities.**

Orange and Grapefruit – Uplifting, stimulating and antidepressant. May help: depression, sluggishness and lack of motivation.

Bergamot – Antidepressant, mood-boosting and balancing. May help: depression, anxiety and winter blues. Bergamot is phototoxic, so exposure to the sun and sunbeds should be avoided for 12 hours afterwards.

Rose – Calming, antidepressant and a general body tonic. May help: insomnia and dry skin conditions.

Frankincense – Mentally stimulating and boosts self-awareness. May help: meditation, concentration and self-reflection.

Sandalwood – Confidence-boosting, anti-inflammatory, sedative and boosts the immune system. May help: low self-esteem, sciatic pain and dry skin.

Tea tree – Antiviral, antiseptic, fungicidal and boosts the immune system. May help: promote healing, reduce swelling and fight off infection.

Eucalyptus – Immune-boosting and a decongestant. May help: sinus problems, coughs and colds, and chest infections. Eucalyptus can produce erythema in some people.

Rosemary – Memory boosting and mentally stimulating. May help: stimulate memory and brain activity, prepare your brain for exams, presentations, speeches, etc.

For stress: Try combining lavender, bergamot and camomile.

For aching muscles: Try using lavender, black pepper and marjoram.

For an energy boost: Try lavender, rosemary and grapefruit or orange.

For depression: Try lavender, eucalyptus and peppermint.

If you're using essential oils for massage, don't have an oil burner, scented candle or perfume in the room as they could interact. Also, don't combine more than three scents in one carrier oil. You should never use an oil if either of you dislike the smell.

Towelling

Several purposes are served by towelling. First, it provides barriers – the person being massaged knows the physical limitations of your massage and that it will not go beyond the barrier of the towel – this is essential to ensure that they can fully relax. Second, towels provide warmth when laid over the body, as the blood pressure lowers during massage and body temperature drops. Third, they provide a feeling of comfort and safety.

Any part of the body that is not being touched should be covered with two or three smaller towels, each one covering a separate part of the body. This method gives you more versatility than if you had one large towel covering the whole body, as you can then reposition the body more easily and it is simpler to change the area you are working on without too much difficulty or upheaval.

As a general rule, the towel is used as a single layer and the top inch or two is either tucked into the edge of any clothing or tucked underneath the rest of the towel to form a

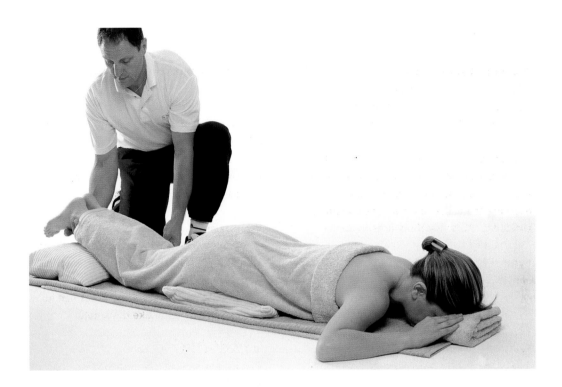

definite edge. For large flat areas like backs and abdomens, lay the towel straight over the lower body; for legs and arms it's often easier to use it at an angle along the joint line.

You will need:
- 2 bath towels for general body coverage
- 2 hand towels for specific areas

The towels should be clean and dry. Because some people are allergic to certain washing powders and fabric softeners, it might be a good idea to use a nonbiological detergent. For added luxury, you can warm the towels on a radiator or in a tumble dryer before use.

Working through clothing
If you want to work through clothing, you can use compression and stretch techniques or small circular massage motions, but you will have to avoid sliding or depth work because clothes will cause friction, restrict movement and prevent good contact with the muscle.

ABOVE **Position the body correctly to boost massage benefits. Place cushions or folded towels under the feet, pelvic area and forehead to provide comfort and protection during the massage.**

The perfect environment
Massage is all about comfort and relaxation, so your surroundings should echo this. Turn down harsh lighting to create a tranquil atmosphere and scent the room with your favourite perfume, incense or aromatherapy oils. Ensure that the person being massaged feels relaxed and comfortable and is not too hot or cold – sometimes being covered with towels can heat the body up too much, so make sure you check how the person feels at regular intervals. Try to make sure you will have peace and quiet, without interruption.

By stimulating all the senses in this way you will magnify the beneficial therapeutic effects of massage on both the body and mind.

You will need:

- Plenty of warm dry towels for covering up massaged areas, keeping the body warm and comforted and preserving modesty.
- Your chosen oil, lotion, cream or talc to provide lubrication, which is especially important on the back because of the large skin area.
- Clean hands and loose, soft clothing so that you feel comfortable and are able to move freely while you massage.
- Soft cushions or pillows to support areas of the body while lying in the optimum positions for being massaged.
- A blanket or thick towel if you are lying on a hard floor.
- A mirror, if required, to check your positioning.
- A glass of water for each person.
- A DO NOT DISTURB sign for the outside of the door if you are likely to be interrupted.

Tips for the masseur:

- Go to the toilet in advance, to make sure you won't have to leave the room mid-massage.
- Turn the lights down low to reduce eyestrain and create an atmosphere. Introduce candles for an alternative and relaxing light source.
- Turn up the heating to ensure the room is warm and draught-free.
- Turn off the phone and any other potential distractions and put on some soft, relaxing, atmospheric music.
- Wash your hands with gently scented soap and warm them.
- Take a moment to focus fully before you start to ease yourself slowly into a calm, centred state of mind. This will ensure that you are ready to give total concentration to the massage.

Tips for the person being massaged:

- Wear comfortable, loose-fitting clothes.
- Remove all bracelets, rings, make-up, contact lenses and glasses.
- Find a comfortable position and be aware of how your body feels.

NOTES

- Test for allergic reactions to creams, oils or lotions and read all the safety guidelines carefully to prevent adverse reactions. If you are worried, the best way to test is to cover a small area of skin on the inside of the arm with the cream 24 hours before you are going to massage and watch for any adverse reactions.
- Check for any contraindications to massage, see pages 12–14, and seek medical advice if you are unsure.
- The person being massaged should allow at least an hour after eating or exercise before having the massage, and avoid stimulants like caffeine in tea, coffee, chocolate and fizzy drinks beforehand.
- Make sure you feel good. You will be in close contact during the time you're giving the massage and infectious or contagious conditions could easily be passed on.
- Cover cuts and scratches on your hands.

Mind-clearing tip

Leave worries and troubles at the door of your massage room and dedicate yourself to the massage. If you find this difficult, use a book to write down all the things that are worrying you and leave it outside the door with your worries. Don't worry about the time you are spending in the massage room either; allow yourself this little treat.

Talk the talk

Take a few minutes to talk to each other about what your expectations are and how you have reacted to treatment in the past. Has the person being massaged ever had a bad or frightening experience? Have they reacted strangely, felt sick, faint or emotional following treatment, or have they suffered allergic reactions to oils, creams or lotions?

Are either of you worried about anything that you should mention? Taking a little time to talk openly will increase the bond between you and give you a platform to clear away worries and troubles before you begin.

BELOW **Massage involves intimate touch, so put each other at ease before the massage begins by talking together.**

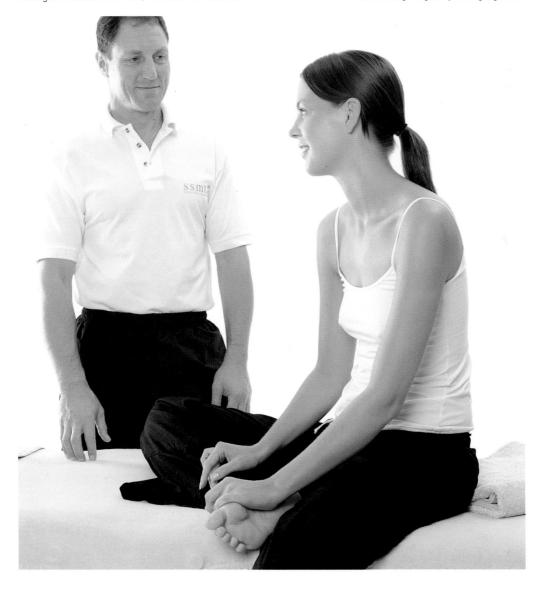

Body therapy
and aftercare

The period of time after massage is very important for ensuring maximum therapeutic benefits for the body and mind. This chapter shows you how to take the best care of your physical and mental states between massages in order to maximize the benefits and ensure that your feeling of well-being lasts.

Massage not only relaxes and unwinds tension, it also acts as a detoxifier, soothes away problems in the body's soft tissues and boosts circulation and lymphatic drainage. But the benefits do not have to stop when the massage is over. Making a few small changes could have far-reaching benefits for your whole health.

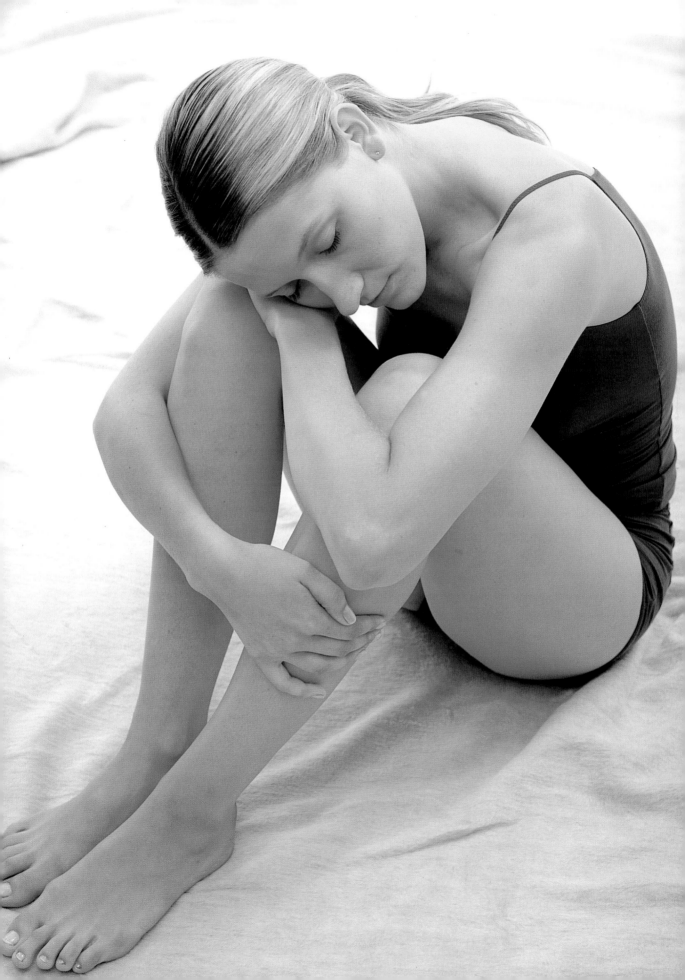

Making the most of massage

Massage can sometimes elicit an emotional response. When toxins and tension trapped in the body are released, fears, anxiety and sadness may come to the surface. Some people feel sleepy, faint or light-headed immediately afterwards and may need a little time to readjust to the pace of normal life. Take care if you're driving right after a massage, as deep relaxation may cause reaction time to slow down. Never drive if you feel light-headed or sleepy; sit quietly or have a snooze and wait until you feel ready to drive.

On rare occasions there may be a physical response like headache, feeling hot, mild nausea or perspiration. However, these symptoms are usually only experienced during the first few massages or in people who haven't had a massage for a long time. They should disappear quickly with rest.

Detoxify

Avoid drinking alcohol or caffeine or smoking for at least 12 hours after to help your body continue the detoxification process. Adding toxins like alcohol or nicotine could adversely affect the process. Regular massage will help your body cope with everyday toxins, and keeping it as free of toxins as possible before and after a massage will help you stay healthy long-term.

Sleep like a baby

One of the major side-effects of massage is a feeling of tiredness – as toxins are released the body can become profoundly heavy. If your body feels fatigued during or after massage, don't fight it. Giving in to tiredness is a luxury we do not often allow ourselves. If you feel sleepy afterwards, it is because your body is telling you it needs to slow down.

Visualization

While the massage is in progress, close your eyes and think of a place that makes you feel comforted, relaxed and calm – it could be a perfect landscape, a gentle lake at sunset or a favourite view – then mentally transport yourself there with all your senses. Think about how the place smells, feels and sounds as well as what you see. While you visualize this special, timeless place, allow your breathing to become deeper and rhythmic and let worries and tension flood away. Take time to bring yourself slowly back to the present, concentrating on what is going on around you, before you open your eyes.

Keep it light

Avoid eating or drinking heavily straight after a massage, or engaging in physical activity. This could divert energy away from vital healing processes toward digestion – steer clear of stimulants like caffeine and stick to water or herbal tea, light snacks and fresh fruit. Make sure you drink enough water to avoid the dehydration that can follow massage. Water keeps the body working efficiently, gives the lymph and circulation systems a helping hand and plumps up skin, making it look and feel fresh and young.

Boost circulation

Slow circulation can affect your body's systems and make the skin dull, dry and flaky. Massage helps circulation but there is also a lot that you can do for yourself in between massages. Use a body buffer or loofah in the shower to rub dry skin off your legs and arms, remembering to work from the extremities towards the heart. Slight redness of the skin is a sign that the blood is flowing strongly to the surface.

Warm down

A post-exercise warming down will help prevent cramp, injury and muscle soreness, as it helps your muscles rid themselves of toxins. Aim for at least five to ten minutes of gentle exercise to end your workout.

Think tall

Good posture can help you get through life without pain and injury. Try to think about how you sit or stand. If you are still for long periods of time – sitting at a desk, cooking or watching television – aim to keep your spine in the neutral position, which will help to reduce stress on the back.

Take a break

Giving a massage can be very draining on your energy levels so, after you have given someone a massage, make sure you take some time to recharge your own batteries. Make sure you drink plenty of water and avoid rushing on to the next thing. Allow your body ten minutes of relaxation and renewal, sitting or lying somewhere quiet and calm.

Vitamin boost

You should aim to eat at least five portions of fruit and vegetables every day to boost your intake of vitamins, minerals and anti-oxidants. Vitamins A, B and C, found in abundance in tomatoes, fruit, leafy green vegetables and watercress, are particularly important for a healthy diet.

Essential nutrients

Fatty acids and elements like zinc and calcium are essential for strong skin, bones, hair and nails. Seafood, leafy green vegetables and nuts all contain these nutritious elements and will help to keep your skin in top condition. Consuming oily fish like mackerel and salmon ensures you have the right building blocks for all-round health.

Antioxidize yourself

Pollution, toxins, alcohol, smoking and stress can lead to a build-up of free radicals in the body, which, if left unchecked, can cause long-term damage. To combat this, make sure you include free-radical busting anti-oxidants in your diet; these are found in fresh fruit and vegetables, garlic, onions and nuts and seeds.

Whole-body massage

The techniques in this section are arranged in sequence so that they can be used to perform a whole body massage if you work your way from start to finish, but they are also designed to stand alone. From this, you can choose to dip in and out to target specific areas, concentrate on a few techniques for a quick fix if you're short of time, or go slowly and follow the techniques through from beginning to end for a total all-over body massage.

All the techniques are explained for one side of the body only; to perform the technique on the other side, simply reverse the instructions and repeat. It is usual for massage therapists to concentrate on one side of the body at a time, working through all the massages on one side before working on the other. The method prevents too much movement around the body and allows the masseur to maintain smoothness and fluidity throughout the massage. The approach here is also more sports-oriented than that of the other two sections, and gives a deeper massage. If you are interested in developing your skills in this area, many health- and sports-affiliated centres and foundations offer courses and workshops on the subject.

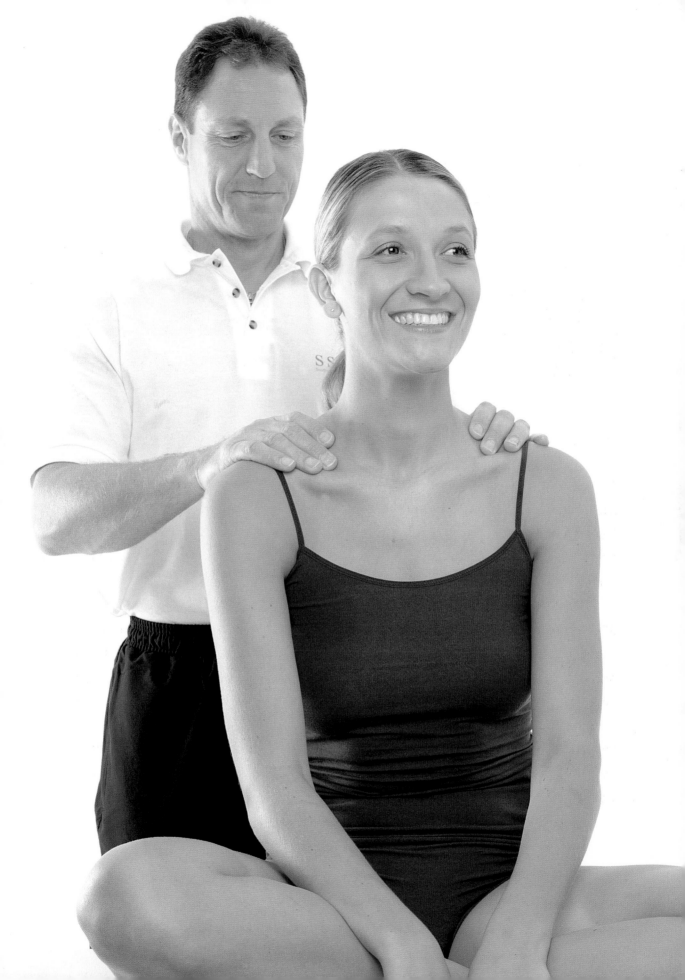

Basic skills
and techniques

Professional therapists spend years perfecting their techniques, but there are a few tips and essentials you can learn in minutes. Getting to grips with massage is hard work unless you know how to do it right, employing your whole body to soothe away stress and tension and promote healing using strong, fluid strokes.

This chapter shows you how to position yourself and the person you are massaging for ultimate benefit and how to use your body-weight to create controlled, smooth strokes. It shows you techniques like effleurage (stroking), petrissage (kneading) and soft-tissue release stretches, the essential ingredients for a professional-style massage.

The positions in this book are designed for you to pick and mix to target problem areas or to follow a whole series for a thorough, all-over massage. Where no specific starting position is given, continue from the previous technique. Massage is intuitive and understanding the basic techniques will enable you to do what is instinctive.

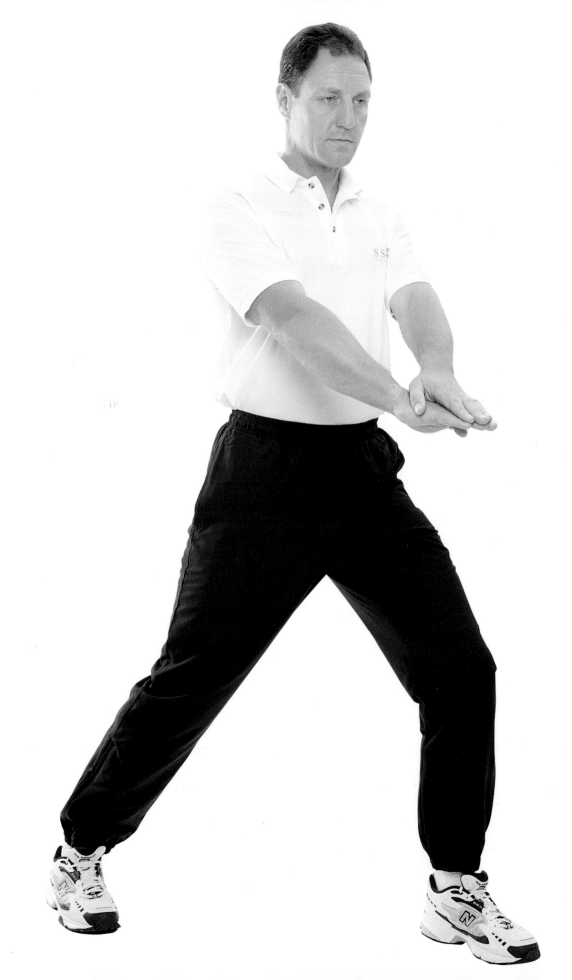

Getting the position right

Professional masseurs have adjustable, transportable couches that help keep the body in a neutral position during massage. To show the perfect massage posture and technique, the procedures explained here assume correct positioning and are described as if a massage bed was being used.

To maximize the benefits of massage, the body must be allowed to totally relax. This means that none of the muscles should be working, the spine and bones should be supported and not stretched, and the head and hips should not be twisted. There are two ways to create a good lying position at home: on the floor and on a bed.

BELOW **The masseur's lower back is straight and his arms are locked.**

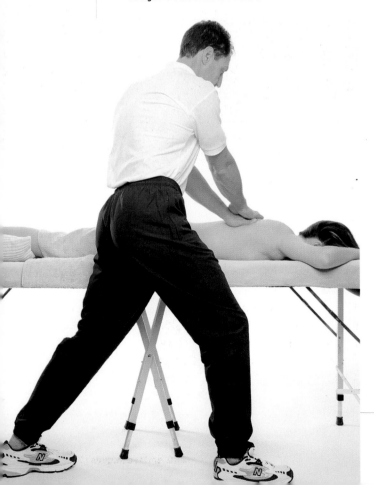

The floor

The floor is usually the best location for a home massage because it is hard and so provides a firm surface for the masseur to push against (a few soft towels or blankets can help to make it more comfortable).

When lying on the back and facing the ceiling (in the 'supine' position), a cushion or pillow should be placed under the knees to reduce pressure on the lower back and a slim towel can be used under the head and lower back for comfort. For lying facing the floor (the 'prone' position), a cushion or pillow should be placed under the hips to raise the lower back and another should be put under the feet so that the knees are bent (see also page 21). The head should be straight, facing the floor and not twisted, and the forehead can either rest on the hands or on a pillow. The arms should be bent at the elbow and resting either side of the head, if they are not forming a platform for the forehead.

Caution: It is most important, for all massage, that the neck is not twisted or cricked. The head should be positioned directly above the spine and the back of the neck lengthened comfortably.

The masseur should kneel (a pillow, towel or cushion can be used) around the body to get into position and use their bodyweight to work the techniques. Sitting cross-legged can be useful when massaging the head and feet.

If the masseur finds kneeling a problem, they may prefer to use a higher surface. If you have a dining-room table, which will take the weight of a body, position the person to be massaged on top of it using the same positions as the floor.

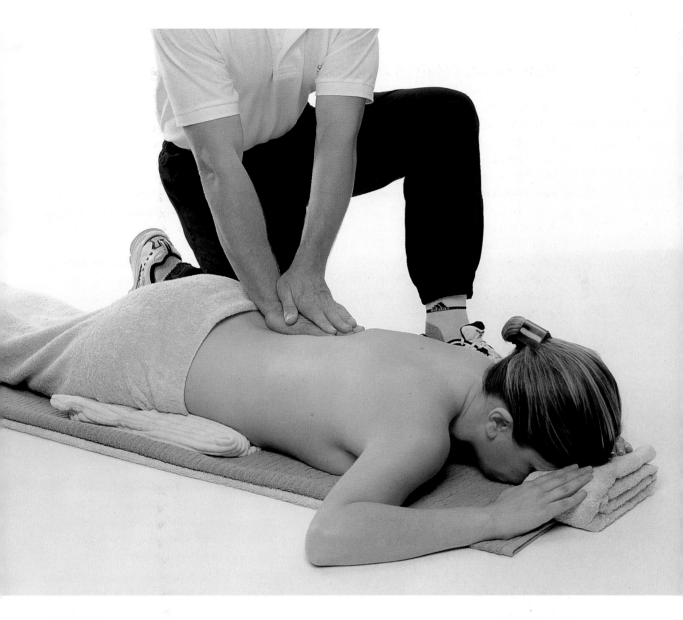

The bed

Beds are not ideal for massage because they are soft, which means the bed rather than the body will move. Positioning is the same as for the floor, but take extra care to ensure that the neck is straight. To massage, come around the side of the bed rather than sitting or kneeling on it. If you have a double bed, massage one side of the body and then move across the bed to massage the other.

ABOVE **If kneeling, the position for the masseur is the same as for standing, with lower arms and back locked.**

Massage is about comfort, both for the person being massaged and the masseur. If there is discomfort or pain, the therapeutic benefits will be lost and you could cause injury or strain. Take the time to create the right atmosphere and find comfortable positions.

Techniques

Massage isn't about having strength in the arms, wrists, hands or thumbs; instead, it is about bodyweight. Much like practitioners of eastern balance arts, such as Tai Chi, masseurs use the weight of their bodies, moving through the hips backwards, forwards and side to side, to create movement. If you watch a professional masseur at work, their back is straight and their shoulders and arms are locked in front of them.

The correct technique is important, not only because it helps you to give the best massage and allows you to control the pressure you are exerting without tiring yourself out, but it also prevents injury and strain, and allows you to relax and enjoy giving a massage as much as receiving one. A masseur who has a good posture does not have to work hard. As long as you are in the right position, the strokes will become smooth, powerful and effortless and the movement instinctive.

For the ultimate comfort of the person being massaged, and to maintain a controlled rhythm throughout the massage techniques, try to avoid removing your hands from the skin while you work. Professional masseurs rarely take their hands off the body, unless it is to add more lotion or oil or to alter their position or the towelling. This constant touch is very important in maintaining and developing a patient-practitioner bond that encourages calm and focuses the massage.

Throughout the massage you should remain aware of your movements. Watch out for any winces, twitches, flinches or movements from the person being massaged that could indicate that you are causing them discomfort or that they are somehow in pain.

Bodyweight balance practice

To get used to using your bodyweight and balance, hold your arms out in front of you, in a circle with your hands together, and sway your hips in order to to move your hands without utilizing your arms. Once you have mastered this, try spreading your feet further apart and, with a smooth lunge, transfer your bodyweight from leg to leg without moving your arms or shoulders. Your back should never bend. If you feel as if you need to bend to exert pressure, bend your knees or move closer to the area being massaged – this should allow you to use the correct technique.

NOTES

- For the comfort of the person being massaged, all techniques require that your nails are short and there are no rough or hard patches on your hands. In addition to this, you should remove all hand and wrist jewellery and watches and have short or rolled-up sleeves.
- The hand of the masseur should always follow the contours of the body, so for some areas, like the forearms and shins, it is sometimes better to use the hand sideways so it fits over the natural curve of the skin.
- If your thumbs, hands, wrists or arms start to ache, it is likely that you are using them directly, instead of using your bodyweight, to exert pressure. To avoid this problem, practise moving around on your feet by using your hips to balance and keeping your shoulders and arms in position without bending them. If you use your weight instead of your muscles, the massage won't feel like such hard work.

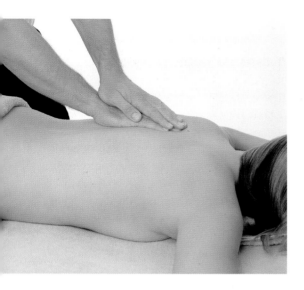

▲ Technique 1: Effleurage

Also known as stroking, effleurage is good for clearing blood, lymph and body fluids, warming up the muscle group and boosting circulation. Using the palm, side or heel of the hand push into the skin and tissues beneath. It can be one- or two-handed and should start slowly, building to the middle of the stroke and tapering off at the end. The strokes should be hard enough to cause some redness and warmth in the skin. Typically, you would start a massage with this, to warm the area for deeper work.

1   Place one hand flat, palm down, with the fingers pointing forwards.
2   Place the other hand over the palm.
3   Lock wrists and elbows.
4   Use your bodyweight to move yourself slowly forwards.
5   DO NOT bend your back – movement should come from knees and hips.
6   Take three or four small strokes and then follow with a single long stroke.
7   For large areas, use a lunge technique. Stand with one leg in front and then transfer your weight to move forwards.

▼ Technique 2: Deep effleurage

This technique is similar to effleurage except that you use the thumbs, which allows a deeper penetration of the body tissues. The basic technique is the same, using the transfer of bodyweight to exert pressure. You are looking for a slight wave of skin in front of the thumb and reddening of the skin in the areas you have worked on; the massage should feel deep, but not painful.

1   Place one hand palm down on the area with the thumb flat.
2   Place the other thumb over the first. For small areas like the arms use a thumb on top, and for large areas like the back and thighs you can place the heel of the hand over the thumb.
3   Lock thumbs, wrists and elbows.
4   Exert pressure through thumbs and, using bodyweight, work away from you.

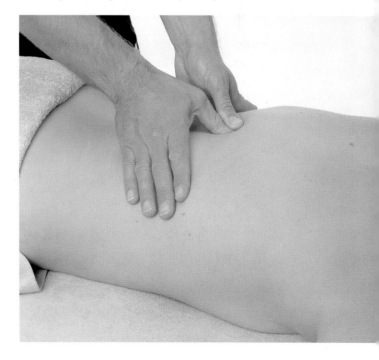

▼ Technique 3: Petrissage

Petrissage employs both hands working in opposite directions to free up problem areas, boost circulation and work deep into muscles (see page 51 for a close-up of the technique).

1. Place both hands palm down, side by side, and lock the thumbs, wrists and elbows in position.
2. Roll your hips right and forwards so that your right thumb moves forward.
3. At the same time, bring the fingers of the left hand back so that they meet and glide over the right thumb.
4. Roll your hips to the left so that your left thumb moves forwards and bring your right fingers back to meet it.
5. Keep both palms on the skin as pivots.
6. Continue to work the rhythm, bringing thumb and fingers together alternately as your hips roll to move your weight.
7. Your shoulders should move with your hips, and should not be still.

▼ Technique 4: Cam and spindle

Cam and spindle is a deep muscle technique for releasing tension and working into the tissues. It employs the knuckles of one hand (the 'cam') and the palm of the other (the 'spindle') working together to penetrate deeply.

1. Make a fist with one hand then join the hands by inserting the thumb of the other hand into the clenched fingers of the fist.
2. Lock your wrists and elbows and, using the outstretched hand (spindle) as a guide and the fist (cam) to massage the muscle, work in small straight motions away from you.
3. To increase pressure, tighten the fist around the thumb and to decrease pressure, loosen the fist.

tip Never cam and spindle over bone; it is a deep technique that could cause harm.

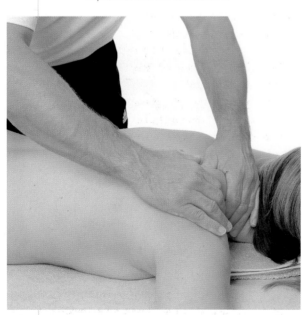

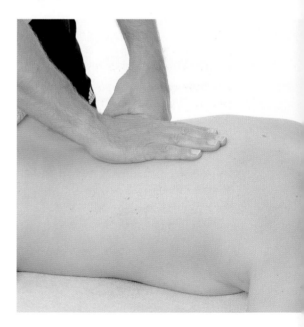

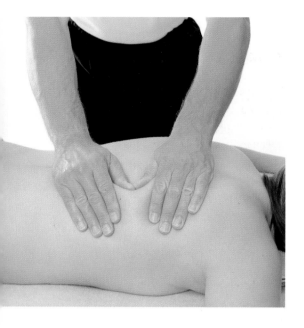

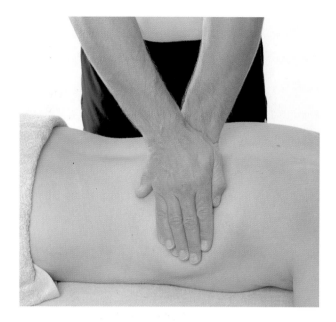

▲ Technique 5: Dermal lifting

Dermal lifting helps to boost circulation into the skin by working the deep layers as well as the surface ones. This technique increases blood flow and stimulates growth and healing.

1   Place both hands palm down on the skin, forming a triangle between your thumbs and fingers.
2   Move your thumbs forwards, using your bodyweight, so that they push into the triangle towards the fingers, raising a wave of skin in front of them.
3   Continue moving the thumbs forwards until a triangle of skin is trapped between the thumb and fingers, then release and work the next area.
4   Work the rhythm by rocking back and forth on your hips to create a controlled movement.

▲ Technique 6: Compression

Compression is one of the most simple massage techniques and also one of the most effective. It stimulates blood and lymph flow and releases tension.

1   Place one hand on the skin with your fingers raised and the heel of the hand prepared to press down.
2   Place the other hand on top of the heel of the contact hand, keeping the fingers relaxed.
3   Using your bodyweight, press down on the area for at least three seconds, and then slowly release the pressure.
4   Move to a new area and create a rhythm by rocking on your hips to produce and release pressure.
5   You should not compress the same area twice.

tip Locking the arms does not mean that they have to be straight; they should be firm but relaxed, and you should move them by using only your bodyweight and not your muscles.

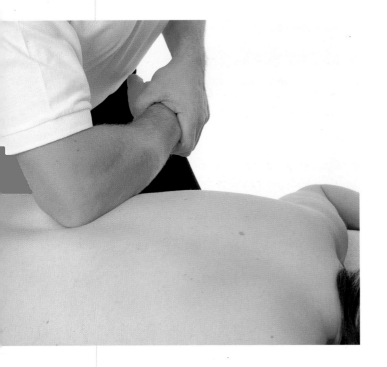

▼ Technique 7: STR (Soft Tissue Release)

STR is a specialized technique used for stretching the muscle fibres using the thumb to exert pressure on the muscle and the other hand to move the muscle into a stretch.

1   Unload the muscle – here the arm is bent at the elbow and the hand supported so the muscle isn't working.
2   Lock the thumb into the muscle – press the flat of the thumb directly into the muscle at the centre of the arm. Use the thumb to stretch the relaxed muscle upwards. Press upwards by moving the thumb 1 cm (½ in) towards

▲ Using other parts of your body

In some cases the hands and thumbs might not be strong enough to exert effective pressure. In this case elbows can be used for deeper penetration.

1   Stand with your elbow by your side, directly under your shoulder.
2   Place one leg in front of you and transfer your weight forward, keeping your elbow under your shoulder.
3   Be aware that although the elbow gives you deeper penetration you lose sensation; it is important to keep going back to using your hands so you can feel the muscle as well.
4   You can also use the forearm, which exerts a broader and therefore more superficial pressure. Do this in the same way as the elbow, placing your whole forearm on the area to be massaged and holding the wrist with the other hand to stabilize the posture.

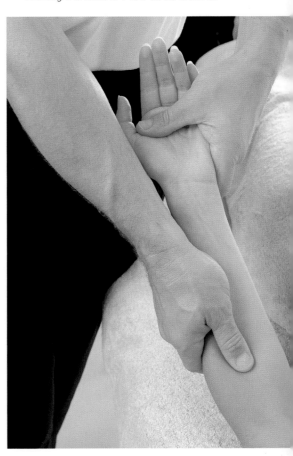

the top of the muscle. This action will stretch the muscle fibres underneath.

3   Load the stretch – keeping the thumb in position, slowly move the muscle into a stretch by moving the wrist downwards to straighten the elbow. Where the thumb is exerting pressure, it will stretch the muscle beneath it.

4   Work into the rest of the muscle – repeat the unload-lock-load-stretch process three or four times, making sure that you work on different areas of the muscle while covering the entire length of the arm, or whatever area you happen to be massaging.

5   Do not work on the same area twice.

▼ Technique 8: Stretch and draw

Stretch and draw combines the long strokes of effleurage with a stretching technique. It is performed towards you for greater control.

1   Position yourself on one side of the body, with your hands on the other side.

2   Form a loose hook with the fingers.

3   Bending your knees, bring your weight backwards, draw the hands slowly towards you, stretching the skin and tissues underneath it.

4   As you come to the end of the stretch and draw stroke, ease off – under control – by straightening your knees.

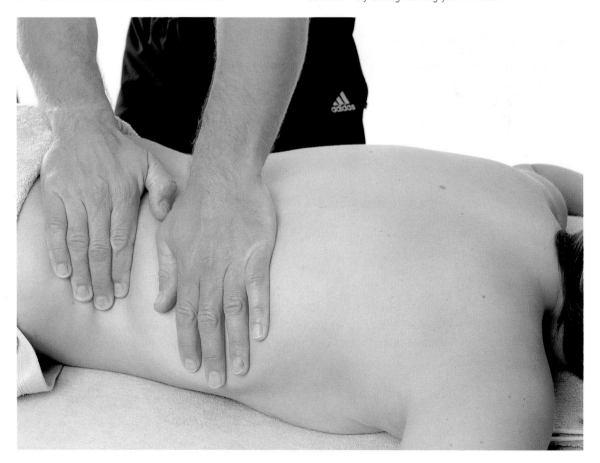

Back, neck and
shoulder massages

Of all the areas of the body, the head, neck and shoulders are the most prone to stress. Everyday stress and activity makes muscles tighten and eyes, jaws and necks tense up. Massage helps ease away tension and stress, boosting circulation and flexibility and preventing stiffness, pain, injury and trauma.

This series of massages shows you how to give a total back, neck and shoulder massage to one side of the body. For an entire session, complete all the massages on both sides of the body, either by exposing the whole back and performing a page at a time on both sides or by concentrating on one side at a time.

The back, neck and shoulders massage series should take about 40 minutes if you follow the sequence here, but you can vary the massage by spending longer or less time on certain techniques or even skipping some altogether. You should always finish with the back relaxation stroke, which will complete the massage.

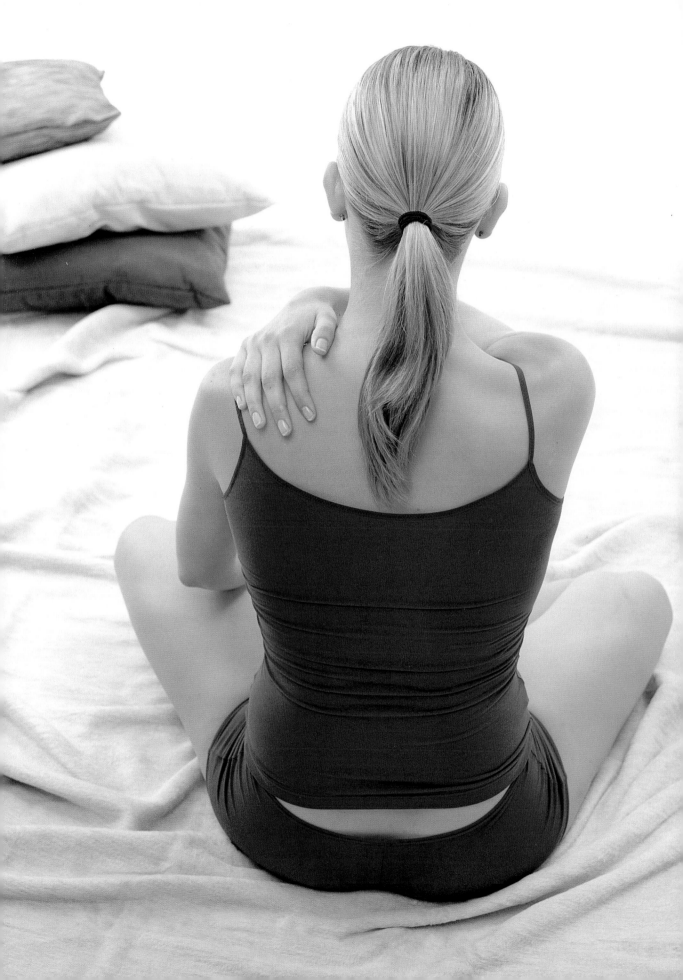

Basic anatomy

In order to understand how best to massage the back, neck and shoulders, the masseur needs to have a basic knowledge of anatomy. The bones and muscles will be discussed here but, it is important to remember that no single thing in our body works in isolation.

Bones of the back, neck and shoulders

The bones of the back, neck and shoulders are balanced on top of the pelvic girdle, a plate of bone at hip level that sits on top of the legs to provide balance and support to the upper body. The spine is composed of bones called vertebrae that sit on top of each other and have a hole running down the middle through which travels the spinal cord and blood supply that provides feeling, nerve control, blood and lymph to the lower limbs.

The top vertebra, which is attached to the occiput bone at the base of the skull, is the only spinal joint that does not move. Together, the vertebrae form a loose S-shape that curves in towards the stomach and lower back, out at the middle back and slightly in again at the neck. When the spine is in this position, the 'neutral position', it supports its own weight with no stress, strain or tiring muscle activity. We work in and towards this position during massage.

The balance of the body comes from the legs. Visualize the bones by working upwards from the pelvic girdle:

Pelvic girdle – A bony plate running across the width of the body to provide strength, balance and support to the upper body.
Sacroiliac joint – Five vertebrae that fuse during puberty to form a strength-bearing joint at the bottom of the spine.

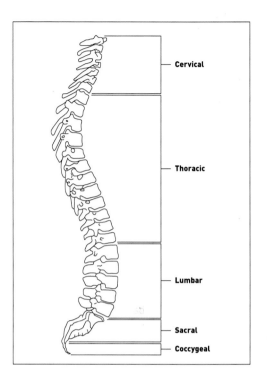

ABOVE **There are 24 moving vertebrae in the spine, with soft tissue discs between each one.**

Lumbar spine – The five largest vertebrae making up the lower part of the back. They form a natural curve, with the apex towards the front of the body (a lordotic curve).
Thoracic spine – The twelve vertebrae, to which the ribs attach, forming the central part of the back. They form slight curve with the apex away from the front of the body (a kyphotic curve).
Cervical spine – The seven small vertebrae of the upper part of the back that form a lordotic curve. The top two form a joint on which the head can pivot.
Clavicles – Two collarbones, one on each side, give stability and movement to the shoulders and attach them to the fixed, stable breastbone (sternum).
Scapulas – The two triangular shoulder blades that attach to and support the arm.

Between the vertebrae are gel-filled discs that allow the bones to move and provide a shock-absorbing casing for the spinal cord. These intervertebral discs account for one-third of the spine length and increase its weight-bearing capacity. It is important not to perform massage techniques directly on the spine as this could cause injury. The vertebrae are used as a guide only to massage the muscles at the sides of the spine. Special care must be taken with the neck vertebrae, which are more mobile and prone to injury.

Muscles of the back, neck and shoulders

The muscles of the back, neck and shoulders perform three tasks – stability to the trunk and upper body through the spine, movement of the head and neck on top of the spine and movement and rotation of the arms.

The main vertical muscles of the back are the paraspinal muscles, which run up either side of the spine to provide support. Two trapezius muscles run across the top of the back to stabilize the shoulder blades. The main muscles in the centre of the back are the latissimus dorsi, which start at the centre of the spine and wrap around and up the back to finish at the sides of the ribcage. Around the sides of the lower back, oblique muscles keep the trunk and abdomen upright. At the lower end of the spine, the large gluteal muscles run down over the bottom and around the hip. These stabilize the pelvic girdle to provide a balancing point for the whole upper body.

Blood and nerve supply

The major blood vessels serving the back, neck and shoulders run down the spine. The carotid artery runs up the side of the neck, taking oxygenated blood to the neck, head and brain, and the jugular vein returns the blood to the heart. The neck and back are the channels for the body's nervous system as the spinal cord runs through the spine.

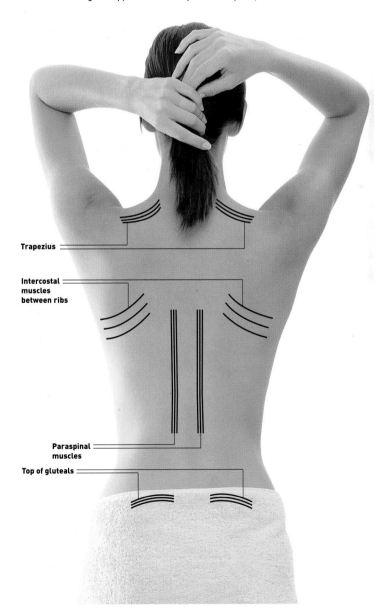

BELOW **The major muscles of the back give support and stability to the body.**

Trapezius

Intercostal muscles between ribs

Paraspinal muscles

Top of gluteals

BEFORE YOU BEGIN this section, make sure that the person to be massaged is lying supine – on their back, facing the ceiling. In each technique where no specific position is given, the person should be lying in the same starting position as described in the previous technique.

tip Remember to use your bodyweight for exerting pressure. If you are finding it difficult to do this, or you can't remember what it feels like, run through the bodyweight balance practice techniques on page 34.

▶ Clavicular effleurage

To ease tension and soreness in the front of the shoulders.

1   Face the left shoulder of the person being massaged.
2   Place the first two fingers of the right hand in the centre of the upper chest just under the collarbone (or clavicle), with fingers facing the right shoulder.
3   Place the first two fingers of the left hand on top and move your bodyweight forwards to move the fingers along underneath the bone, finishing at the shoulder.
4   Rock backwards, dragging the fingers lightly over the skin surface, and repeat several times on both sides.

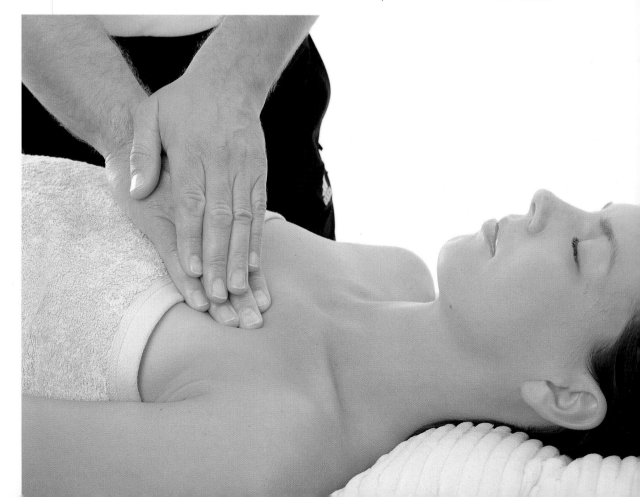

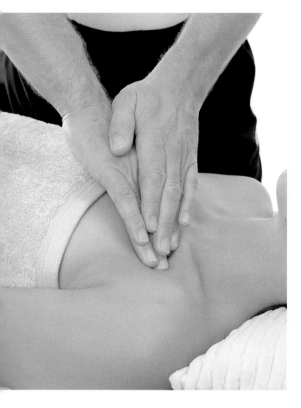

▼ Sternal and clavicular chest stretch

To stretch out the chest muscles, which may be tight due to stress or bad posture.

1   Stand to the right facing the shoulder.
2   Pick up the right arm by the wrist so it is level with the shoulder, pointing towards the ceiling, and support it.
3   Place the heel of your right hand into the side of the chest and push gently while you bring the arm down. Maintain pressure until the elbow is level with the shoulder.
4   To stretch through the chest, pick up the arm by the wrist with both hands. Step backwards and let the arm drop until it is level with the shoulder.

◄ Sternal effleurage

To ease tension in the chest.

1   Place four fingers of the right hand as before, with the left hand positioned palm down over the fingers.
2   Starting centrally, work all four fingers along the line of the collarbone, lightening the stroke towards the end and then back lightly over the skin.
3   Repeat several times on both sides.

Deep effleurage of the chest (optional)

1   Position as above, but this time use the thumb of the right hand, covered by the thumb of the left. Perform a deep stroke across the chest from the centre to the side of the shoulder.

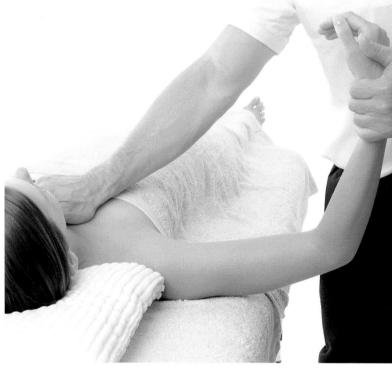

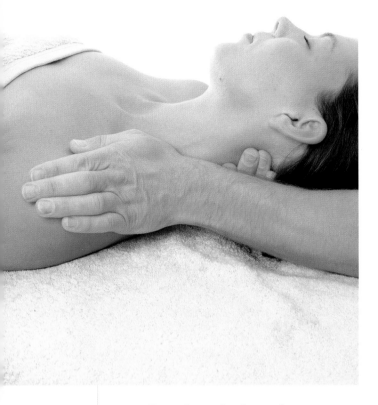

▼ Transverse neck effleurage

To work deeper and further into the neck muscles.

1   Position yourself as previously but this time, instead of using the heel of your hand to stroke down the neck, use your thumb to stroke in a downward motion from the front of the neck to the back.
2   Start with your thumb at the base of the ear and draw the thumb down over the side of the neck, working your way down the neck in three or four parallel strokes.

▲ One-handed neck effleurage

To drive out tension from stress and bad posture, from the sides of the neck.

1   Position yourself behind the head, facing down the body.
2   Cup your right hand under the neck, cradling the neck in your hand and allowing the head to rest on it.
3   Bring the fingers of your right hand gently towards you, bringing the right ear down towards the right shoulder and exposing the left side of the neck.
4   Place the heel of the left hand on the top of the neck and slide it away from you, towards the top of the shoulder. Remember to keep the right hand very still as it supports the head.

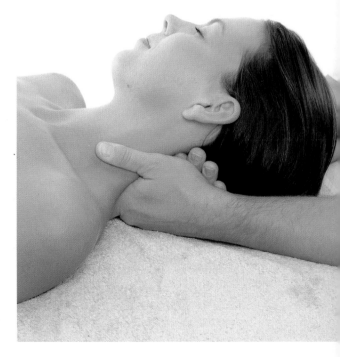

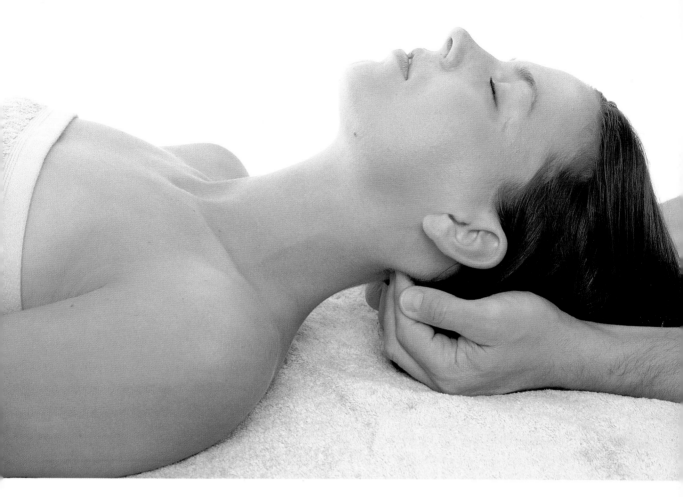

▲ Occiput pressure release

To relieve pressure, tension and stress from the muscles at the base of the skull, which can cause headaches, neck and back pain.

1   Position yourself behind the head facing down the body as before.
2   Cup both hands under the head and cradle the weight in your hands. Have your fingers at the base of the skull, under the ridge of bone (the occiput).
3   With the ends of your fingers, make small gentle circular movements around the base of the skull, being careful not to apply too much pressure.
4   Work your way around the whole bottom of the skull from the centre to the base of each ear and back again.

BEFORE THE NEXT technique, direct the person being massaged to turn onto their stomach so the massage can be performed with the body lying prone (facing the floor).

Occiput deep effleurage

To work further into the occiput.

1   Face the left side of the neck. The head and the neck should be in line.
2   Place your right thumb in the centre of the neck at the occiput.
3   Using the rest of your right hand to stabilize the thumb, stroke down along the ridge of bone towards the base of the ear. Take care not to press too hard, if the person feels any pain, or altered sensation in or around the eyes, you must stop immediately.

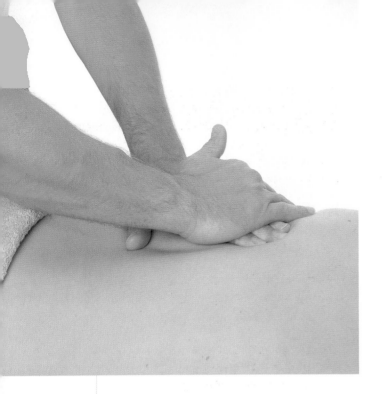

▼ Spinal thumb effleurage

To work deeper into the spine muscles.

1   Place your right hand on the bottom of the spine with the thumb and fingers at right angles. Lay the thumb beside, but not on, the spine on the side nearest to you, and the fingers pointing up the spine.
2   Place the left thumb on top of the right thumb and work your way up the back, exerting enough pressure to form a slight wave of skin in front of your thumb.
3   Instead of working up the back in one long stroke, which could force you to bend your back, work in three or four shorter strokes to cover the whole length, with overlaps between strokes. To move forwards, perform a lunging motion with your left leg and shift your bodyweight smoothly onto it.
4   Remember to keep your hands lightly on the skin between strokes to maximize relaxation potential.

▲ Spinal four-fingered effleurage

To relax and release tension in the spine before starting deeper techniques.

1   Position yourself at the middle of the left side facing the opposite shoulder.
2   Place the first two fingers of your left hand beside the spine on the side closest to you, on the ridge of muscle that runs up beside the spine (the paraspinal muscles).
3   Cover these fingers with the palm of the other hand and work up the paraspinals to halfway. While doing this, you should be pressing hard enough to create a slight wave of skin in front of your fingers.
4   In this way work your way up the back in three overlapping strokes: make one stroke from the bottom to halfway, then one from a quarter of the way to three-quarters, then one from halfway to the top, tapering the stroke on the shoulder in a controlled way without allowing the stroke to fall off the shoulder.

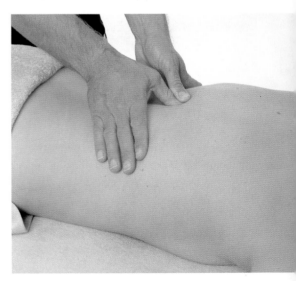

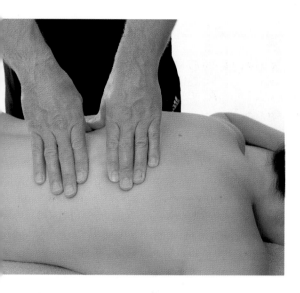

▲ Transverse thumb effleurage away from the spine

To stretch the spinal muscles away from the spine and reduce tension caused by bad posture.

1 Face the lower back.
2 Starting at the bottom of the back, place your right thumb on the side of the spine nearest to you (beside the spine, not on top of it).
3 Place your left thumb on top of the right and stroke towards you, finishing in a controlled way before your thumbs drop off the side.
4 Place your thumbs at the side of the spine about 5 cm (2 in) further up and repeat.
5 Work your way up the spine in this way, moving up every 5 cm (2 in) or so after each separate stroke, to finish at the shoulder blade.

tip If your thumbs begin to get tired while performing the effleurage techniques here, make sure that they are locked in position with no bending of the hand or wrist. Remember to use your bodyweight for exerting pressure.

▼ Circular shoulder effleurage

To reduce pressure and tension which can build up in the shoulders due to stress and bad posture.

1 Face the left shoulder.
2 Put your right hand palm down, fingers towards the head, next to the spine on the side furthest from you.
3 Raise your fingers slightly and stroke the heel of the hand up the spine until it reaches the neck.
4 Move the hand sideways on to the top of the shoulder in a circular motion and finish the stroke with control, just before the heel of your hand falls off.

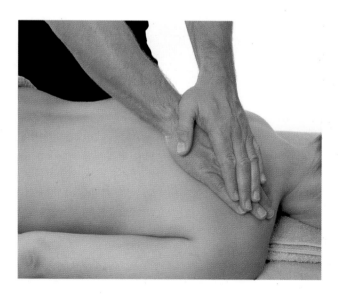

▼ Spine to shoulder blade effleurage

To release tension in the shoulder blades.

1. Face the left shoulder.
2. Reach over and place the flat of your right thumb at the nape of the neck on the opposite side of the body and cover it with the left forefingers.
3. Using the fingers of your right hand as a guide, make a straight stroke down from the base of the neck towards the top of the shoulder.
4. Move your thumb to the starting point, shift down 2.5 cm (1 in) and make a second stroke parallel to the first.
5. Repeat the downward movement between strokes and finish halfway down the shoulder.

Neck to shoulder blade effleurage

To work deep into the postural muscles at the side of the neck to reduce tension and increase movement.

1. Position yourself at the left of the neck with your body inclined towards the feet of the person being massaged.
2. Reach over and position your right thumb just below the hairline on the right side.
3. Cover your right thumb with your left thumb and make a gentle stroke down the neck towards the top of the shoulder, ending the stroke where the shoulder bone meets the arm.

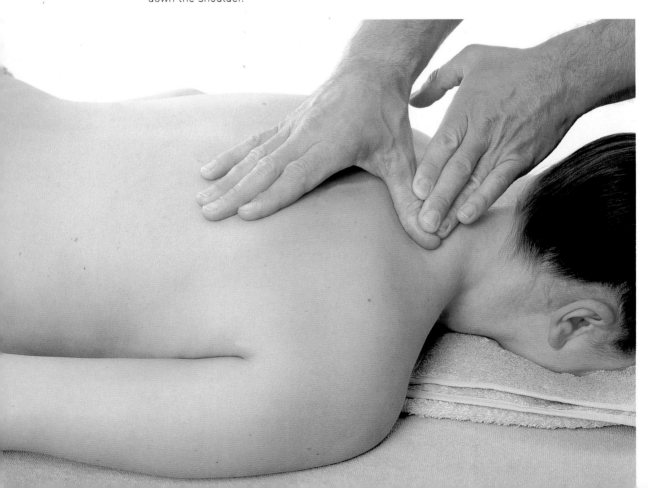

▼ Shoulder petrissage

To work deep into the postural muscles at the top of the neck to reduce tension and work away muscle knots.

1   Position yourself at the left of the neck with your body inclined towards the head.
2   Reach over to the right side of the neck and place your left hand on the side of the neck and your right hand at the bottom of the neck, where it curves into the shoulder.
3   Petrissage this area, starting very gently, bringing the left thumb to the right fingers and the right thumb to the left fingers.

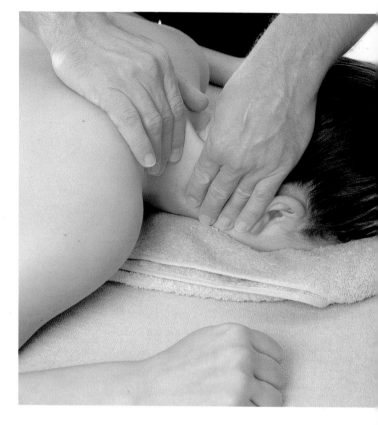

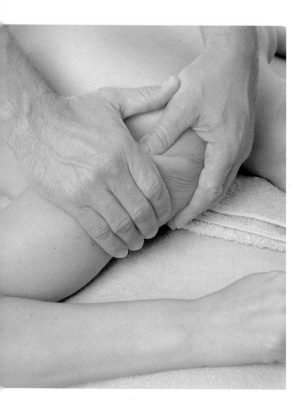

▲ Neck petrissage

To work deeply across the muscles of the neck.

1   Position yourself to the left side of the neck.
2   Reach over the body and place both hands gently on the opposite side of the neck.
3   Using gentle movements, bring alternate fingers and thumbs together to petrissage the muscles at the side of the neck. Take care not to exert too much pressure in this area. If in doubt, ease off.

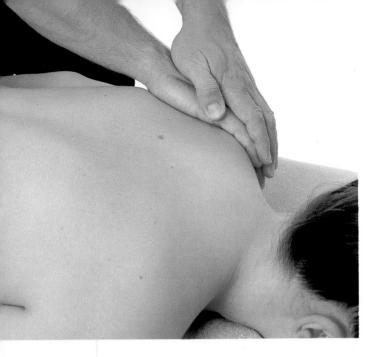

▲ Neck stretch and draw

To pull the shoulders away from the neck to reduce bunched up muscle tension in this area.

1   Position yourself at the left side of the ribs with your body facing the head.

2   Place your right hand on top of the shoulder so that your fingers disappear over the edge at the front of the shoulder, towards the arm.

3   Form a loose hook with your fingers so that you feel the shoulder underneath them.

4   Lock the fingers in place and gently draw the hand back, over and across the skin, using your bodyweight to perform the movement. Keep all parts of your hand in contact with the skin at all times, gently releasing the hooking of your fingers as your hand moves backwards.

5   End the stroke when your hand lies flat on top of the shoulder and the fingers are no longer hooked.

▼ Spine to central shoulder blade effleurage

This technique and the next one – the lower shoulder blade effleurage – work deep to increase postural flexibility.

1   Gently place the left arm by the side of the body, then position yourself on that side facing the head.

2   Use your whole hand to grasp the fleshy circular area that lies on top of the shoulder and raise until you see the shoulder blade lift up off the back. Remember not to bend your back.

3   Hold this position with your left hand and use the flattened fingers of your right hand to stroke in and around the edges of the shoulder blade. The thumb of your right hand should trail after the fingers around the contours of the shoulder blade.

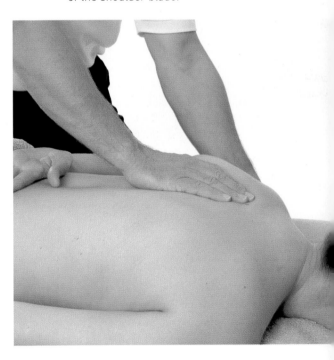

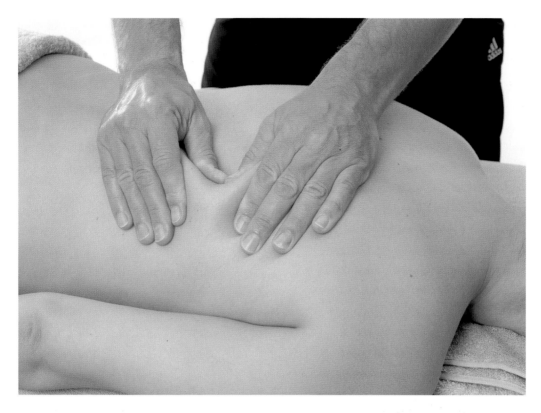

Lower shoulder blade effleurage

1 Face the right ribcage.
2 Reach over to the other side of the body with your left palm and cover it with your right, positioning the two palms face down at the bottom of the shoulder blade just the other side of the spine. Do not touch the spine.
3 Following the line of the ribs, stroke along the bottom of the shoulder blade, finishing the stroke as it tapers off the side of the body.

▲ Dermal lifting of the middle back

To boost circulation to the thick skin at the centre of the back in order to stimulate nerves and boost skin health.

1 Position yourself at the left side facing the middle of the back.
2 Place the flats of both thumbs on the opposite side of the body, off the spine.
3 Using the thumbs and first fingers of both hands, alternately pick up and drop sections of skin, working smoothly to create a lifting rhythm, taking care not to pinch the skin.
4 The movement should feel fluid and smooth, not jerky or painful. Work your way down from the spine towards the side of the body and sideways towards the lower back.

▼ Dermal rolling of the middle back

To work into the deep levels of the skin to boost circulation.

1   Make sure you have lubricated the skin as dermal rolling is a high-friction technique.
2   Place both hands on the opposite side of the body with the thumbs placed flat along the ridge of muscle that runs next to the spine and the fingers of both hands forming a triangle that points towards the side of the body.
3   Lift and roll the skin in this triangle, working side to side and forwards and backwards to cover the whole middle back area down to the lower back and up to the shoulder blade.

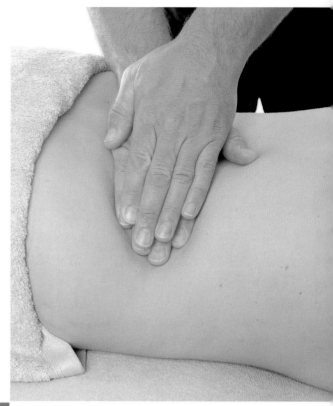

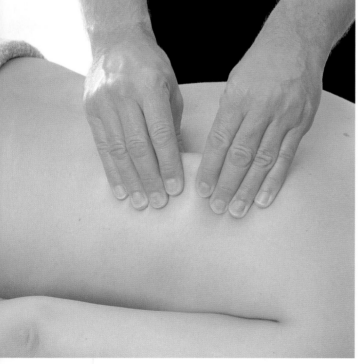

▲ Lower back effleurage

To ease pain and tension in the lower back and prepare for deeper massage.

1   Face the left lower back.
2   Place your right palm down on the V-shaped bone at the bottom of the spine, with the heel of your hand against the V and your fingers pointing away, towards the opposite side.
3   Place your left palm down, so that it covers your right hand.
4   Slowly start to press down with the palms and stroke away from you towards the top of the hip, easing off when you reach the hip.
5   At the end of the stroke, drag the fingers lightly across the skin to the starting position and repeat.

▼ Deep thumb lower back effleurage

To work deep into the lower back.

1   Face the left lower back.
2   On the side closest to you, place your right thumb just in front of the V at the bottom of the spine, with the fingers at right angles to the thumb.
3   Place your left thumb over the right. Stroke gently down towards the top of the hip (towards you), releasing the pressure to finish the stroke smoothly and returning the hand to the starting position. Maintain a light pressure on the skin so that you don't break contact.
4   Repeat several times, applying slightly more pressure each time for deeper and deeper effleurage.

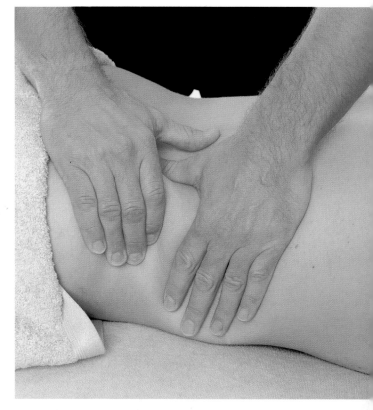

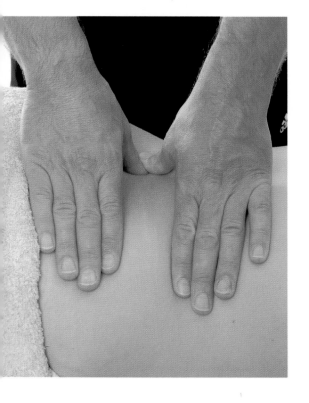

▲ Lower back petrissage

To boost circulation in the skin and muscles of the lower back.

1   Face the left middle back.
2   Bend your knees and place both hands on the other side of the spine with fingers facing away from you, down towards the side of the body.
3   Petrissage, bringing alternate thumbs and fingers together using your bodyweight to create a rhythm.
4   Work your way from the spine down towards the side of the body. Then move down towards the bottom of the back and repeat the movement.

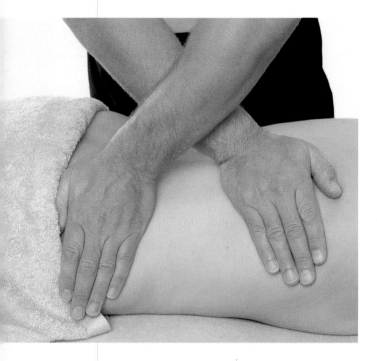

▲ Lower back stretch (with crossed arms)

To stretch the muscles of the lower back and release tension from bad posture.

1 Face the left lower back.
2 Cross your arms over each other and place the hands palm down in the middle of the lower back. The little fingers should be together and the heels of the hands next to, but not touching, the spine.
3 Push your bodyweight down and, as you do so, allow the hands to spread apart, stretching the skin beneath.
4 Continue the stretch as far as you feel comfortable with crossed hands, or until the lower hand reaches the bottom of the back. Then straighten your knees and lift up your body (to reduce the pressure going through your hands) to end the stretch in a controlled manner.

▼ Transverse draw around hip

To work away tension and knots in the muscles that lie at the side and centre of the lower back.

1 Bend your knees, straighten your back and rock forwards to allow you to lean over the body without stretching or bending your back.
2 Place the left palm on the side of the hip, with the fingers facing towards the front of the hip and make a loose hook with the ends of the fingers. You should be able to feel the front of the hip in your fingers.
3 Place the right hand on top of the left hand for strength and stability.
4 Lock the arms and wrists in position. This is very important for stretch and draw techniques because they involve

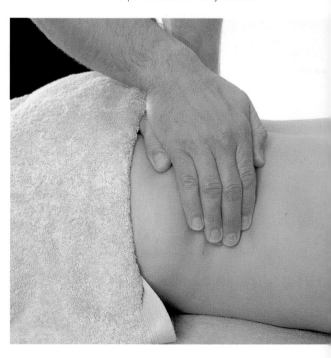

quite a lot of bodyweight transfer, which can cause back problems if not performed correctly.

5   Rock backwards and upwards, straightening your knees and controlling your bodyweight transfer, and draw the hands around the hip towards the V-shaped bone at the bottom of the spine. Gradually loosen the hooked fingers as they travel around to the centre so that by the time the heel of your hand arrives at the bottom of the spine, the palm is flat. Repeat once more.

6   Take a step up towards the head and repeat the draw, this time finishing at the base of the ribs instead of at the bottom of the spine.

►Cam and spindle of lower back

1   Position yourself on the left side of the lower back.

2   Place your right palm down over the spine, with the thumb at right angles facing the head.

3   Make a fist with your left hand around the thumb of the right hand without moving it.

4   The left hand should not come into contact with bone at all. Be very careful; this is a deep massage technique that could cause problems if performed incorrectly.

5   Step forwards with your right leg and lunge forwards onto it very slowly, beginning to work the cam and spindle away from you. Use the right hand as a guide and the left hand to produce a deep massage. Release the pressure as your hands taper off the back.

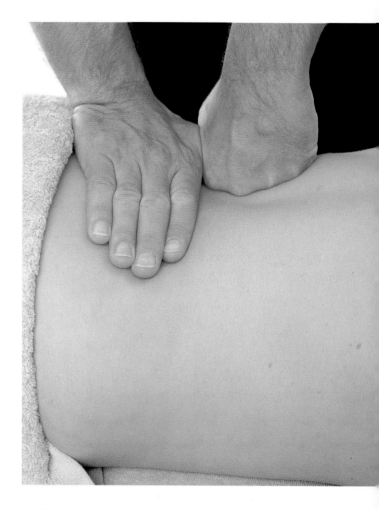

6   **Variation:** For a deep massage of the paraspinal muscles, you can perform a cam and spindle technique working your fist up the muscles at the side of the spine, from the bottom of the back towards the shoulders. Take care to avoid applying pressure on the spine – deep techniques are for massaging muscles only.

▼ Transverse draw of gluteals

To ease tension and knots in the muscles at the top of the buttocks.

1. Face the left lower back. You will need to work in a straight line over the top of the buttocks, rather than arcing over the lower back as in the transverse draw on pages 56–57.
2. Bend your knees, straighten your back and rock forwards to allow you to lean over the body without stretching or bending your back.
3. Place the right palm on top of the hip with the fingers facing towards the front and make a loose hook with the ends of the fingers.
4. Place your left hand on top of your right hand for extra strength and stability. Lock the arms and wrists in position.
5. Rock backwards and upwards, straightening your knees and controlling your bodyweight transfer, and draw your hands around from the hip and over the top of the buttocks towards the V-shaped bone at the bottom of the spine, gradually loosening the hooked fingers as your hands travel around to the centre of the buttocks.
6. By the time the heel of your hand arrives at the bottom of the spine, the palm should be flat over the bottom of the back. Repeat once more to complete.

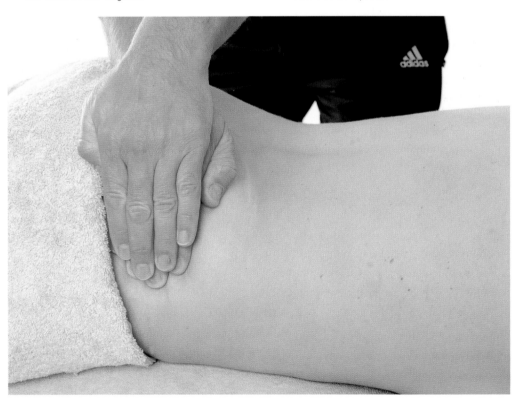

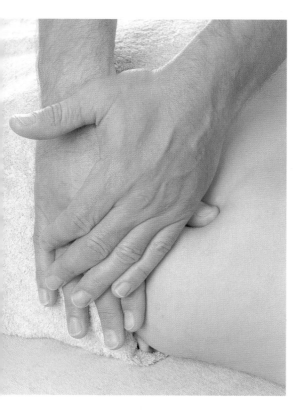

▼ Cam and spindle of top of buttocks

To reach into the deepest levels of the soft tissues that underpin the lower back.

1   Bend your knees, straighten your back and rock forwards to allow you to lean over the body without bending.
2   Place your left hand on the opposite side of the base of the spine so that the thumb points towards the feet and fingers point towards the side.
3   Make a fist with your right hand around the left thumb, so the knuckles of the right hand sit at the top of the buttock.
4   Using small, deep strokes, work your way around the top of the buttocks towards the side of the hip.

▲ Single thumb stroke of top of buttocks

To work deeper into the sitting and standing muscles.

1   Bend your knees, straighten your back and rock forwards to allow you to lean over the body.
2   Place your right thumb on the V at the bottom of the spine with the fingers pointing towards the side of the body.
3   Cover the right thumb with the heel of the left hand and make a deep stroke over the top of the buttocks, towards the hipbone.
4   Remember to keep your back straight as you finish the stroke on the side of the buttock, by the hip, and draw it back, keeping in soft contact with the skin. Repeat once more.

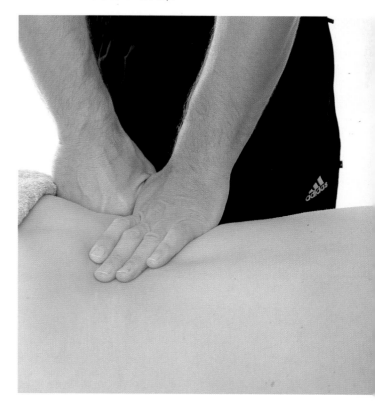

▶ Complete back relaxation stroke

To finish off the back, neck and shoulder massage by using relaxing strokes to ease away any remaining residual tension in the muscles and soft tissues. It also encourages regeneration and healing within the skin, as well as using a caring touch to boost self-esteem and inner peacefulness.

These steps should be performed as one big movement down the spine and back up again. However, to extend the feeling of relaxation, the steps can be performed separately as a four-step process that can be followed with the complete stroke.

1   Position yourself at the head of the person being massaged, looking directly down the body. Because this is a warming-down relaxation process, a lighter touch should be used than for other massages.

2   This stroke requires a lot of body movement, so before you start, position yourself in a lunge position so that you can shift further backwards and forwards without strain or stretching. (For a floor alternative, try kneeling on one knee and placing the other foot on the ground. This allows you to move forwards and backwards smoothly.)

3   Place your hands either side of the spine at the base of the neck, just on top of the shoulders, raise up the fingers of both hands and make a single stroke straight down the spine with the palms of the hands, finishing at the bottom of the spine with the heels of the hands touching the top of the buttocks.

4   When the heels of your hands touch the top of the buttocks, twist the hands slightly so that the fingers face inwards and the palms face out towards the hips.

5   Push your hands out towards the hips, with the palms leading and the fingers following, in a curved motion that reaches down the sides of the back at lower back level.

6   Using your palms to lead the fingers, bring the hands up the back and closer together so that they lightly touch each other at the level of the shoulder blades. Remember to use your own bodyweight to bring the stroke back towards you, rather than the muscles of your hands, arms or shoulders.

7   Using the palms to lead the hands away from each other, bring the stroke out over the shoulder blades and trace a small circle around the top of the shoulder, bringing your palms on top of the shoulder.

8   When your palms reach the top of the shoulder, shift your bodyweight again to go forwards and move the palms towards the outside of the ribcage at chest level, fingers forward. Finish the stroke by lightly bringing your hands off the skin.

9   Repeat the stroke several times, as required.

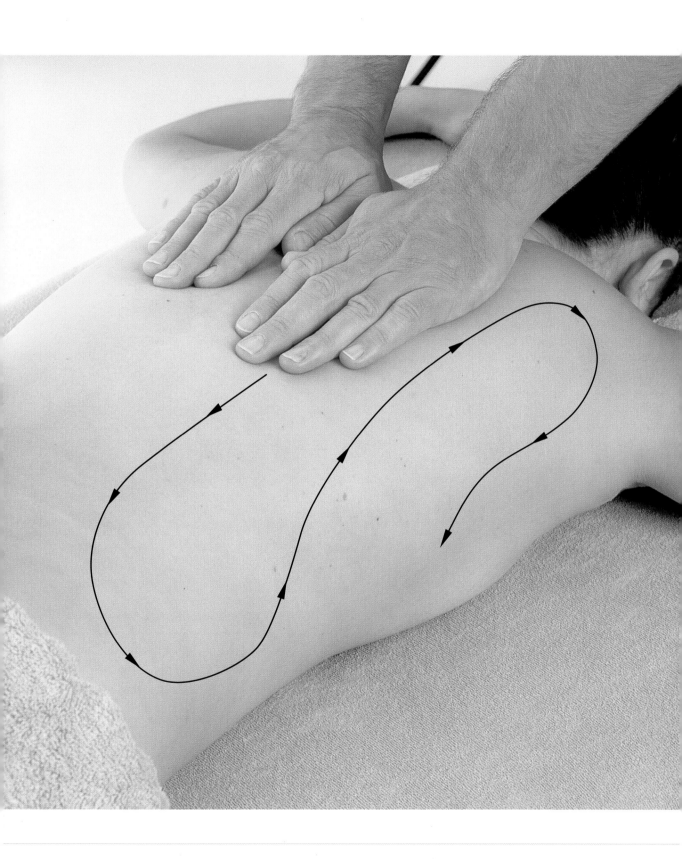

Leg and arm
massages

This chapter will show you how to give a total arm and leg massage to treat tired limbs, boost the flow of blood and lymph back to the heart and encourage the renewal and rejuvenation of cells. Unlike the back, neck and shoulders, where the main benefit of massage is to relax tension held in postural muscles and drive away muscle fatigue and tiredness, massage in the arms and legs is also useful for helping the circulatory and lymphatic drainage systems.

The total arm and leg massage should take about 40 minutes, but you can pick and choose techniques to highlight specific areas or just concentrate on the upper or lower limbs, which take about 20 minutes each to do. You should start with a clearance technique (see pages 66–7) and finish with limb vibrations (see pages 76–7 and 89) to relax any residual tightness in muscles. Because the muscles of the legs and arms lie near the surface you can develop your own intuitive touch by responding to what your hands encounter.

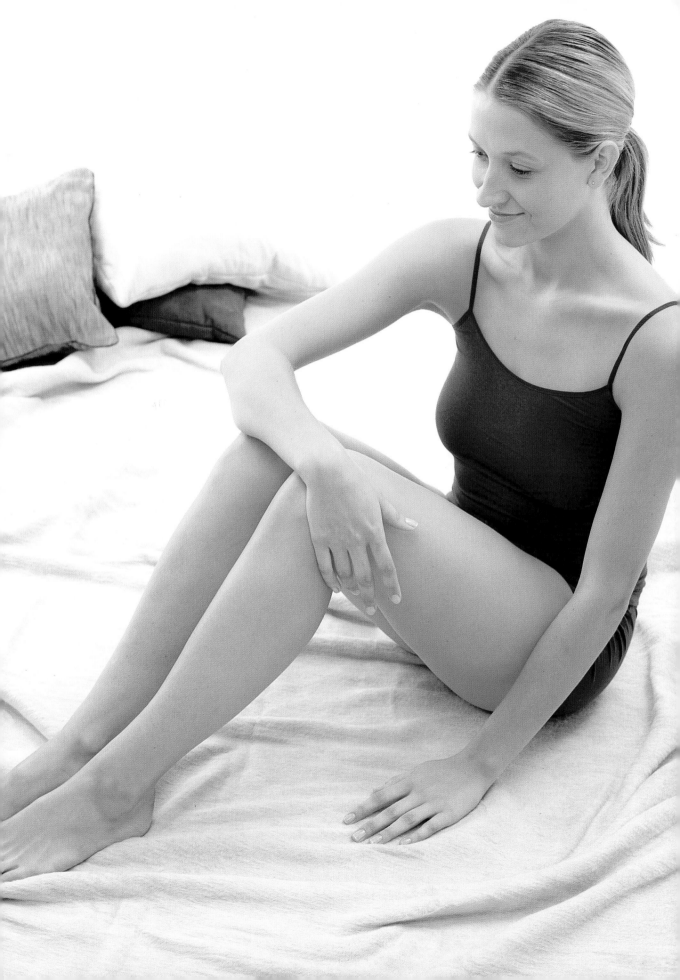

Basic anatomy

The limbs undergo different stresses and strains to the rest of the body because they are the most flexible. Thick arteries and veins run to and from the heart to our limbs. A complex system of nerves control feeling, muscles give a wide range of movement in all directions, and sensory receptors in the skin respond to minute fluctuations in touch, temperature and positioning. Massage benefits all these systems and is particularly good for boosting fluid drainage and return of blood from the extremities.

The difference between the arms and legs is that the legs are weight bearing and the arms are not. Because of this, the muscles in the arms and legs have slightly different qualities – the legs are built for strength and balance while the arms are designed for controlled and complicated movements.

The arms
Bones

The arm hangs from the shoulder joint, a ball and socket that is held in place by the muscles of the shoulder. The long bone at the top of the arm, which runs from shoulder to elbow, is called the humerus. At the elbow joint, this is attached to the two bones of the forearm, the ulna and radius. At the wrist, the ulna and radius attach, via a network of ligaments and tendons, to the hand bones.

Muscles

Each of the major muscle groups contains several individual muscles that work together to take the arm through its whole range of movement. Massage of the arm not only prevents blockage in the muscles but also reduces swelling, decreases tension and boosts circulation in and around tendons

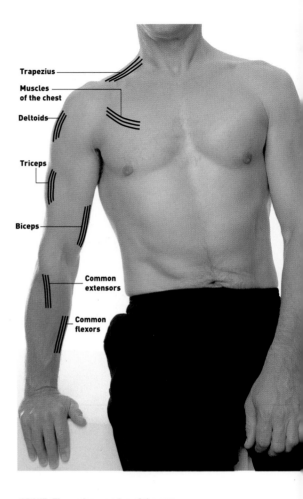

ABOVE **The major muscles of the arm benefit from massage to keep them supple and at a full range of movement.**

to increase efficiency, power and flexibility. Several major muscle groups of the arm, arranged in opposing (antagonistic) pairs, are responsible for movement:

- The muscles in the chest contract to bring the shoulder forwards.
- The trapezius muscles that run from the back of the shoulder across the back, contract to bring the shoulder backwards.
- The deltoid muscles on top of the shoulder, and curving over the arm, contract to bring the arm upwards.

Labels on image: Trapezius, Muscles of the chest, Deltoids, Triceps, Biceps, Common extensors, Common flexors

- The muscles in the underarm contract to bring the arm down.
- The biceps at the front of the top arm contract to bend the elbow.
- The triceps, which are opposite the biceps at the back of the arm, contract to straighten the arm.
- The common extensors, on top of the forearm, contract to raise the fingers of the hand and extend the wrist.
- The common flexors, at the bottom of the forearm, flex the wrist bring the fingers up.

Blood and nerve supply

The major artery of the arm, the brachial artery, runs through the shoulder and down to the elbow where it branches into two through the lower arm. The veins follow the same path, in the opposite direction. The brachial nerve runs through the shoulder into the top of the arm and the medial and ulnar nerves supply the whole arm with motor control and sensation.

The legs

Our legs bear the body's weight and give us balance and movement. This means that, unlike the arms, which can maximize their dexterity, the legs have to be strong and very secure. To do this, the legs are made up of thick, strong bones, large muscles that can bear a huge load, joints filled with shock-absorbing cartilage and flat, strong feet and ankles to maximize balance.

Bones

The legs start at the hip, which is a ball and socket joint that fits neatly inside a hole in the pelvic girdle. The femur, the large, long bone at the top of the leg, runs from the hip to the knee, where it becomes wider and meets the tibia, the large bone that runs

down the centre of the lower leg, and the fibula, the smaller bone that allows the lower leg to carry more load as it twists and moves over the ankle. At the ankle, the tibia and fibula meet to join up with the bones of the foot in a joint that relies heavily on ligaments.

BELOW **By keeping the leg muscles flexible and strong, the joints of the knees and ankles are supported.**

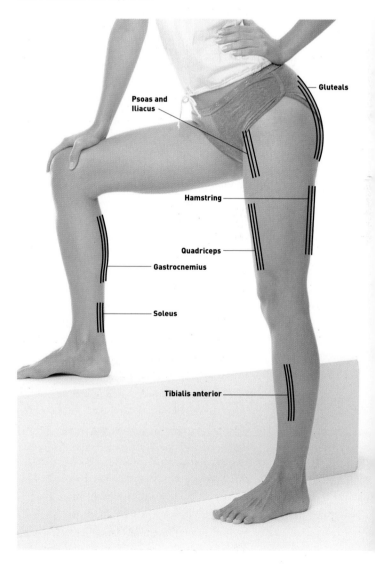

Muscles

Just like the arms, the legs contain several major muscle groups, each performing specific functions and working with each other to extend and to facilitate the range of movement.

- The gluteal muscles run from the lower back to the thigh, forming the major muscle groups of the buttocks. When these muscles contract they pull on the femur to straighten the leg from the hip.
- The psoas and iliacus muscles run down the front of the hip from the side of the body; they bend the leg from the hip.
- The hamstring muscles at the back of the thigh contract to bend the knee.
- The quadriceps muscles at the front of the thigh contract to straighten the knee (a sheet of strong tendonous tissue called the iliotibial band runs down the outside of the thigh to help stabilize this movement).
- The muscles at the back of the calf, including the gastrocnemius and the soleus, contract to point the foot.
- The muscles of the shin, including the tibialis anterior, contract to bring the toes towards the shin.

Blood and nerve supply

It is important to understand the location of nerves before beginning massage. The major arteries serving the leg run through the centre of the hip, travelling down the middle of the thigh (femoral artery) and through the back of the knee (popliteal artery) before branching out into the lower leg and foot. The major nerves (sciatic nerve, femoral nerve and peroneal nerves) run down from the bottom of the spine through the hip and branch out to cover the muscles and skin surface.

Lymphatic drainage

The arms and legs hold the major lymphatic drainage systems of the body, which carry lymph and fluid to be dealt with in the lymph glands. This body system serves to reduce swelling and drain fluid from the limbs and is particularly important for people who spend long periods standing upright, as gravity can cause collections of fluid in the lower limbs.

Massage boosts lymphatic drainage in several ways; first, application of pressure and strokes can reduce blockages and free up sticky channels; second, the act of stroking upwards actually 'pushes' fluid up the lymph vessels; and third, the general increase in circulation that follows massage helps fluid transfer in individual cells and tissues. Because of the dramatic effects massage can have on lymphatic drainage, it is important that it is performed correctly. As such it can give your body a massive boost; used incorrectly or in the wrong order it can cause blockage, fluid build-up and pain. Massage should work from the top down, using upward strokes. This means that:

- The individual strokes of the massage should always move in an upward direction, from the extremeties towards the heart, to push lymph and fluid upwards.
- Clearing techniques should start at the top of the limb and work downwards, clearing the lymph from the top to avoid fluid build-up.
- Even though the massager starts at the top, the techniques stroke upwards.

RIGHT **When performing a massage to enhance lymphatic drainage, work from the hands and feet towards the heart, following the arrows as shown here.**

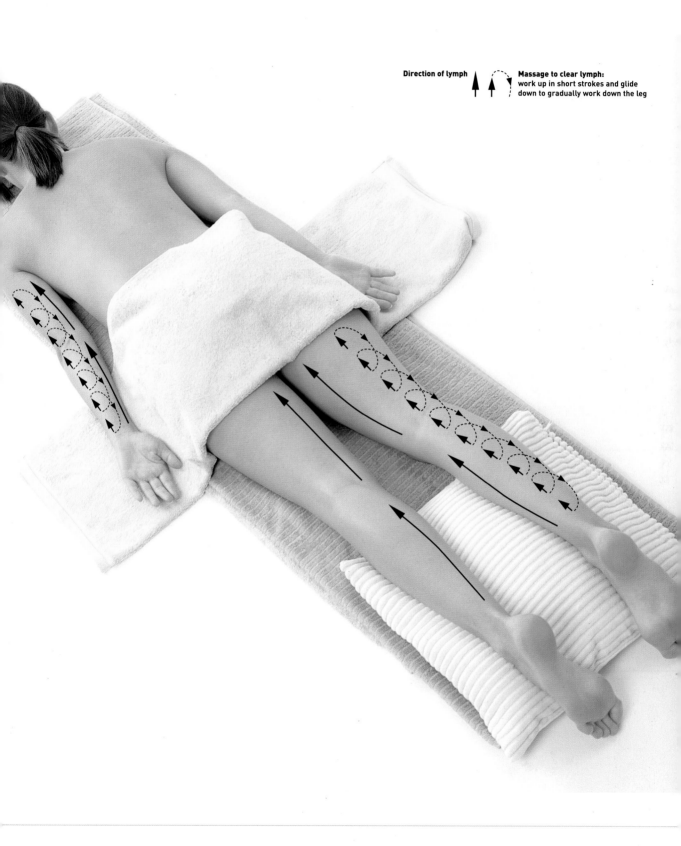

Direction of lymph ↑ ↑ **Massage to clear lymph:**
work up in short strokes and glide
down to gradually work down the leg

BEFORE THE NEXT technique, make sure the body is lying supine – face up.

▼ Front of shoulder effleurage

To ease tension in the postural muscles at the front of the shoulder, especially good for people who work at keyboards.

1   Face the left side of the person's chest.
2   With your left hand, lift up and support the arm so that it lies out at a ninety-degree angle to the body, elbow slightly bent.
3   Place your right thumb on the front of the shoulder where it meets the arm.
4   Make a stroke up from the shoulder towards the collarbone, stopping gently when your thumb reaches the bone.

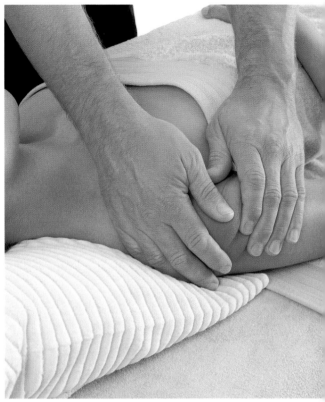

▲ Top of shoulder petrissage

To reduce stress and postural tension on top of the shoulder and into the neck.

1   Face the left shoulder at an angle to the body.
2   Place both hands on top of the shoulder so that the palms cover either side.
3   Petrissage by bringing thumb and forefinger together at the same time as exerting slight pressure downwards, pressing hard enough to produce a redness, and a slight torquing of the skin as your hands move over it.

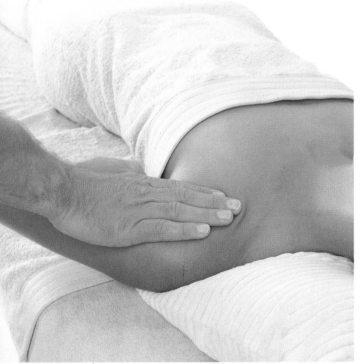

▼ Bicep effleurage

To stimulate flow of blood and lymph in the upper arm and boost circulation.

1   Face the left arm.
2   With your left hand, pick up and support the forearm so that the elbow is slightly bent, and the inside of the upper arm – the bicep – is exposed.
3   With your right hand, form a slight curve around the upper arm at elbow level (your thumb should be close to the elbow) and then allow your fingers to fall and relax so they conform to the shape of the arm.
4   Make a firm stroke up the arm towards the shoulder, leading with the outside edge of the palm, until you reach the crook of the arm.

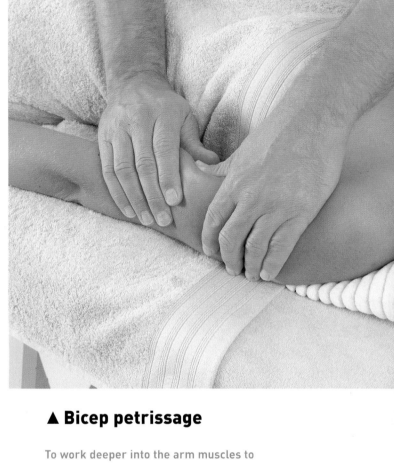

▲ Bicep petrissage

To work deeper into the arm muscles to reduce tension.

1   Place both hands on the top of the arm at the elbow and petrissage in an upward direction, working slowly towards the shoulder.

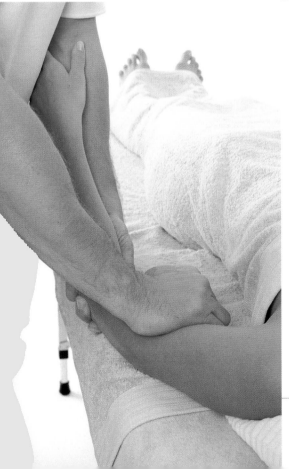

tip It is important to remember that the movement of your hands to petrissage should come from a rolling action in the hips and legs. The arms and shoulders should remain locked in position in a relaxed posture.

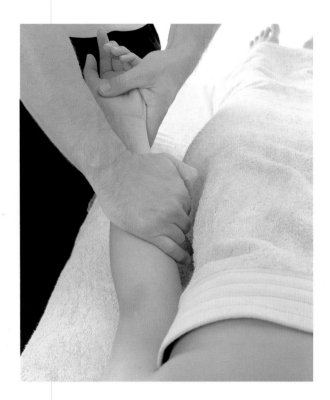

▲ Inside of forearm effleurage

To encourage the flow of lymph and blood away from the hand towards the heart and to boost circulation in the lower arm.

1   Face the bottom of the left arm.
2   With your left hand, raise the arm by the hand so that it is bent, and the wrist and hand lie directly above the elbow in a vertical line with muscles relaxed.
3   With your right hand, form a conformable shape over the top of the forearm at the wrist and make a firm stroke down towards the elbow
4   Repeat the stroke at both sides of the forearm, moving about 5 cm (2 in) in either direction to cover the whole forearm in three strokes.

▼ Palm stretching

To reduce stress and strain in the muscles and soft tissue of the hands and increase flexibility.

1   Face the left hand.
2   With both hands, pick up the hand so that the palm faces up, towards the ceiling, with your fingers at the back of the hand and your two thumbs resting in the middle of the palm touching each other.
3   Slowly draw the thumbs apart, at the same time as flexing the hands slightly back and outwards, so that you stretch the palm out as the thumbs move away from each other.

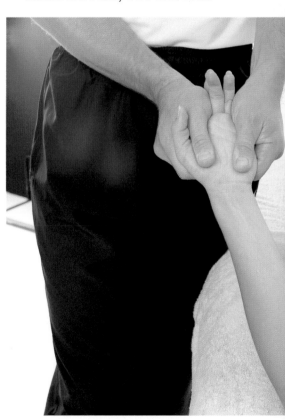

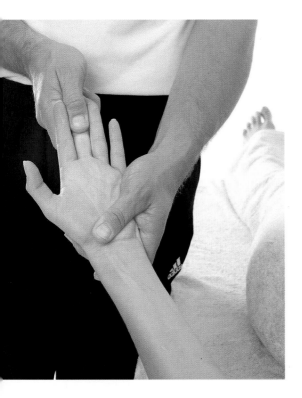

▲ Finger drawing

To ease away tension held in the hands.

1   With your left hand, support the
    forearm so that the elbow is bent
    and the arm muscles are relaxed.
2   Place the right hand over the first
    finger of the hand so the thumb points
    down the hand and the fingers curl
    loosely around the back of the finger.
3   Draw the finger out by exerting a
    slight pull as you draw your hand
    down the finger, with the thumb
    working down the inside of the finger
    and the fingers down the outside.
4   At the same time as you draw the
    finger out, move the hand up and
    down in a rocking motion to maximize
    the relaxation and stretch benefits.
5   Work your way down the fingers,
    repeating the process for each finger.

▼ Base of thumb petrissage

To work deep into the large muscles at
the base of the thumb.

1   Place your right hand into the hand
    so that the creases between thumbs
    and first fingers lie touching each
    other. Adjust your position by moving
    your hand up and down until your
    thumb sits flat on the fleshy part
    at the base of the thumb and your
    fingers support the area behind the
    base of the thumb.
2   Move your thumb in small circular
    clockwise movements around the
    base of the thumb so that it works
    into the muscle.

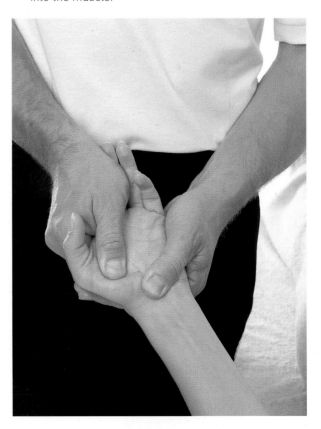

▼ Back of forearm effleurage

To stimulate the flow of blood and lymph up the forearm and clear fluid blockages.

1   Face the left hand of the person being massaged.
2   With your own left hand, pick up the arm by the hand so that it is bent and the wrist and hand lie vertically above the elbow with muscles relaxed.
3   With your right hand form a conformable shape over the top of the forearm at the wrist and along one side of the forearm – the cupped shape of the hand should follow the contours of the forearm.
4   Make a firm, slow stroke towards the elbow. Do not allow the wrist to bend.
5   Repeat the stroke at both sides of the forearm, moving about 5 cm (2 in) in either direction to cover the whole forearm in three strokes.

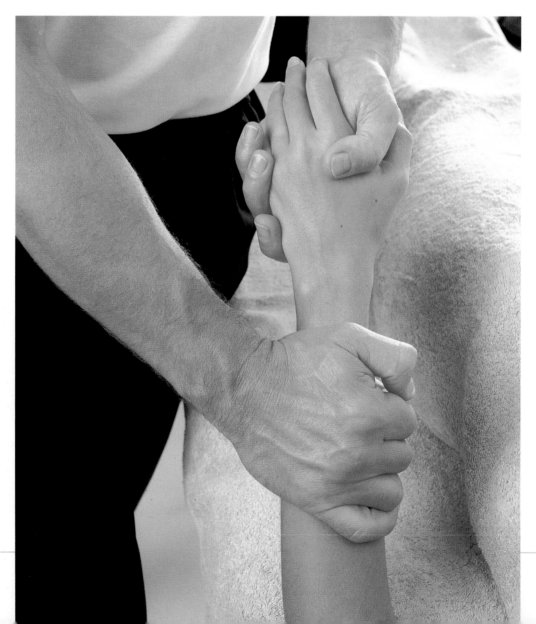

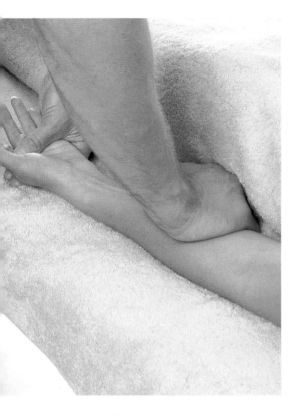

▲ Anterior forearm compression

To work into the muscles of the forearm to help reduce muscle tension and release toxins.

1   Using the heel of your hand, press down for a few seconds at the wrist end of the forearm, then release the pressure and move up 3–5 cm (1–2 in).
2   Continue this, pressing, releasing and moving up until you have covered the whole back surface of the forearm and reached the elbow.

▼ Forearm STR

To stretch specific parts of the muscles of the forearm.

1   Position yourself by the left forearm.
2   With your left hand, extend the hand to contract the muscle on top of the forearm. It should be extended but not stretched and should feel comfortable.
3   With your right hand, push the thumb directly into the muscle on top of the arm with a downward movement.
4   Move the thumb upwards (towards the elbow) by about 1.5 cm (½ in), so that you stretch the muscle slightly underneath it.
5   Lock the thumb in position and, slowly and gently, move the hand back down.

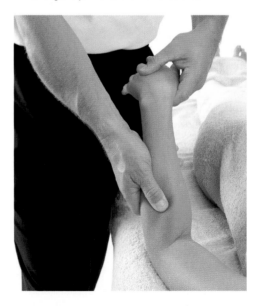

tip The point of contact where the thumb meets the muscle might be a little sore because this is a deep technique that stretches the muscle. It should not be painful except for a mild feeling of discomfort or tenderness where the thumb is in contact. If it causes pain or soreness, stop immediately and move on to another massage.

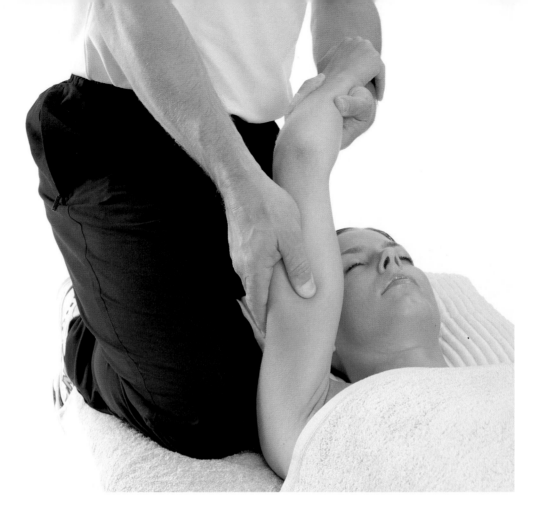

Bicep petrissage

To work deep into the muscles of the top of the arm to boost circulation and release tension.

1 Face the left elbow.
2 Place both hands on the top of the arm at the bicep, with palms of hands on top of the arm and the fingers pointing downwards.
3 Grasping the skin and exerting a gentle downward pressure, bring alternate thumbs and fingers together to petrissage the bicep muscle.
4 Move the petrissage around so you cover the whole area between the elbow and the shoulder.

▲ Tricep STR

To target specific parts of the muscle for localized stretching.

1 With the left hand, hold the forearm straight up in the air without lifting the shoulder – straighten, do not stretch.
2 Push the thumb of your right hand, directly into the muscle at the back of the arm (the tricep) near the back of the elbow. Lock the thumb in place and, keeping the same pressure, move it down towards the shoulder so that the muscle is locally stretched.
3 Keeping the thumb in place, stretch further by using your left arm to bend the arm at the elbow, releasing your thumb as the hand gets to the shoulder.
4 Repeat several times as you work your way towards the armpit.

BEFORE THE NEXT technique, direct the person being massaged to turn face down.

▼ Tricep effleurage I

To encourage the flow of lymph, blood and toxins away from the back of the arm.

1   Face the right side of the person being massaged.
2   Using your left hand, grasp the forearm and bend the elbow inwards.
3   Place your right hand over the tricep at the back of the arm, with the palm of the hand facing downwards and the side of the hand at the elbow forming a contour over the arm.
4   Stroke your hand towards the shoulder, using the palm to produce pressure on the tricep.

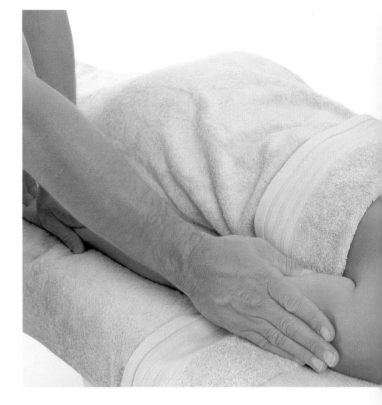

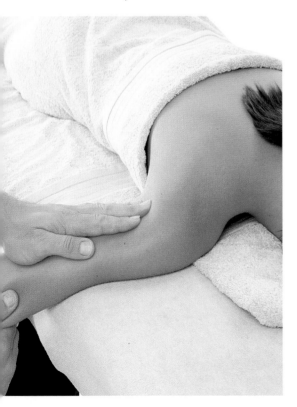

▲ Tricep effleurage II

To work away tension and toxins from the upper arm.

1   Face the right ribcage with your body at forty-five degrees to the arm.
2   Bring the arm down so that it lies palm up by their side.
3   Place the thumb of your right hand on the tricep at the elbow and make a long stroke down towards the shoulder. Use the thumb to exert pressure and allow the fingers to form a contour around the arm shape.
4   Move your hand slightly to left and right and repeat the stroke.

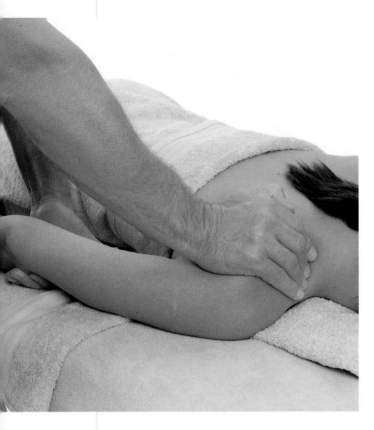

BEFORE THE NEXT technique, direct the person being massaged to turn onto their back so that the massage can be performed with the body lying supine – face up.

▶ Complete arm shake for relaxation

To relax the muscles at the end of the massage and to encourage all the tissues and fibres of the arm to work together to reduce toxins and tension and to boost relaxation, regeneration and healing. The arm shake should be used following all arm massages.

1   Stand slightly apart from the body at hip level, facing at an angle to the body so that you look directly towards the shoulder.
2   Using both hands, grasp the sides of the wrist and hand and lift the arm about 10 cm (4 in) so that the elbow and upper arm are supported and the shoulder is not lifted off the ground.
3   Using both arms together, make gentle up and down movements to shake the whole arm in a relaxed and controlled motion, starting with larger movements that get smaller and smaller until they stop.

▲ Back of shoulder effleurage

To ease tension in the postural muscles and stimulate circulation.

1   Lie the arm, palm up, by their side. Place your left hand in the crook of the elbow and lift about 5 cm (2 in) to reveal the shoulder blade.
2   Place the palm of your right hand flat on the top of the arm by the shoulder with your fingers pointing towards the shoulder. Lift the fingers slightly and stroke with the palm towards the top of the shoulder and into the shoulder blade, stopping level with the armpit.
3   Repeat several times, pushing harder each time.

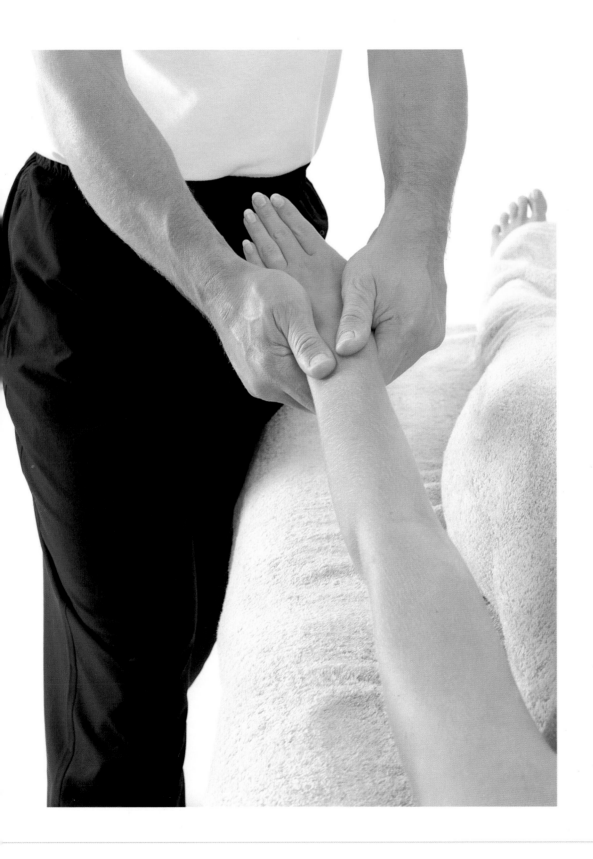

▼ Rolling compressions working down the thigh

To prepare the muscles in the front of the thigh for deep massage by clearing lymph, fluid and toxin build-up.

1   Position yourself halfway up the left thigh facing up towards the head.
2   Place both hands, palm down on the top of the thigh with fingers slightly raised and the right hand a fraction higher up the thigh than the left.
3   Press with the heel of your right hand, hold for a few seconds and release.
4   Repeat with the left hand, then move the right hand down and repeat, pressing and releasing with alternate hands all the way down the thigh to release tension.

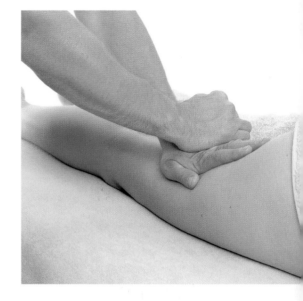

▲ Heel of hand thigh compressions

To clear more toxins, lymph and tension.

1   Place your left hand palm down, fingers raised, in the centre of the thigh, 5 cm (2 in) below the groin.
2   Place the right hand on top of the left so that the heel of the right hand is directly above the heel of the left.
3   Lock your wrists so they do not move.
4   Make a deep stroke of about 7.5 cm (3 in) using the heel of your hands to apply pressure in an upward direction.
5   Move down 15 cm (6 in) and make another stroke, the same length as the first and ending where the first began.
6   Continue to work down the thigh, making deep strokes of about 7.5 cm (3 in) in length all the way down. The strokes should not overlap and should end where the previous one began.
7   Once you reach the soft muscle on top of the knee, move your hands to the top inside of the thigh and repeat. Do the same for the outside of the thigh.

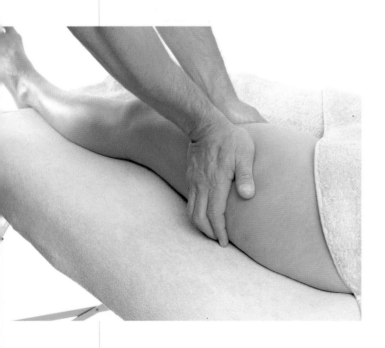

▼ Thigh effleurage I

To encourage the flow of lymph away from the leg and boost circulation.

1 Position yourself beside the left knee facing towards the head.
2 Place your left hand over the fleshy muscle on top of the knee so the side of your hand faces up towards the head and your thumb lies alongside the fingers nearest to the knee.
3 Assume the lunge position and place your right hand over the top of your left hand, slightly further back towards the knee so the last two fingers of the left hand are not covered.
4 Lunge forwards and make a single stroke up from the knee to the top of the thigh, pushing down with the side of your hand and allowing your hand to follow the contours of the thigh to maximize the point of contact. Finish the stroke at the top of the thigh.

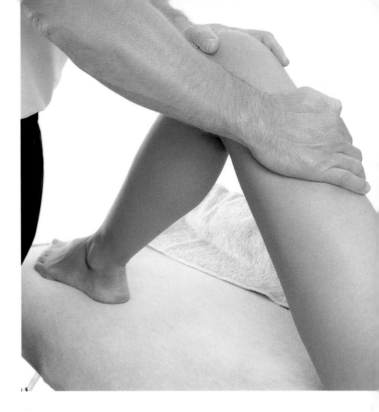

▲ Thigh effleurage II

To release deep tension contained in the thigh muscles.

1 Bend the knee and put the foot flat on the bed or floor surface to stretch the thigh muscle.
2 Steady the leg with your left hand.
3 With your right hand lying across the thigh, make a single stroke up from the knee to the top of the thigh, pushing down with the side of your hand and allowing your hand to follow the contours of the thigh to maximize the point of contact.
4 Finish the stroke at the top of the thigh in a controlled manner.
5 Replace the leg to its lying position, with the knee straight or slightly bent.

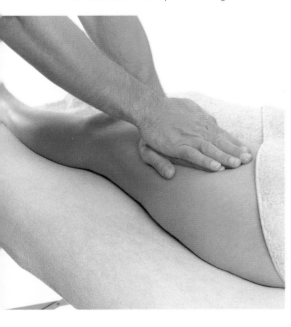

tip While performing this technique, do not touch the kneecap itself. Start above the knee and work gently upwards.

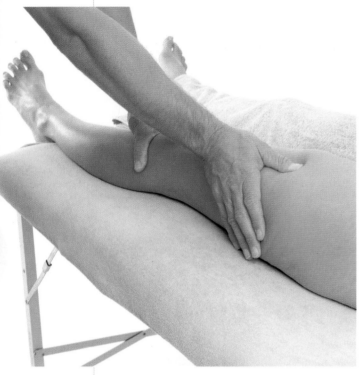

▼ Thigh petrissage

To work over the whole thigh to boost circulation to all muscles and soft tissues, as well as to encourage the regeneration of the skin and the release of tension.

1 Face the right thigh.
2 Reach over and place both hands next to each other palm down on the left thigh just above, but not touching, the knee with fingers and thumbs forming a loose triangle.
3 Bring alternate fingers to thumbs to petrissage and move up the thigh, working from the knee to the hip up the outside of the thigh.

▲ Deep effleurage of thigh

To work deep into the thigh muscles targeting specific areas for circulation and regeneration.

1 Place your right hand on the thigh, just above the knee, so that the fingers point down the outside of the thigh towards the head and the thumb rests on top of the thigh.
2 Make a deep stroke upwards in a straight line, continuing up the centre of the thigh from the knee to the hip. Use your fingers to guide the stroke.
3 Repeat the stroke from above the knee a further four times, twice on the inside of the thigh and then twice on the outside. Do not go over the same part of the thigh twice.

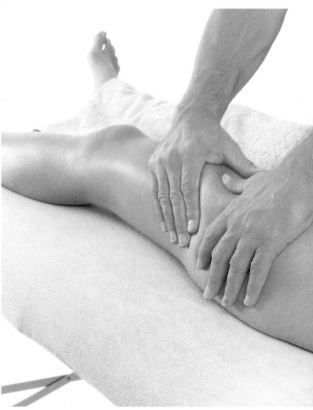

▼ Ankle to knee effleurage

To boost the flow of lymph, to increase circulation and to ease away tension.

1   Position yourself about halfway down the left shin.
2   Place your left hand over the very bottom of the shin, just above but not on the ankle, with the side of the hand facing up towards the head and the thumb on the side nearest the foot.
3   With the heel of your right hand, lunge forward to make a single stroke from ankle to knee. Finish underneath the knee without touching the kneecap.
4   Repeat several times, moving to the outside and inside of the shin.

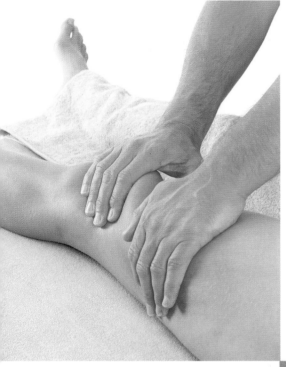

▲ Transverse draw of knee ligaments

To work across the knee ligament, which can become tight, and to free up tension in the centre of the leg.

1   Reach over with your left hand and form a loose hook with fingers, at the bottom of the thigh above the knee.
2   Place your right palm on top of the left hand, lock wrists, arms and shoulders.
3   Pull with the left hand while applying pressure down through the palm with the right to stretch the knee ligaments under your fingers, work in an arc to finish on top of the thigh about 5 cm (2 in) higher than where you started.
4   Move about 5 cm (2 in) up the leg and repeat the draw parallel to the first one, continuing to move up and repeat until you reach the top of the thigh.

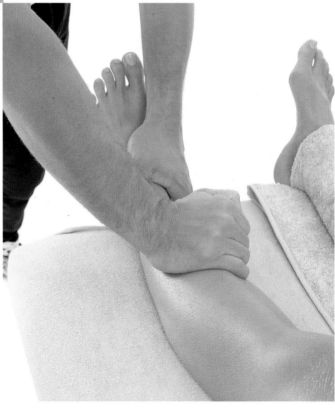

▼ Shin STR

To target specific areas of the shin muscle, easing away stresses and strains and boosting flexibility.

1   Using the left hand, flex the foot so that the toes point to the ceiling and your palm supports the foot sole.
2   With your right thumb, press into the centre of the muscle that runs down the front of the shin, just to the side of the bone, and lock the thumb in position. Then move upwards towards the knee while still exerting pressure.
3   Use the left hand to bring the foot slowly to a point, while keeping the right thumb in position to increase the stretch.
4   Repeat several times over the muscle; do not press into the same area twice.

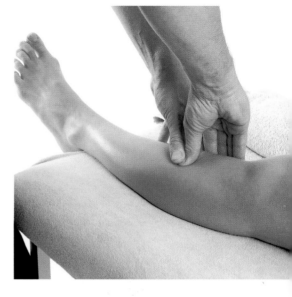

▲ Transverse glide across front of shin

To work deeper into the muscles at the front of the shin, which are prone to tension, to ease away fibrous build up and separate it from surrounding tissues to clear away toxins.

1   Place your thumbs pointing towards you beside the shin bone on the muscle that runs up beside the shin, just below the knee. Your fingers should be pointing down the inside of the lower leg.
2   Dropping your bodyweight, make a single stroke down towards you, pulling the shin directly away from the shinbone. Stop the stroke when you feel your thumbs coming off the edge of the shin.
3   Move down about 5 cm (2 in) and repeat the stroke, working towards the ankle, until you have covered the whole shin.

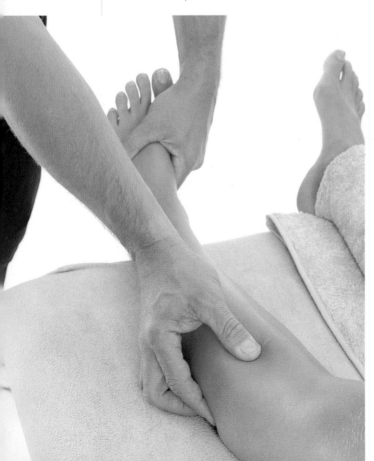

▼ Draw of front of foot

To work into the muscles, ligaments and tendons of the foot in order to stretch and ease tension.

1   Position yourself by the left foot facing the head.
2   Grasp the ankle with your right hand so that the thumbs sit on top of the foot and the fingers and palm support the sole. Hold the shin steady with your left hand.
3   Lock your wrists, arms and shoulders in position and rock back on your feet, pushing apart with your thumbs at the same time so your right hand stretches the foot sideways while your left stretches it lengthways.
4   Repeat several times to stretch out the ligaments and tendons of the foot.

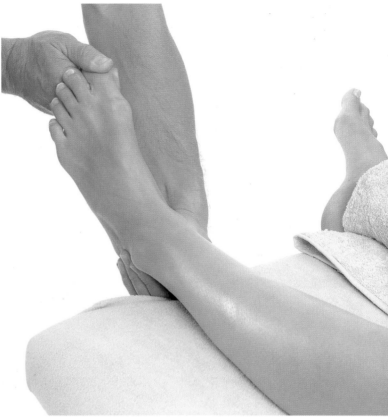

▲ Toe stretch

To work into the toes for nervous stimulation to boost balance and skin regeneration.

1   With the left hand, support the left foot at the heel, lifting it about 5 cm (2 in).
2   Place the right thumb on top of the base of the little toe and curl your right index finger underneath the toe at the base.
3   Slowly and gently draw the toe out, using the finger as a pivot and the thumb to stretch the toe out over the top of it.
4   Repeat for each toe.

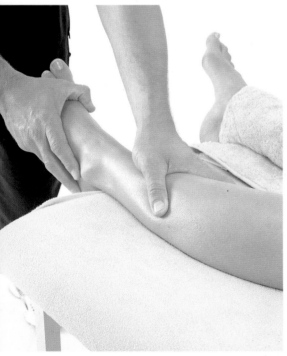

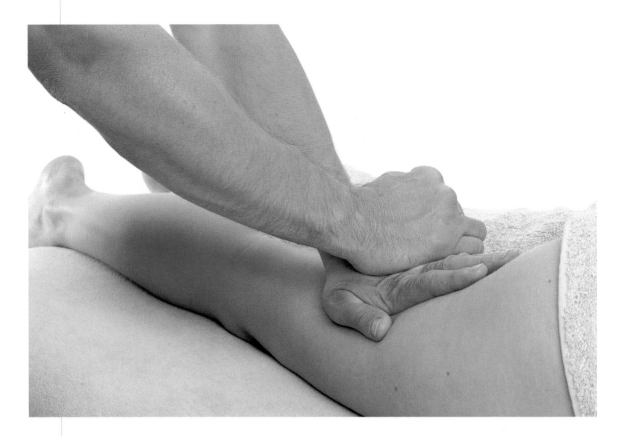

BEFORE YOU BEGIN the following techniques, direct the person being massaged to turn onto their stomach so that the body is lying prone (facing the floor).

▲ Heel of hand working down hamstrings

1 Position yourself beside the left thigh facing the head.
2 Place your left palm on the centre of the thigh, 5 cm (2 in) below the bottom, with fingers slightly raised.
3 Place the right hand on top of the left so that the heel of the right hand is directly above the heel of the left.
4 Lock your wrists together. Make a deep stroke of about 7.5 cm (3 in) using the heel of your hands to apply pressure in an upward direction.

5 Move the hands down 15 cm (6 in) and make another stroke (this stroke should be the same length as the first and should end where the first began).
6 Continue to work down the thigh in this way, pushing upwards but working downwards to clear the lymph, making deep strokes of about 7.5 cm (3 in) in length all the way.
7 Stop compressions BEFORE you reach the soft triangle behind and above the knee (the location of the leg artery, which should never be massaged).
8 Move your hands to the top inside of the thigh and repeat. Repeat again for the outside of the thigh.

tip After the first stroke with your hands, you can do this with your forearm. Get close to the body with your shoulder over the leg. Bend your elbow directly under your shoulder, hold the left wrist with the right hand and stroke up using the forearm.

▼ Hamstrings effleurage I

1 Position yourself by the left knee facing the head of the person being massaged.
2 Place your left hand palm down on the bottom of the hamstrings (avoiding the soft fleshy triangle at the back of the knee where the main leg artery is located). Place it sideways so that the thumb is nearest the knee, and cover it with your right hand.
3 If you are at a massage table or bed, move one of your legs forward to give you a stable base to lunge onto, and lunge forward, making a stroke up the thigh towards the head.

▼ Cam and spindle of the hamstrings

1 Form a fist with your left hand. Place it knuckle down on the the back of the thigh, 7.5 cm (3 in) below the buttocks.
2 Place the thumb of the right hand inside the left fist and the palm of the right hand flat on the outside of the thigh with fingers pointing to the head.
3 Use the right hand as a guide and the left fist for pressure, make a short stroke up towards the head.
4 At the end of the stroke move about 15 cm (6 in) down the thigh and repeat, continue down the thigh. Stop before you reach the soft triangle at the back of the knee.

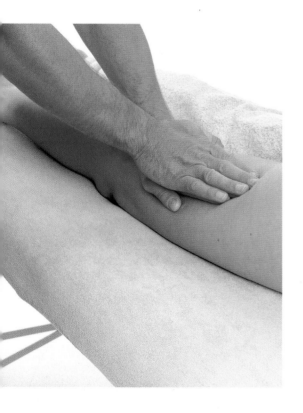

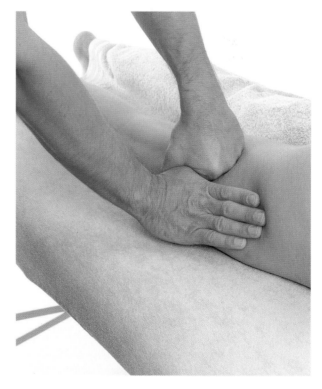

▼ Hamstrings effleurage II

1 Place your left thumb on the bottom of the hamstrings (avoid the soft fleshy triangle at the back of the knee) and cover it with the right thumb.
2 Move one of your legs forward to give you a stable base to lunge onto and lunge forward, making a deep thumb stroke up the thigh towards the head.
3 Repeat several times to the left and right of the original stroke, taking care not to cover the same area twice.

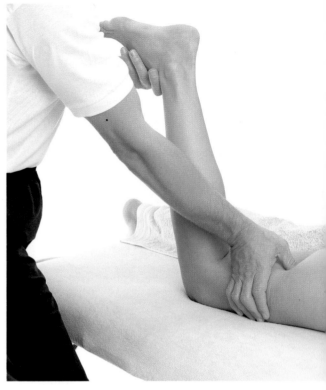

▲ Hamstrings STR

1 Position yourself by the left hamstrings facing the feet.
2 With your left hand, pick up the foot so that the knee bends and the foot points straight up towards the ceiling.
3 Put the right thumb into the hamstring muscle about halfway up the leg and shift it backwards up to the head about 5 cm (2 in) to put the muscle on a stretch.
4 Using your left hand for control, slowly drop the foot so the knee straightens and the hamstring is stretched.
5 Repeat several times, working the whole thigh but carefully avoiding the fleshy soft triangle above the back of the knee.

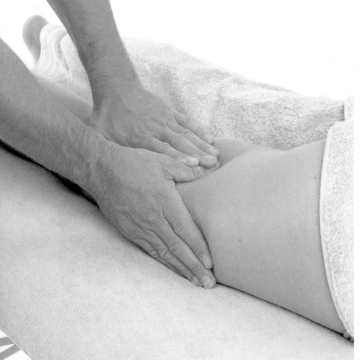

▼ Rolling compressions of the calf

1. Position yourself by the left calf facing the head.
2. Place both hands palm down on top of the calf below the knee with the fingers slightly raised and the right hand slightly higher up than the left.
3. Press down with the heel of your right hand, hold for a few seconds and then gently release.
4. Repeat with the left hand and then move the right hand down and repeat, pressing and releasing with alternate hands, working the whole way down the calf to the ankle.

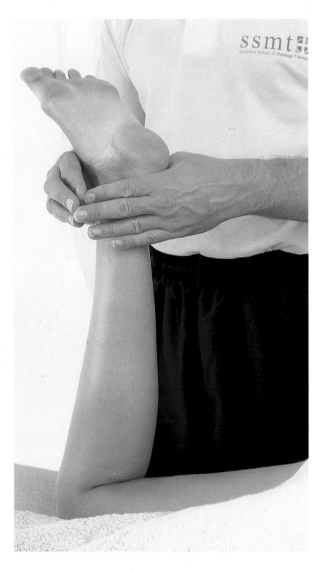

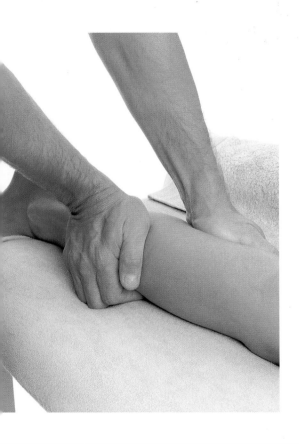

▲ Side calf vibrations

1. Position yourself by the left knee and pick up the foot, bending the knee so that the foot points to the ceiling.
2. Use both hands to form a loose circle with fingers and thumbs around the ankle and let the foot rock in this circle to gently vibrate the calf muscle.

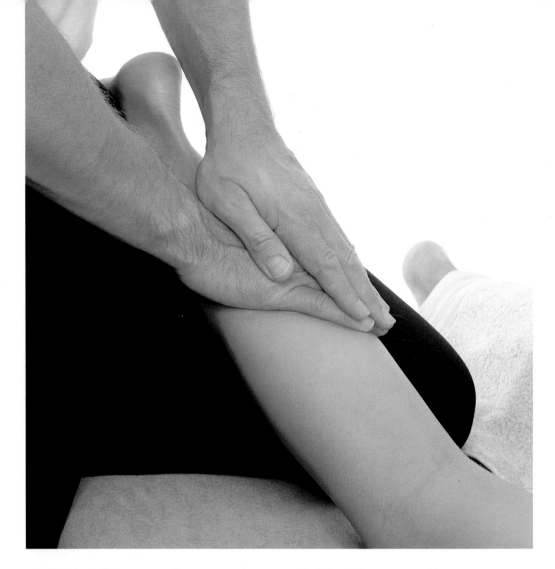

▲ Calf effleurage I

1 Position yourself by the right calf facing the head. Arrange the leg so the knee is bent and the calf is resting on your knee, a towel or a cushion – the foot should be higher than the knee and hip.

2 Put your right hand over the calf at the ankle, with the outside of the hand facing towards the knee, and cover it with the left hand.

3 Firmly stroke up the calf from ankle to knee, finishing in the crook of the knee.

Calf effleurage II

1 Place your left thumb just above the ankle with the outside of the hand facing up towards the knee. Cover the thumb with the right hand so that the last two fingers of the left hand are not covered.

2 Make a firm stroke up the calf from ankle to knee, finishing in the crook of the knee.

▶ Sole of foot effleurage

1 Position yourself by the right foot.
2 Put both thumbs on the sole of
  the foot by the toes, and support the
  underside with the palms and fingers.
3 Make a deep stroke with your thumbs
  down from the toes towards the heel.

▼ Knuckle kneading to sole of foot

1 Support the front of the foot with
  the left hand, and then place the
  right hand in a loose fist on the sole
  of the foot.
2 Using the knuckles, knead into the
  sole, working up from heel to toes.

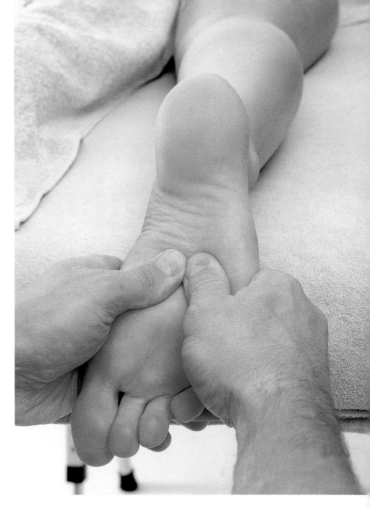

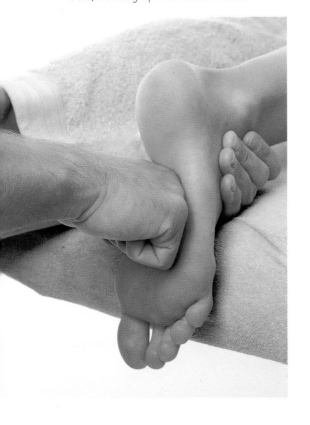

Complete leg relaxation vibrations

1 Hold the foot with one hand under the
  heel and one hand on top of the foot.
2 Tighten your grip slightly and arrange
  your hands so that they hold the foot
  secure at the ankle and no twisting is
  possible.
3 Shake your hands gently up and
  down to produce a vibration up the
  whole leg.
4 Repeat with a side-to-side motion of
  your hands for total relaxation.

Abdominal
and rib massages

The midpoint of our body holds the key to many of our vital life processes. It is often this area that responds to stressful situations in our lives and holding the trunk in tension can cause problems with digestion and other vital processes. Not only does the abdomen contain the digestive system which absorbs nutrients and energy from the food and water we consume, but it also holds the kidneys, liver, spleen and, in women, the reproductive organs.

Massage boosts circulation and removes blockages and toxins from abdominal soft tissue, as well as helps the gut to work efficiently by giving the movement of its contents a helping hand. This chapter shows you how to massage the abdomen to ease problems with digestion, dissolve away muscle tension and get rid of breathing problems and rib stiffness. Working through the techniques from beginning to end will take around 15 minutes.

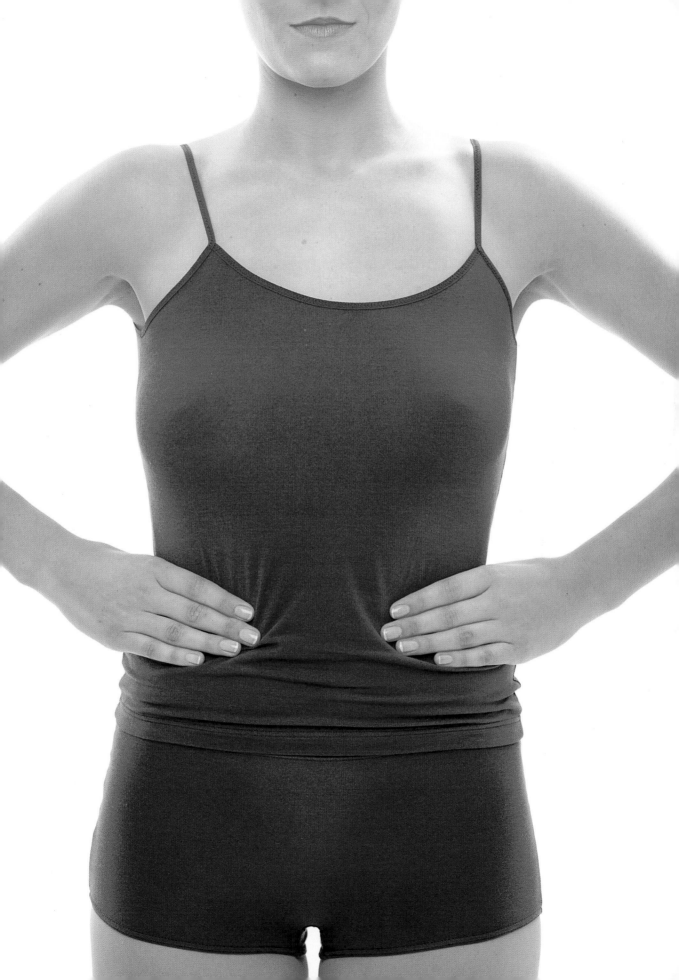

Basic anatomy

The abdominal cavity is home to much more than just the stomach. The liver, kidneys, reproductive organs and the lower half of the digestive tract are all securely contained here, so massage can be very beneficial for general health and well-being.

The digestive system

Food is broken down into an easily digestible form in the stomach, and then travels into the small intestine, where nutrients and

BELOW **Be aware of the position of the internal organs, diaphragm and colon in the abdomen when massaging.**

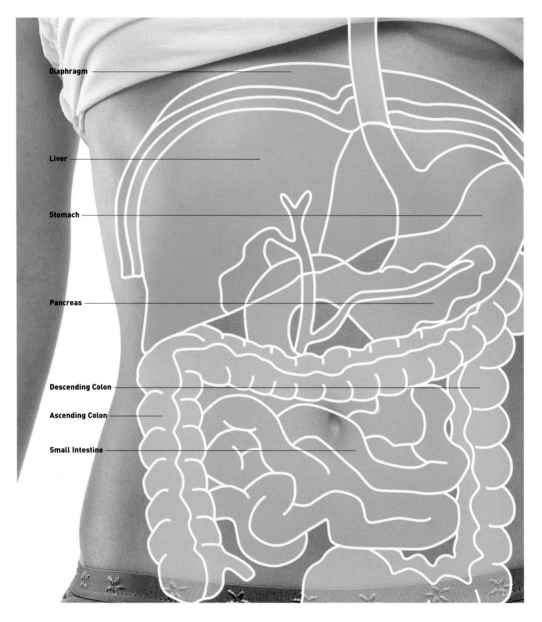

Diaphragm

Liver

Stomach

Pancreas

Descending Colon

Ascending Colon

Small Intestine

energy are absorbed. The small intestine is composed of a tube that runs from the ribs to the lower abdomen in twisting rows. The food travels down this until it reaches the end, near the right hip. It then enters the large intestine, which is where the last stages of digestion and most of the water absorption take place. The large intestine has three main parts – an ascending arm which runs up the right side of the body from the front of the hip to the bottom of the ribcage, a small part which runs across the bottom of the ribcage and a descending arm which runs from the ribcage down the left side, finishing above the left hip and emptying into the rectum.

Food travels through all parts of the intestine by a motion called peristalsis, which is a contraction of the circular muscle of the

NOTE

It is very important when massaging that the strokes never oppose the movement of food through the gut, as this could cause blockage, toxin build-up and digestive problems. Clearance strokes should move from the right hip up towards the ribs, across and down the left side, following the direction of the large colon. Abdominal massage should never use too much force as it could damage important organs underneath the skin – it should be firm but soft and should certainly never cause any pain or discomfort.

vessel walls. In some sections, such as the ascending arm of the large colon, this muscle activity is working against gravity. Massage in these areas can help to increase the efficiency of the digestive processes.

The ribs and diaphragm

The ribs, and the intercostal muscles that allow them to move against each other, are vital for efficient functioning of the body. When we breathe in, the diaphragm – a strong but thin sheet of fibrous material that sits under the ribcage – is forced down into the abdominal cavity and the ribcage expands, forcing oxygenated air into the lungs. When we breathe out, the ribs collapse back, the diaphragm is sucked into the chest and the air in the lungs is expelled. Breathing problems can be debilitating and upsetting, but massage of the intercostal muscles and the bottom of the ribcage helps to release any build up of tension and toxins that can affect breathing. The soothing strokes also deepen breathing and encourage relaxation.

Finding the right position

Positioning for abdominal massage is different to that for other types because it is important that the abdominal muscles are relaxed and not put on a stretch. Sometimes when we lie flat on our backs the abdomen can be stretched, decreasing not only comfort but also the efficiency of the massage. To make sure the abdomen is perfectly relaxed, the person being massaged should lie on their back facing the ceiling, with a pillow under their head to raise it up slightly (but keeping the neck straight). Another pillow should be placed under the knees so the legs are bent slightly at the hip and the curve of the lower back is just in contact with the floor. This should free up the abdominal muscles from doing any work, allowing them to relax.

Unlike the techniques for the back, neck, shoulders, arms and legs, these abdominal massages cover the whole area, so there is no need to repeat them on the other side.

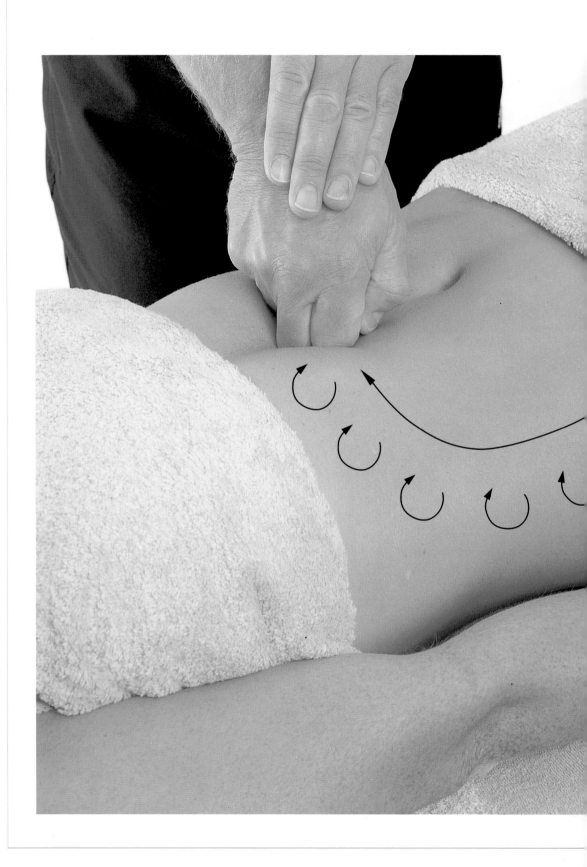

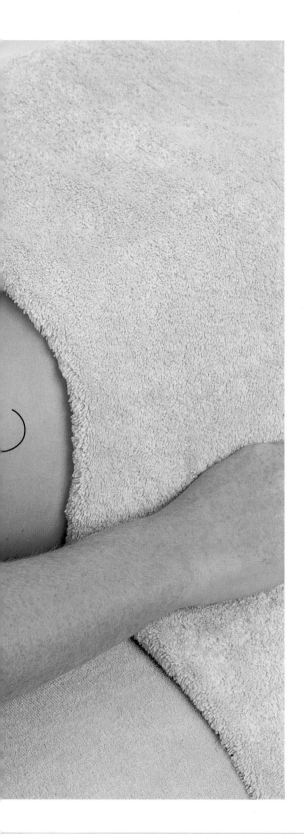

BEFORE THE FOLLOWING techniques, make sure the person being massaged is lying supine – face up.

◄ Clockwise circular stroking

1 Position yourself by the abdomen, facing the head of the person being massaged.
2 Place your right hand lightly on the abdomen just above the right hip and form a very loose fist so that the knuckles are in contact with the skin.
3 Taking care not to press too hard, work your fist in a small clockwise circle at the right hip, ending the stroke slightly above the position you started in.
4 Move up towards the head about 5 cm (2 in) and repeat the circular stroke (remember to go clockwise).
5 Work your way slowly and gently up the right side of the abdomen to the bottom of the ribcage, across the lower ribcage and down the left side of the abdomen towards the left hip, finishing just above the left hip, level with your starting position.

tip This helps to clear the digestive tract so it is important that all strokes work clockwise and from the right hip up and around to the left, following the direction of the intestine. This stroke must be done before any other abdominal massage.

▼ Alternate hands effleurage

1 Face the left side of the abdomen of the person being massaged.
2 Place both hands palm-down on the abdomen above the right hip with the fingers touching the skin.
3 Using the fingers of the left hand to create light pressure, make an n-shaped stroke in an anticlockwise direction travelling up towards the ribcage on the right side.
4 Make another stroke further up the right side and work your way around the bottom of the ribcage and down towards the left hip, keeping the finger strokes light.

▼ Deep stroking around the bottom of ribs

1 Place your right hand palm-down at the top of the abdomen under the ribcage, so that you can feel the bones at the bottom of the ribcage with the side of your fingers. Cover your right hand with your left hand.
2 Working alongside and just under the bottom of the right side of the ribcage, make deep strokes towards the left side of the body, using the bottom of the ribcage as a guide.

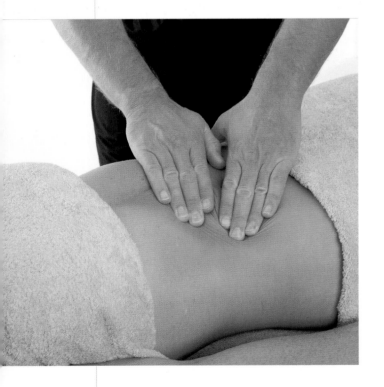

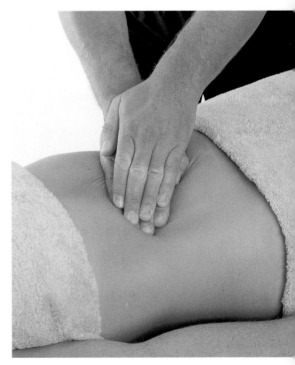

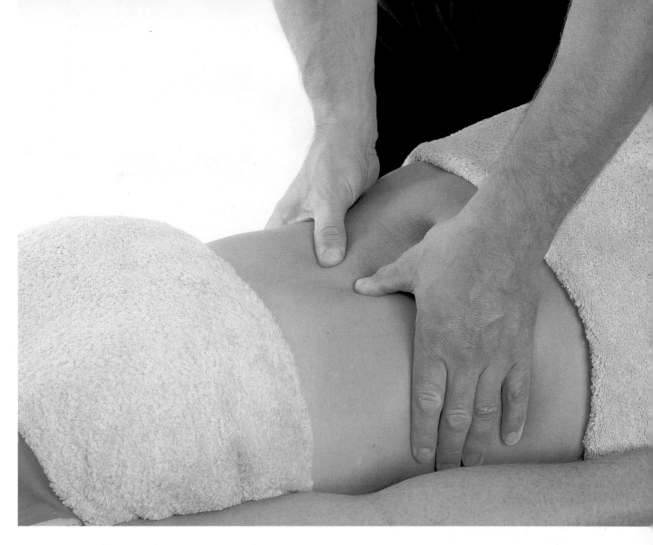

▲ Interactive abdominal compression

1 Position yourself at the left hip, facing the head of the person being massaged.

2 Place your left hand around the side of the body above the hip with the fingers pointing down the side of the body and the thumb positioned so that it sits on top of the abdominal muscles (about 5–7.5 cm (2–3 in) in from the side of the body). Place the right hand in the same position on the opposite side.

3 Ask the person being massaged to bring their head up, using the abdominal muscles, so that they are looking directly down between their feet without twisting or strain.

4 Press your thumbs into the abdominal muscles, then push them upwards and lock in position.

5 Ask the person being massaged to slowly drop their head backwards in a controlled way until the muscles are completely relaxed.

6 Release the thumbs, move a little further up the abdomen and repeat as many times as required until you reach the bottom of the ribcage. Take care not to cover the same area twice.

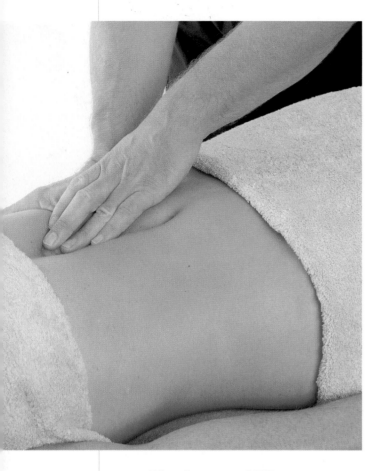

▼ Deep finger rib effleurage

1   Place the right hand on the right side of the ribs, allowing the fingers to fall between the lower ribs at the side.
2   Place your left hand on top of the right fingers and make a stroke, with the fingers staying between the ribs, up towards the centre of the chest.
3   When you reach the centre of the chest, turn the hand over and continue the stroke with the fingers leading the palm down towards the left side (towards your body).

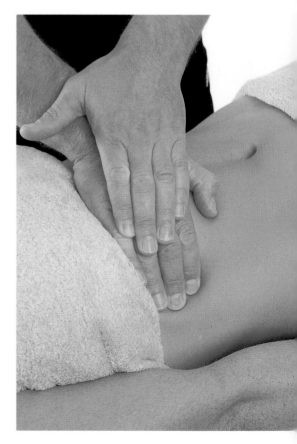

▲ Diaphragm STR

1   Place the right thumb about 10 cm (4 in) away from the centre of the chest just under the bone of the lower rib. Support the thumb using the fingers of your left hand.
2   Ask the person to take a deep breath in, and then as they breathe out push firmly, but not too hard, with your thumb up and under the ribs. Ease off as the out-breath finishes.
3   Repeat twice more, asking them to take longer to breathe out each time.
4   Repeat on the other side.

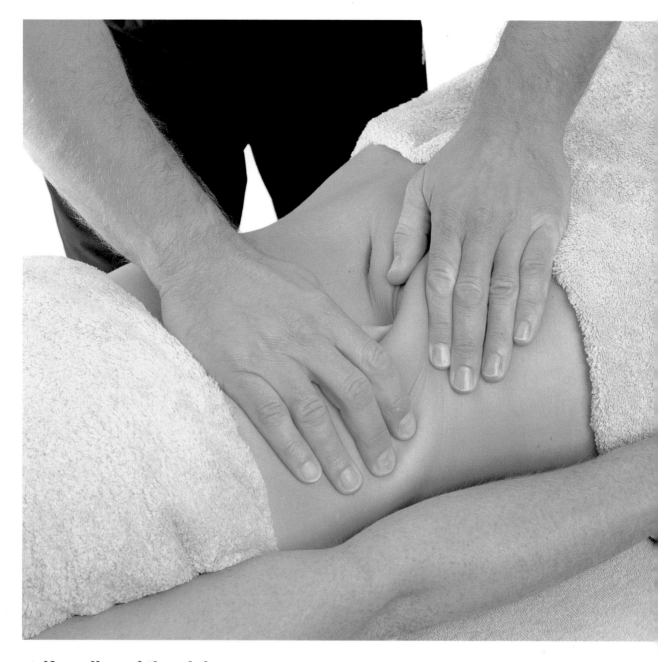

▲ **Kneading of the abdomen**

1   Reach over to the abdominal muscles at the side opposite to you. Place your palms flat on the abdomen with the fingers pointing downwards and your thumbs pointing roughly at each other.

2   Petrissage, bringing alternate fingers and thumbs together to work opposite directions, around the whole side of the abdomen.

3   Move to the opposite side of the body and repeat the steps to massage the other side of the abdomen.

Self-massage
techniques

It is not always possible to find a willing and suitably skilled friend, partner or family member to give you a massage. However, that does not mean you can't still treat yourself to the boost in well-being, relaxation and tension release that it offers. This chapter shows you how to massage yourself to soothe stress and to treat a range of common injuries and conditions. It gives you a quick and easy way to deal with lifestyle problems such as stress, bad posture and sore muscles, as well as common complaints such as breathing difficulties, headaches, digestive problems and poor flexibility. This self-treatment chapter will also show you a few easy-to-reach acupressure points through which you can boost your mood, relieve tension and beat insomnia.

The intuitive side of massage is very important here as you learn to listen to your body and to work into areas of tension and stress with your own hands, easing away pain and distress.

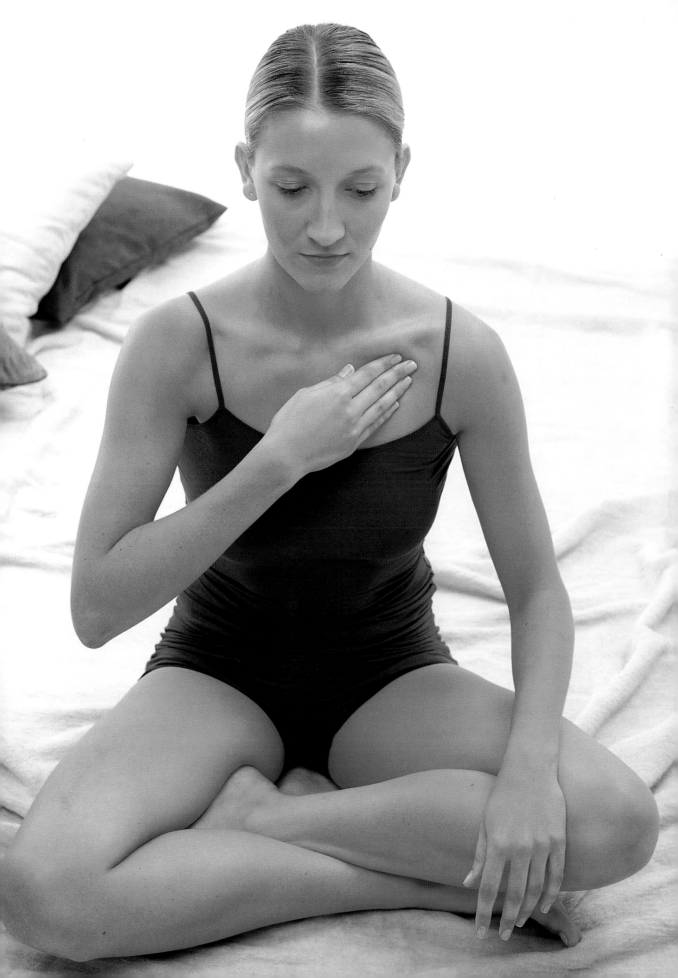

Preparation and tools

Massage soothes, calms and relaxes stressed, tense and tired bodies and boosts overworked minds, but all too often it is not available when we need it most – sitting at a desk, after a gym workout or at home. The great advantage of learning to heal yourself with self-massage is that you can use it any time, anywhere. You don't need to wait for an appointment; just clear your schedule for half an hour and you can reap the beneficial effects of massage when you feel the need.

Tools

There are a variety of self-massage tools that can help you reach hard-to-get-at areas of your body for total tension release.

Chinese balls – Available from oriental shops and some complementary medicine centres, Chinese hand balls are a fun way to keep your hands and fingers flexible. To use them, hold two balls in the palm of a hand

BELOW **Chinese balls can be rolled in the palm of the hand to relieve stress and encourage suppleness.**

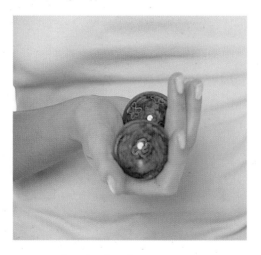

NOTES

- Stay relaxed, centred and calm. The beneficial effects of the massage will be diminished and even lost if you enter into this personal time in a stressed, frenetic manner.
- Before you start, take at least three long, slow, deep breaths, closing your eyes and concentrating on how the self-treatment massage will benefit your mental and physical states.
- Don't massage or exert pressure if you feel pain in any area.
- Remember to avoid danger zones, such as the soft areas of the eyes, the sides of the neck and the soft triangle above the knee at the back.
- If you are pregnant, or think you might be pregnant, be aware of the possible effects of massage and steer clear of massaging the stomach and lower back. Also avoid the use of essential oils or mediums that may contain them.
- Make that sure your clothing is loose and comfortable and that you occupy a position that allows your back to assume the neutral position, with the neck and head comfortable, supported and not twisted or cricked (see also page 32).
- If you are closing your eyes during the massage, make sure you can't be disturbed – even if it means locking the door or disconnecting your phone.
- Most importantly, never feel guilty about taking a few minutes out to boost your physical and mental state – it is always time worth spending. Learning to give your body and mind what they need allows you to be focused, centred and efficient when you return to daily life.

and circle them around each other using your palm and fingers. Some versions have a musical chime to help relax the mind.

Rubber stress balls – These malleable balls can be squeezed and moulded in your hands to work the muscles and relieve tension.

Massage pegs – Massage pegs fit around the knuckles of the hand and have a roller or ball attached to them for massaging specific points of the body. They can be used for providing light or deep strokes to muscled areas like the thigh, forearm and calf, but care should be taken in bony areas and around joints.

Spiky balls – Soft, spiky rubber balls can help you release tension in your back, neck and shoulders by providing a soft, textured

tip For each of the self-massage techniques, you should start in a relaxed, comfortable position that allows your body to enjoy the massage and your mind to concentrate on the task.

pressure to the muscles. They are most effective if you lie on the floor and place them under your back, neck or shoulders, rolling yourself on top of them in a slow, controlled way to target problem areas and release muscle tension. They can also be rolled under the feet and between the hands.

Foot rollers – Foot rollers are designed to target tension and muscle tiredness in the soles of the feet. Sit in a chair with your foot flat and roll it forwards and backwards over the roller to relieve pain and stiffness.

BELOW **Rollers for the hands and feet can be used to target stiff and sore areas.**

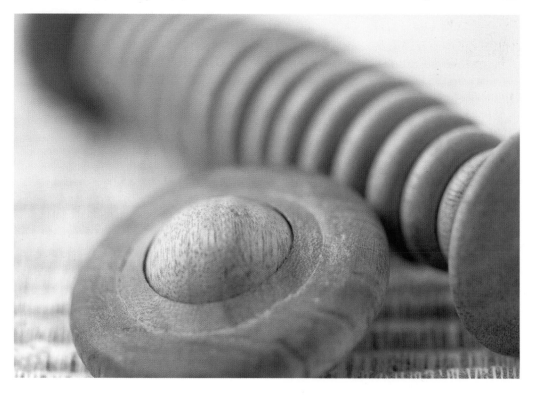

THE FOLLOWING TECHNIQUES help to relieve the pain and pressure of headaches, migraines and sinus problems.

▼ Temple massage

To relax the eyes, forehead and scalp, reducing stress and soothing away the pain of tension headaches.

1   Place the flats of your thumbs on the temples. They should sit comfortably in the dip between the outside of the eyebrow and the hairline.
2   Exert gentle pressure on the temples and move the hands simultaneously towards the eyebrow in a circular motion, working from the hairline towards the eye, past the eyebrow and back up towards the hairline. Make sure you cover the whole space of the temple with your fingers.
3   Continue this circular movement for at least a minute, closing your eyes and concentrating on releasing tension in the forehead and eyes.

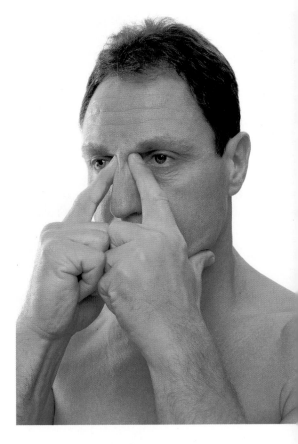

▲ Circular sinus compressions

Soothes and revitalizes tired and stressed eyes to reduce headache pain and release tension.

1   Place the first fingers of each hand either side of the top of the bridge of the nose, the area where it curves up into the eyebrow.
2   Using gentle pressure, make circular motions on both sides, closing the eyes as you do this.
3   Repeat these circular motions for at least a minute.

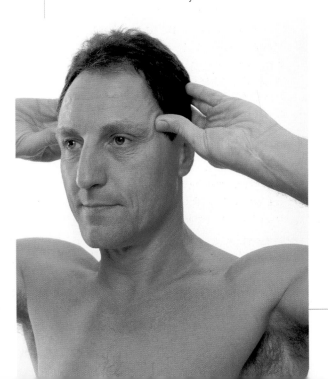

▼ Occiput thumb compressions

1 Place the flats of the thumbs behind the bottom of the ears under the skull bone (which will feel round under your thumb) and reach your fingers to the crown of your head.
2 Trace the line of the bottom of the skull around towards the spine until you reach a soft area under the skull – about 5 cm (2 in) around from the spine. This area is called the occiput.
3 Gently press the thumbs into the occiput and make small circular motions, working upwards closer into the spine and then downwards nearer the ear.
4 Continue these circular occiput compressions for at least a minute.

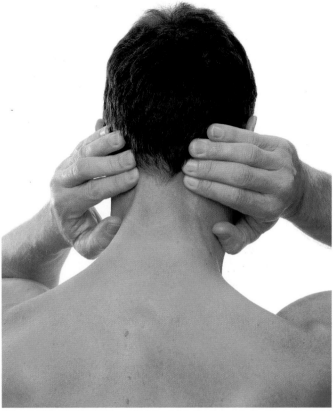

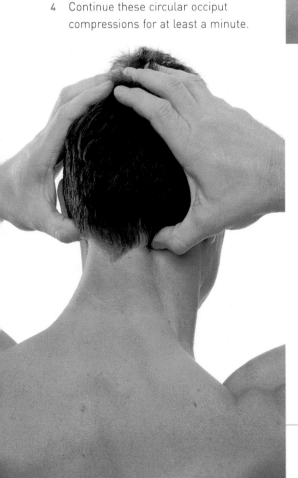

▲ Occiput draw

1 Position both palms to touch the skin on the side of the neck, cupping the ears and with the fingers reaching up towards the occiput.
2 Exert pressure on the occiput with the first two fingers, drawing them across the edge of the spine towards the ear. Palms should rest on the sides of the neck.
3 Bring your chin down and in so the neck is stretched throughout the draw.
4 Stop the draw when your fingers reach the area behind the ears and repeat the whole movement several times.

tip A major cause of headaches is tension and stress stored at the top of the neck, where it meets the skull at the back of the head, the occiput. This massage releases tension to soothe away pain and stress in this area.

Ice massage

This technique is designed to reduce inflammation and pain through the application and soothing massage of ice. Always wrap ice up in a soft material or it could cause cold burns to the skin.

1   Prepare an ice pack by wrapping up several ice cubes in a linen towel or an absorbent cloth. Alternatively buy a ready-made pack.
2   Rub the ice pack gently on the back of your neck, the base of your skull and the forehead and temples, using slow circular movements to soothe away inflammation.
3   Never continue the massage for longer than five minutes – the maximum time for ice massage in this area.

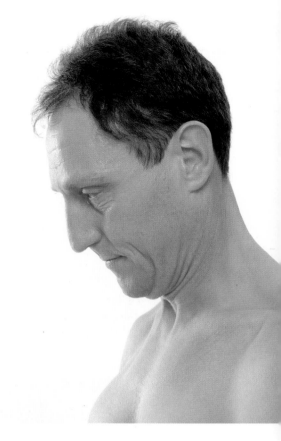

▲ Chin to chest stretch

A simple way of releasing tension stored in the muscles at the back of the neck that can be performed anywhere and at any time.

1   Slowly drop your chin down so that you are looking at the floor, without allowing your back, neck or shoulders to bend or curve.
2   Still looking at the floor, bring your chin back towards the neck so that you form a double chin. This stretches out the back of the neck.
3   Release and re-stretch several times, making sure that your shoulder and back stay upright and your chin is tucked well in to the front of the neck.

▶Ear to shoulder stretch

Another simple but highly effective self-stretch for the neck, to reduce tension and stress in the muscles.

1   Sit up straight with your back upright, facing straight ahead with your chin level. This is the neutral position.
2   Slowly and gently allow the head to drop sideways so that the ear meets the shoulder. Do not twist the head – your eyes should look straight ahead the whole time and your face continue to look directly in front of you.
3   As your ear drops towards your shoulder, you should feel a stretch in the other side of the neck. Hold the stretch for at least 30 seconds before slowly raising the head back to the neutral position.
4   Repeat on the other side.

A continuation of this stretch is to move the head slightly forwards at an angle in order to allow the stretch to move further into the back of the neck:

5   Begin in the neutral position. Move your face a quarter turn to the right so that you are facing about 45 degrees in front of you.
6   Keeping the head steady, drop the right ear towards the top of the shoulder as before, feeling a stretch around the back and side of the left side of the neck and into the top of the shoulder. Hold for 30 seconds.
7   Repeat on the left side, ear to shoulder, remembering to sit upright in the neutral position at all times to avoid twisting the neck.

tip Remember to always return to the neutral position between stretches to ensure that the neck does not twist, strain or bend.

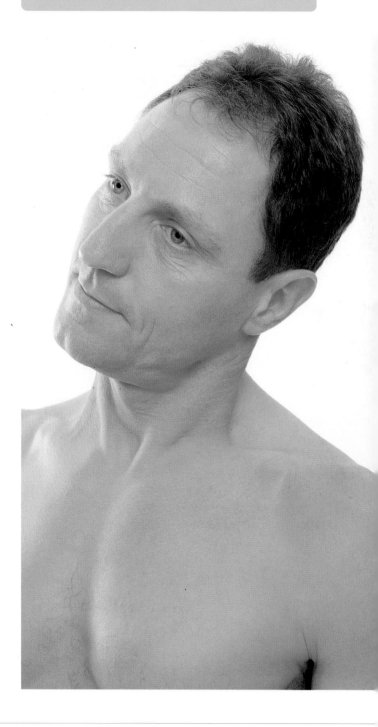

LOWER BACK PAIN can be very painful and is often due to poor posture or long hours of desk work. The following techniques can help to relieve this problem.

▼ Seated stretch with the hands between feet

To release tension in the lower back.

1 Sit up straight in a chair, facing straight ahead with your knees apart and a space of at least 1 m (3 ft) in front of you.
2 Put your arms out in front of you and slowly bend over so your head moves down between your knees and your hands travel back under the chair.
3 Stay in this stretch for several seconds before slowly returning to a sitting position.

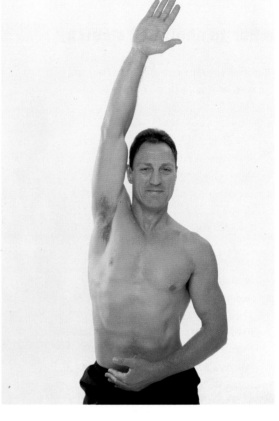

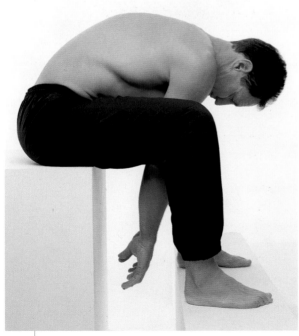

▲ Seated side stretch

To free up tension in the ribs, ease breathing and encourage relaxation, as well as stretching out the lower back by enlarging the space between vertebrae.

1 Sit up straight in a chair, facing ahead with your chin level.
2 Imagine there is a piece of string attaching your left shoulder to the ceiling. Raise your right hand straight up over your head, taking care not to squeeze the neck, and reach up as far as you can on this imaginary string.
3 Release, return to neutral and repeat a further two times breathing out as you reach upwards.
4 Repeat on the other side.

▼ Self-massage of gluteals

A deep technique to ease tension in the base of the back.

1   Stand up straight and face directly ahead, with your feet hip-width apart.
2   Pull yourself up from the chest as if you were being held up by an imaginary harness (this stops pressure being put on the lower back because of sagging).
3   Place your hands on the hips with the thumbs reaching into either side of the lower back where it meets the buttocks. The fingers should rest towards the front of your body.
4   Using circular motions, massage the muscles at the top of the buttocks with your thumbs.

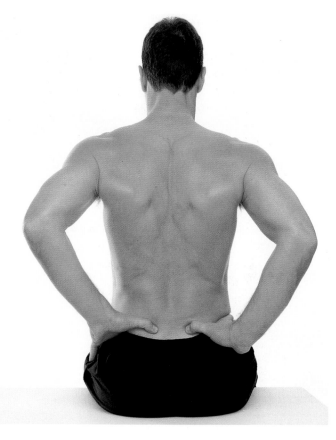

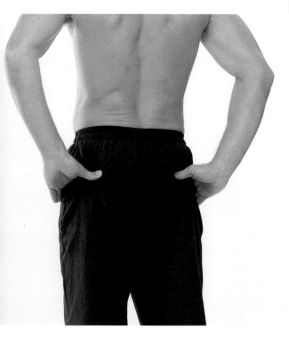

▲ Self-massage to base of spine

A simple massage technique to ease tension at the bottom of the spine and boost posture.

1   Place your hands on the lower part of the back, palms on hips, and the thumbs spread around the back facing towards each other.
2   Massage the muscles around the lower back (avoiding the spine) with the flats of your thumbs, using circular motions to cover the whole lower back.

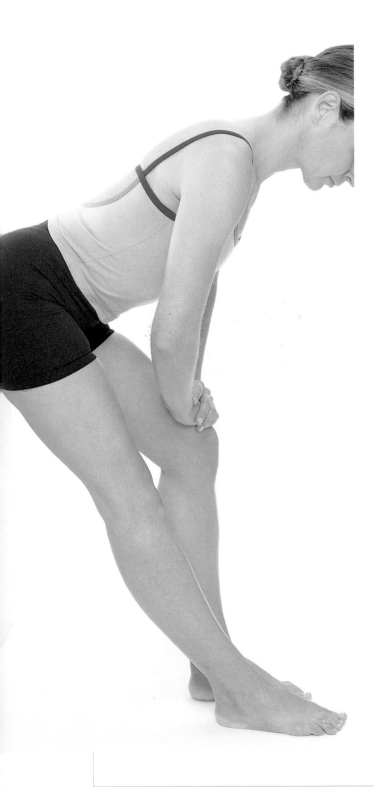

SITTING AT A DESK for hours can make the hamstring tight and stiff. These techniques will help stretch them out again.

◄ Seated hamstring stretches

To ease pressure on the lower spine by stretching out the hamstrings.

1   Sit straight on the edge of your chair facing ahead with your feet flat on the floor and your knees hip-width apart.
2   Straighten your left leg and rest the heel on the floor so that it sticks out straight in front of you.
3   Keeping your back straight and your chin in a straight line with your head (not jutting out), lean forwards over the outstretched leg until you feel a stretch in your hamstrings.
4   Hold the stretch for at least 30 seconds and repeat on the other leg.

Seated pelvic tilts

To stretch the lower back and reduce tension caused by bad posture.

1   Sit up straight with the buttocks pushed to the back of a chair and slide one hand into the curve of your lower back with the palm outwards.
2   Using the muscles in your lower abdomen and pelvis and taking extra care not to move the top of your body, which should remain totally still from the waist upwards, push your lower back against your hand and hold it there for several seconds.
3   Release the lower back and perform the stretch two or three times.

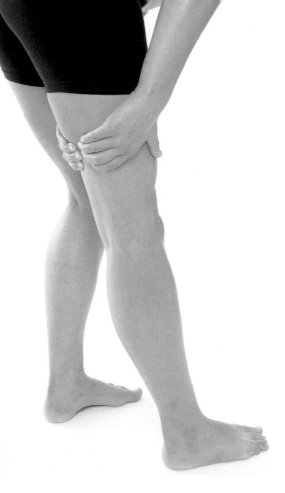

▼ Hamstring STR

To further stretch the hamstrings and release more tension.

1 With your back straight, bend from the waist, reaching your hands around the back of your thigh.
2 Bend the knee and push two fingers of each hand (touching each other to form one point of contact) into the muscle. Push in and up towards the buttocks to stretch the hamstring.
3 Work in the stretch by slowly straightening the leg and repeat the process several times for each leg. Work around the whole thigh, but avoid the area above the knee.

▲ Standing hamstring massage

To reduce stress in the hamstrings from over- or under-use. This simple massage technique is best performed in the shower, though it can also be used when standing normally.

1 Take your weight onto one leg with the other leg slightly bent and placed in front of you.
2 Making sure that your back stays straight, bend over from the waist so your hands reach around the back of the front thigh without stretching the shoulders, arms or back.
3 Use the fingers of both hands to knead the muscle of the back of the thigh, taking care to avoid the soft area just above the knee.
4 Repeat for the other leg.

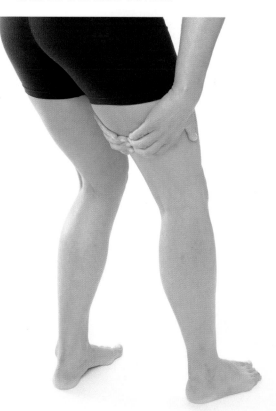

JOINT PAIN can be debilitating, but the following massages can help by boosting blood flow to the affected joint.

▼ Top of shoulder massage

To reduce tension caused by repetitive work at a desk and bad posture.

1   Place four fingers of the right hand at the midpoint between the left shoulder and neck.
2   Use a circular motion to work well into the muscle.
3   If required, work deeper by forming a hook with the fingers and drawing them to the front of the body.

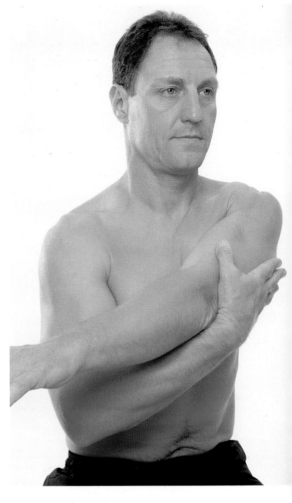

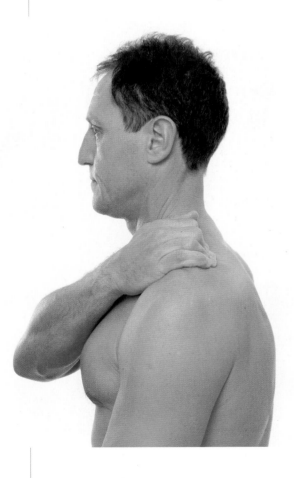

▲ Shoulder stretch across the body

To stretch out tension in the back of the shoulder and the upper arm.

1   While seated, straighten your left arm out in front of you.
2   Place the right hand across the body so the wrist touches the outside of the left arm above the elbow.
3   Looking straight ahead, use the right hand and arm to bring the left arm, still straight, across the chest to stretch out the shoulder.

▼ Deep thumb stroke of the forearm

To relieve tension in the forearm, wrist, elbow and hand.

1   While seated, place the right hand on a flat surface, such as a desk or tabletop.
2   Place the left thumb on top of the right wrist and work up towards the elbow using small strokes.
3   As a continuation of the massage, you can also work transversely, across the forearm from side to side, to work deeper into the muscle.

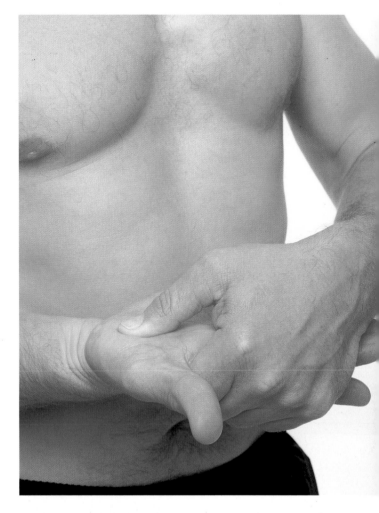

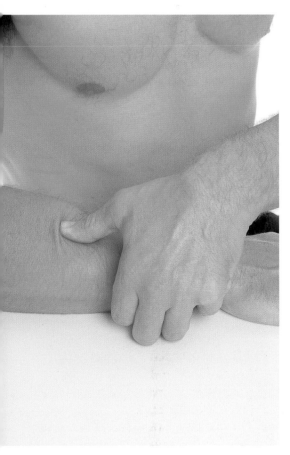

▲ Kneading the base of the thumb

To reduce tension in the hands.

1   Place the right palm upwards with the left thumb on the large pad of muscle at the base of the right thumb.
2   Using circular motions to reduce tension, work the thumb, in small strokes, from the hand to the wrist.

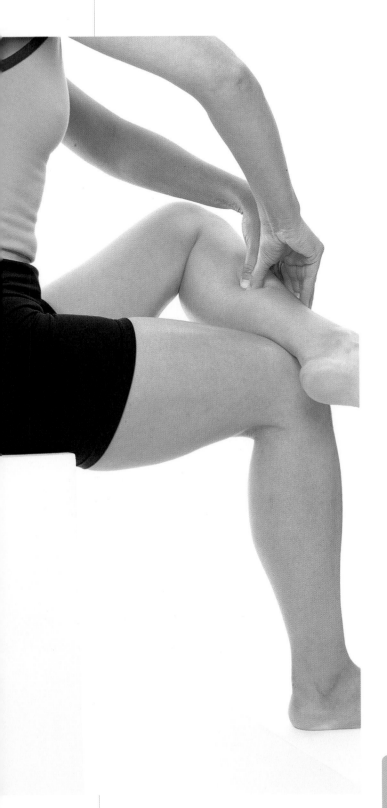

FITNESS WORKOUTS, particularly those that involve running, walking or cycling, can work the muscles of the legs very hard. You should always warm down to allow your muscles a period of gentle exercise to release toxins and reduce next-day stiffness.

These massages will help you avoid problems following a workout by targeting areas that commonly develop stiffness and soreness.

Shower self-massage

The heat and steam from the shower will boost circulation to muscles and increase the dilation of blood vessels, which can help with muscle soreness.

1   Use a hand-held showerhead to work into muscled areas like the shoulders, back, neck, thighs and calves. Make sure the temperature isn't too hot, as this can shock the skin and tissues.

◄ Compression and draw of the calf

To work out tension and blockages in the calf muscles after exercise.

1   Sit with your left foot crossed over so that it rests on the right knee.
2   Place both hands around the lower leg with thumbs facing towards you.
3   Push both thumbs down from the shin towards the floor, drawing the muscle away from the shin in a slow and controlled movement.

tip For deeper tension release, you can add active movement to this compression and draw technique. Start with the toes flexed up towards the shin and then slowly release them so they point ahead as you complete the draw.

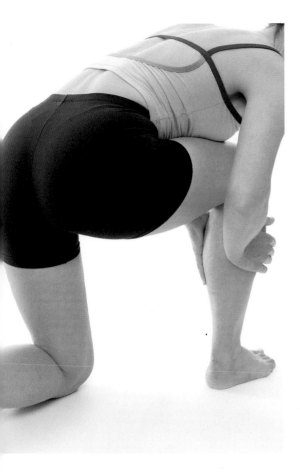

▼ Double finger draw up the shin

To reduce tension in the lower leg, particularly after walking, running, stepping or cycling.

1   Position yourself on the floor with one shin vertically in front of you.
2   Lean forwards and place the first two fingers of each hand together on the outside of the ankle joint.
3   Slowly draw your fingers up the outside of the shin towards the knee.
4   You can choose to add active muscle movement by pointing and flexing the foot as you make a second stroke.

▲ Self-compression of the calf

To get rid of toxin build-up and fluid blockage in the calf after a vigorous workout.

1   Kneel on your left knee with your right foot flat on the floor.
2   Lean forwards and place the heel of the right hand on the bottom of the right calf, as low as you feel comfortable.
3   Press into the calf muscle and hold for several seconds.
4   Move about 5 cm (2 in) up and work your way up the calf to the knee. Do not go over the same area twice.

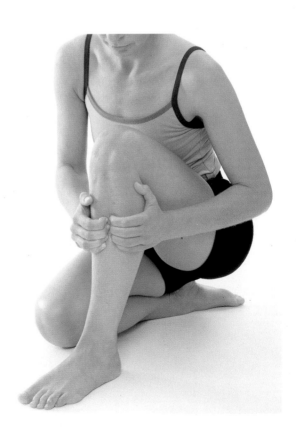

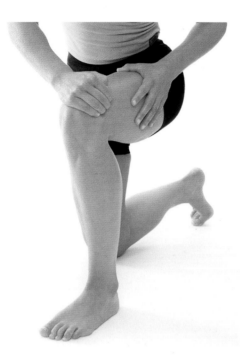

▼ Deep strokes to top of the calf

To reduce tension and pain around the top of the calf and knee.

1. In a sitting position, place both hands on either side of the calf with the thumbs at the top of the calf about 5 cm (2 in) below the knee.
2. Work both thumbs up towards the knee in deep strokes. Do not go above the crease at the back of the knee.

THESE POST-WORKOUT massages are performed in a sitting or kneeling position. You should never massage if you feel pain or discomfort anywhere in your body, or if there is any swelling or injury to the area you are treating.

▲ Transfrictional glide over the sides of the knee

To reduce tension on the knee joint following running and walking.

1. Kneel on your right knee and place the right hand over the left knee, with the fingers to the outside of the knee.
2. Working in a small, circular movement with your fingers, cover the area to the outside of the knee avoiding the kneecap.
3. For deeper contact, try adding a squeezing motion or working with the thumb.

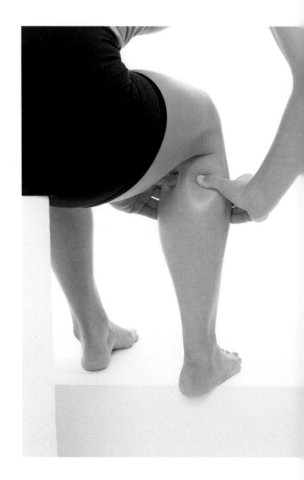

▼ STR knee

To stretch out localized areas of the thigh muscles and to release tension in the knee. Particularly good following a run or a hilly walk.

1   Sit upright and place the right thumb on the left thigh above the knee and the left thumb on top of it.
2   Straighten the leg, bringing the foot off the ground to knee level.
3   Press the thumbs into the muscle of the thigh and bring them back to your body, locking and loading the muscle.
4   Slowly lower the foot to the floor, keeping the thumb pressure constant, to deepen the stretch.
5   Move the thumbs up about 5 cm (2 in) and repeat up the whole thigh, taking care not to STR the same area twice.

▼ Calf stretch, medial and lateral

To stretch out tight calf muscles, boost toxin disposal in the lower leg and reduce stiffness.

1   Stand facing a wall, about 30 cm (1 ft) away from it.
2   Place the heel of your foot on the floor in front of the wall and the ball of your foot against the wall so that the toes point up towards the shin.
3   Keeping the leg straight, bring the thigh and the knee towards the wall to stretch the calf. Hold the stretch for at least 30 seconds.
4   To spread the stretch further into the calf, move the heel a little to the right of centre and repeat the stretch, then repeat about 5 cm (2in) to the left. Note that your toes stay in the same place for all three stretches, it's only your heel that moves sideways.

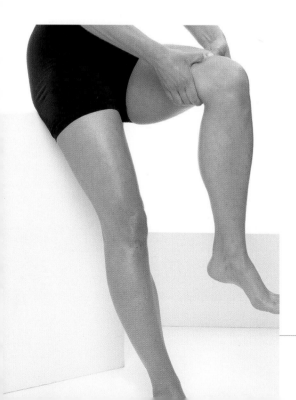

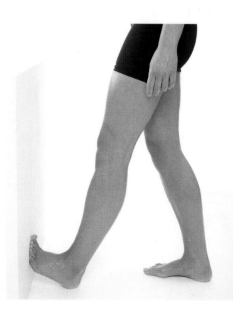

THE FOLLOWING TECHNIQUES target areas that are particularly affected by tension.

▼ Anterior chest massage

To reduce tension across the front chest, to free up breathing and loosen the neck.

1. Place the four fingers of your right hand on the left side of your chest.
2. Starting at the centre of the chest, move the fingers in a circular motion working out towards the shoulder.
3. Breathe in and out slowly as you perform the massage, deepening the strokes lightly as you breathe out.

▼ Anterior neck stretch

To work further into the chest and front of the neck.

1. Use four fingers in circular motions as before, but this time turn your head to the right so that you stretch out the muscles and ligaments at the front of the neck.

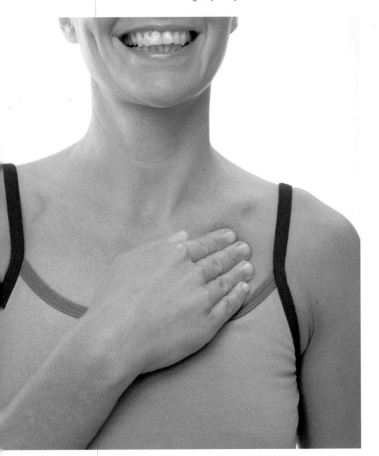

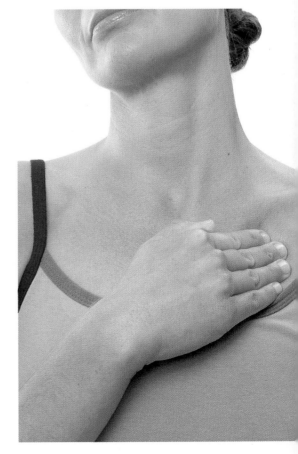

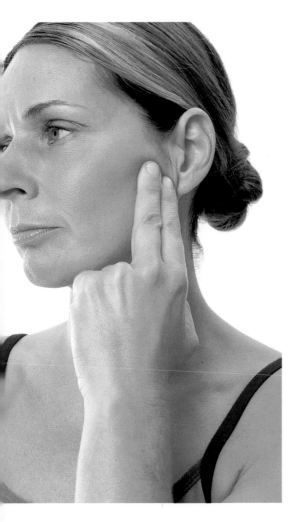

▲ Two finger massage to base of jaw

To relieve tension in the jaw and sides of the face.

1   Place the two fingers of the left hand together on the jaw so that the first finger fits into the bony area in front of the earlobe.
2   Using small circular motions, work the thumb lightly into the jaw area, keeping the contact broad and being careful not to press too hard. The jaw should move slightly to the side.

▼ Scalp tension buster

To reduce tension held in the scalp and to boost relaxation.

1   Spread out the fingers and thumbs of both hands and place them at either side of the head, with the thumbs above the ears and towards the back of the neck.
2   Work the fingers and thumbs in small circular motions.
3   After a few seconds, move the hands so that they cover a different area.
4   Breathe deeply in and out to enhance the relaxation.

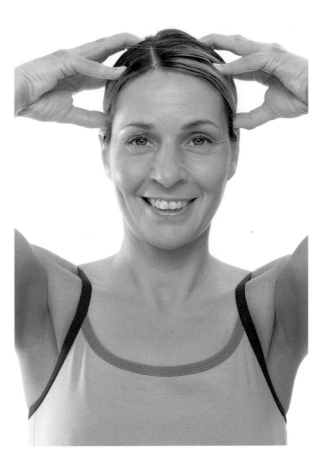

THE FOLLOWING TECHNIQUES help to aid common abdominal problems.

▼ Period pain

Helps to combat menstrual pain, as well as soreness due to muscle cramp.

1   Sit or stand with your lower back free.
2   Place your hands on your hips with the thumbs on the lower back at hip level on either side of the spine.
3   Move the thumbs in small, light circular motions into the pressure points of the lower back. Stop if you feel any discomfort.

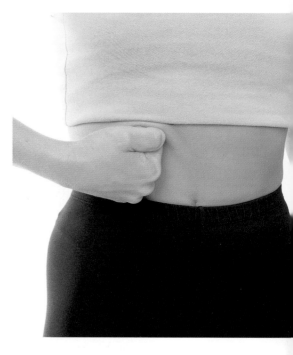

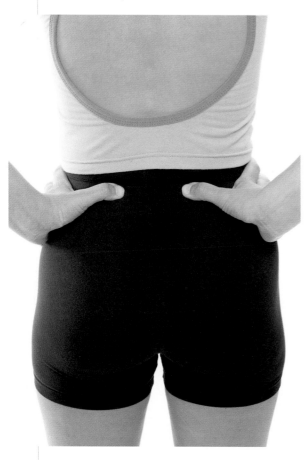

▲ Wind pains

To reduce pain caused by the build up of wind in the abdomen by releasing trapped air and boosting digestive flow.

1   Find a quiet spot where you won't be embarrassed if wind escapes.
2   Stand or sit comfortably.
3   Form a loose fist with your right fingers (so that the palm stays flat but the fingers are curled) and place it at the front of the right hip.
4   Use loose circular motions in a clockwise motion to follow the line of the large intestine, working up the right side to the ribs, across the bottom of the ribcage and down towards the left hip.

Using acupressure

One or two fingers should be used to stimulate each acupressure relief point using constant pressure. Circular massage movements should not be used. Initially, keep the pressure light and constant for 30 seconds, then repeat the compression with more pressure if required. Each compression should be held for 30 seconds.

Acupressure point 1

An instant mood-booster point to help fight depression and lift the spirit. This is found where the thumb and forefinger form a V. Use the opposite thumb to push into the area.

Acupressure point 2

A tension-relief point, good for relieving tension headaches, boosting concentration and relieving tired eyes. Found in the occipital hollow where the bottom of the skull meets the neck, either side of the spine. Use the thumb to gently press either side of this area.

Acupressure point 3

A stress-relieving point that is good for reducing anxiety and tension. Found at the top-centre of the forearm in the large muscle just below the crease of the elbow.

Acupressure point 4

A metabolism-boosting point, good for chest and eye problems and boosting general circulation and metabolism. Found on top of the foot, roughly in line with the middle two toes and directly over the arch.

Acupressure point 5

An immune-boosting point, good for combating fatigue and depression. Found on the inside of the ankle above the foot between the Achilles tendon and the anklebone.

Acupressure point 6

A point for pain relief, tension release and mood-boosting. Found on the back, in line with the kidneys. Sit up straight in a chair and form a fist with each hand. Place the fists behind your back, level with the elbow, and lean back gently to stimulate the point.

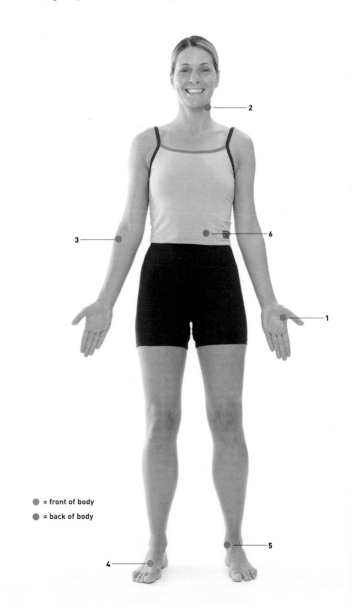

● = front of body
● = back of body

Hand and foot
massage

An understanding of the positive effects of massage on our physical and psychological health can help you adapt your sequence of movements to ensure maximum benefits for yourself and your massage partner. Before you begin to massage hands and feet it is important to appreciate how they are an integral part of the whole body and cannot be viewed in isolation from all the systems and structures that make up each individual.

Hands help us to communicate with others and express our creativity. Yet we reward them by soaking them in strong detergents and exposing them to the harshest of weather. Feet enable us to walk, run and jump for joy. Yet we cram them into ill-fitting shoes and expect them to bear our full body weight for hours on end. It is no wonder that skin becomes dry and cracked, joints start to stiffen and ache, and the blood circulation to the extremities slows down. Hands and feet deserve care and attention – and respond surprisingly quickly to a therapeutic touch. The palms of the hands and soles of the feet contain thousands of sensory nerve endings, making them among the most sensitive parts of the body.

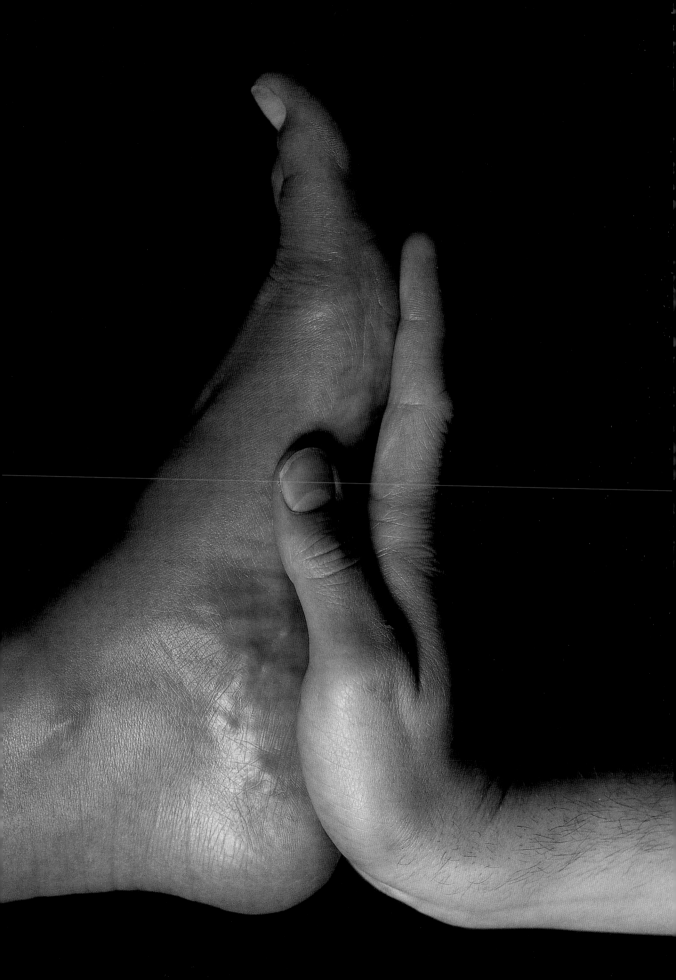

Preparing
for massage

Massage is a basic, nurturing instinct. Massage has also been described as one of the oldest forms of healing. Since ancient times, people all over the world have used the natural therapeutic power of touch in their everyday lives. Once you have learnt a few simple techniques, you can use your natural skills to give a safe and effective hand or foot massage to family and friends.

Massage is likely to bring many benefits. However, before you begin your massage, it is essential to set time aside to discuss any relevant health issues or concerns. You need to know your massage partners state of health so that you are prepared for any problems that may arise during the massage, and how to deal with them.

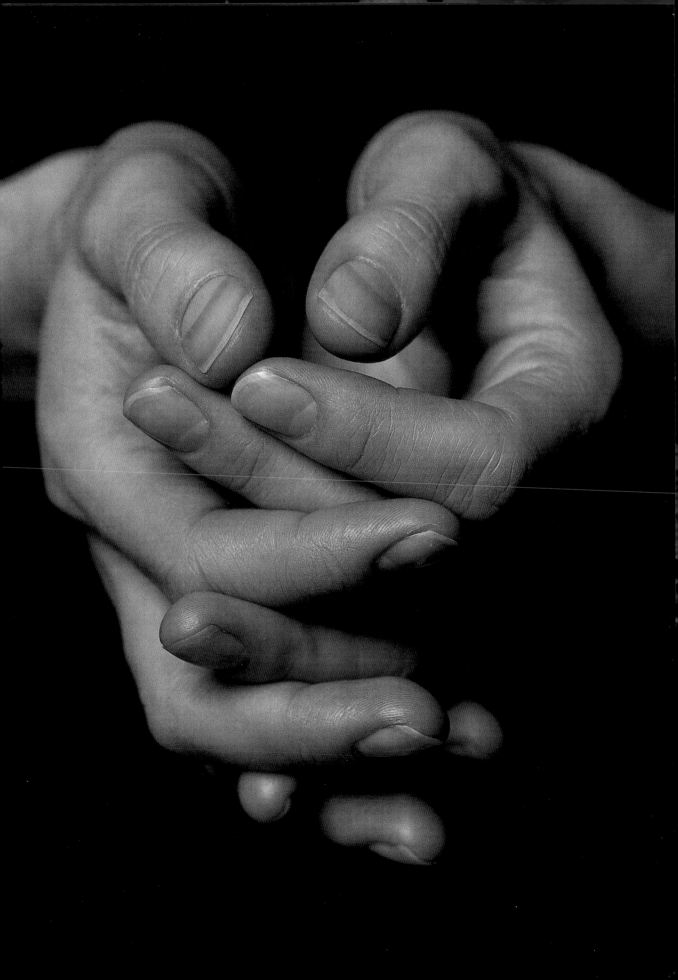

Check hands and feet

Hand and foot massage is generally considered to be a safe, non-invasive therapy that is suitable for most people. However, it is important not to launch straight into action without being aware of safety guidelines. At the start of your massage, always observe hands and feet – through vision and touch. Firstly, check for any conditions that may make massage inadvisable or where you need to take extra care. Then look for signs that may reflect your massage partner's state of health. These are not always accurate, but they do help to make you aware of the possibilities so you can adapt your massage accordingly or seek advice from your massage partner's doctor.

Colour

Check the colour of the palms and soles, fingers and toes. A fleshy, pinkish colour indicates good circulation and balanced body systems. A very pale colour usually shows lack of blood flow to the extremities, which may be due to a drop in body temperature or general tiredness. Blue or purple hands and feet are a sign of poor circulation and possibly high levels of medication. A red colour may indicate chronic stress and high blood pressure.

Temperature

Hands and feet should be pleasantly warm to touch. Coolness may indicate poor circulation and listlessness. when palms and soles feel very hot, this may be a sign of weight problems, high blood pressure, anxiety or burning anger.

Skin condition

Skin tissue should be soft and supple. Look for any signs of hard or cracked skin. This may indicate a lack of adequate protection from detergents or the elements, poor posture or ill-fitting shoes.

Tension

Relaxed hands and feet indicate a relaxed person. If they feel tense, then chances are your partner is too.

Moisture

The skin on the soles and palms should not feel too dry or too moist. If the skin is very dry. this suggests a lack of fluid and poor circulation. If it is very damp, it could indicate high levels of stress and anxiety, a weight problem or unsuitable footwear.

Flexibility of joints

If wrists and ankles are stiff, this may be associated with an injury or a joint condition such as arthritis. Special care should be taken when massaging.

Condition of nails

Healthy nails are pinkish in colour with a smooth surface and slight sheen. Poor circulation is usually indicated by a blue or purple tinge and brittle nails. Very thick, pitted nails may be a sign of a skin disorder, while horizontal ridges often appear after an illness or trauma.

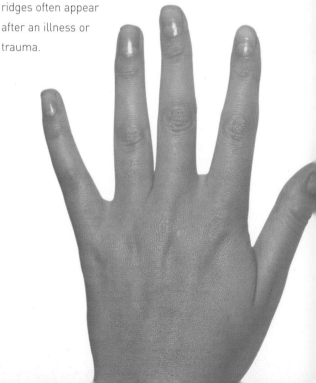

Muscles, bones and other structures

Hands and feet are capable of an amazing variety of movements. This efficiency is entirely due to a highly sophisticated structure of bones, muscles, and other structures, such as the ligaments and tendons in the wrist, hand, ankle and foot. These work together to enable us to control movements. Bones form the body's framework offering support and shape to structures such as hands and feet. Where movable bones meet they form joints. Different types of joint allow varying degrees of movement.

Muscles and tendons

Muscles are attached to bones on either side of a joint by fibres of tough connective tissue, known as tendons. Muscles exert a pull on the tendon, which moves the bone and any weight it is carrying.

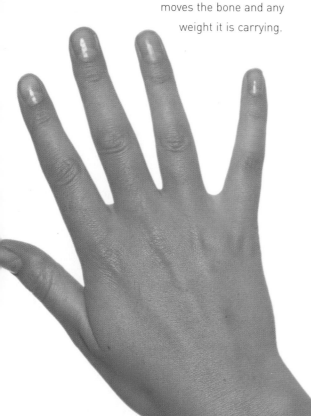

Muscles and tendons work in pairs to facilitate movement. One set of muscles and tendons acts to raise a bone, while the other set relaxes to allow the movement to take place – and vice versa. The tendons in the hands and feet are long and enclosed by slippery synovial sheaths, which enable them to slide when the fingers or toes bend. As we grow older, tendons and ligaments tend to shorten and tighten, which leads to stiffness and poor mobility.

Ligaments

Bones are bound together at joints by extremely strong bands of fibrous tissue known as ligaments. The ligaments bend as the joint bends, but as they only have limited ability to stretch they are able to prevent excessive movement between two bones. The term 'double-jointed' means that in some people the ligaments can stretch more than usual.

Muscles and blood supply

Muscles have their own blood and lymphatic vessels. As the muscle relaxes, oxygenated blood flows in to nourish the tissues; as the muscle contracts, deoxygenated blood is forced out, carrying away impurities and metabolic waste products. If muscles are over-worked or tense, the local blood and lymph circulations are impeded, which leads to a shortage of oxygen and a build-up of waste products. This situation adversely affects the efficiency of the muscle, leading to muscle fatigue, soreness, discomfort, aching and transient pain.

Muscles and bones of the hand

The hand is a wonderfully versatile structure. It is strong enough to grasp and carry heavy objects, yet is capable of the precision and flexibility needed to make highly involved movements, such as writing or turning a door handle. Each hand is made up of 27 bones. There are:

- Eight carpals, which are irregularly shaped, and placed in two rows of four to form the wrist.
- Five metacarpals, which extend from the wrist to the fingers and make up the palm of the hand. The metacarpal in the thumb is the most mobile.
- Fourteen phalanges – two in the thumb and three in each of the fingers.

The forearm is made up of two long bones – the radius and the ulna – which stretch from the elbow and work with the bones of the wrist to allow a wide range of movement.

There are few muscles in the hand itself. Some muscles lie on the outer edge of the palm and at the base of the thumb. Small muscles between the metacarpal bones enable the fingers to move from side to side. But the main muscles used in hand movements are situated in the forearm and connected to the fingers by long tendons. Muscles in the lower arm enable the palm to turn upward or downward, the wrist to rotate and the fingers and thumbs to curl and straighten. Movement is aided by joints, or knuckles, in the fingers and thumb, which help make the hand so flexible.

Tendons are attached at one end to the arm muscles and at the other to bones in the fingers and thumb. When the appropriate muscles contract, they pull on the tendons and so bend or stretch the fingers or thumb. The tendons are bound to the wrist by a strong ligament just above the wrist joint.

Muscles and bones of the foot

The foot supports the weight of the body and acts as a powerful lever to move the body forward when walking or running on different surfaces. The foot, combined with other senses, also helps us to maintain balance.
These tasks are facilitated by a complex arrangement of bones, ligaments, tendons and muscles. The bones of the foot are positioned in a similar lay-out to those of the hand but the foot is a stronger and less flexible structure. The foot is made up of 26 bones.

TRY THIS OUT

To watch the tendons in action, place your hand palm down on a flat surface. Now raise your fingers and thumb. You will be able to see the five tendons along the back of the hand working to straighten your fingers. To see the reverse action, hold your hand out with your palm facing upward. Pull your sleeve back so you can see your forearm. Move your fingers toward the palm, one by one. Again, you will be able to see tendons working to close the fingers.

There are:

- Seven tarsals, which are irregularly shaped bones forming the ankle. The largest tarsal, the calcaneus, makes up the heel.
- Five metatarsals, which stretch between the ankle and the toes, and form the body of the foot. The metatarsal on the inside of the foot is the thickest and strongest, carrying the most body weight.
- Fourteen phalanges – two in the big toe and three in each of the other toes

The bones and joints of the foot are arranged to form dynamic arches – two along the length of the foot, and one across the foot – between the ball of the foot and the heel. If you look at a footprint made by a normal, healthy foot you will see that only the outside of the foot touches the ground. The arches of the foot, which are maintained by strong ligaments and muscles, support the foot, absorb shock and provide leverage when walking, running and jumping. The height of the arches determines the shape of the foots. When the muscles and ligaments become strained and stretched, the arches may begin to weaken, which eventually leads to a condition known as 'flat feet'.

The lower leg is made up of the two long bones – the tibia and the fibula – which work with the bones of the ankle to allow a wide range of movement in the foot.

There are few muscles in the foot. The main muscles are in the sole of the foot and help to bend and spread the toes. The big toe is controlled by its own muscle as it plays such an important role in walking and maintaining balance. Small muscles on the top of the foot straighten and lift the toes. The main muscles are connected to the bones of the foot by long tendons. The ankle joint is supported by strong ligaments. When the appropriate muscles contract, they pull on the tendons and so stretch or bend the foot and toes. Muscles at the front of the leg help bend the foot upward at the ankle and straighten the toes; while muscles at the back of the leg lift the heel upward and curl the toes downward.

The Achilles tendon, situated at the back of the heel, is the strongest tendon in the whole body. It is attached at one end to the calf (gastrocnemius) muscle and at the other to the calcaneus, the largest bone in the foot, which forms the heel. This thick tendon is clearly seen when you stand on tiptoe or point your toes.

How massage helps muscles, tendons and ligaments

Hand and foot massage can help promote the health, strength and flexibility of muscles, tendons and ligaments.

- The increased flow of blood and lymph brings fresh supplies of nutrients and oxygen to muscles and joints and removes waste products and excess fluid. This helps improve joint mobility and reduces the stiffness, tiredness and aches so often caused by standing or long periods of repetitive hand movements.
- The increased blood supply and frictional heat creates warmth in the area which encourages relaxation, so bringing pain relief.

Hand and foot massage techniques

Massage of any kind can be classified as the manipulation of the body's soft tissues – the skin, fat, muscle and connective tissue such as tendons and ligaments. It involves a series of movements using your hands. Each movement is applied in a particular way with the aim of having a specific therapeutic effect on the area being massaged.

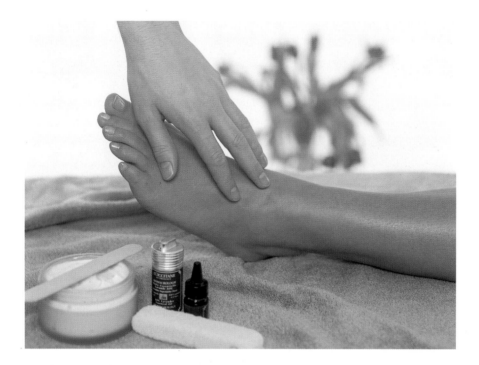

As Hippocrates wrote in around 460–375BC, 'rubbing can bind a joint that it is too loose and also loosen a joint that is too hard'. Massage can be stimulating or sedating. It can be performed gently or vigorously. So, it is necessary to know the effects and benefits of different 'rubbing' or massaging movements before you begin. The main movements used in hand and foot massage are: stroking, effleurage, kneading and tapping.

Stroking

Your hands and feet have nerve endings that respond to touch by sending signals to the brain and influencing the way you feel, both mentally and physically. The impact of stroking shows that touch does not have to be deep to be beneficial. Soft stroking helps soothe and calm the sensory nerves, sending waves of pleasure throughout the body. It has an almost soporific effect and can be used at any time during the massage to help relax your partner. Faster, more energetic stroking is energizing and revitalizing, and a great way of pepping up the circulation to warm your extremities in chilly weather.

A hand or foot massage begins with gentle stroking to spread the oil or cream, and familiarize both giver and receiver with the sensation of skin to skin contact. It is used to calm and relax between more vigorous movements, and again at the end of the massage to bring it to a relaxing conclusion. Gentle stroking is a slow, light and superficial gliding movement, your hands and fingers are supple and slightly cupped so they mould naturally to the bends and curves of the part being massaged. It is a smooth, rhythmical and repetitive action that is beneficial for both giver and receiver. Indeed, studies show that stroking a pet is an effective way of reducing stress levels and improving general well-being – and giving a massage can be an equally rewarding experience.

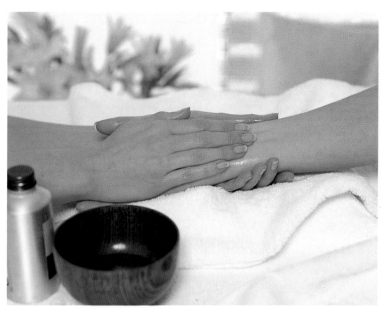

Feathering is a form of gentle stroking that has an almost instant calming effect on the sensory nerve endings. Feathering can be used at any time between movements and is often used as a final stroke to conclude the massage. It is particularly beneficial when massaging someone who is elderly, frail or anxious, and it is effective with babies, too. Use the tips of your fingers to stroke the skin very lightly and softly as though massaging it with a feather. Release your touch very, very slowly at the end of each stroke so that your hands float smoothly away.

Effleurage

This movement is the basis of any massage. The name is derived from the French word 'effleurer', which means 'to skim over'. It is a similar movement to stroking but is generally a firmer, smoothing action. Slow effleurage with a light or moderate pressure flows on naturally from gentle stroking and helps prepare the area for subsequent deeper massage movements. Once the soft tissues start to relax, you may choose to use more energizing strokes with a faster action and deeper pressure. Effleurage is a useful linking movement between different strokes. And, if you are unsure what to do next, try a few effleurage strokes. You can give a pleasurable massage by using effleurage strokes alone.

Effleurage strokes are usually directed towards the heart, so helping to boost the flow of deoxygenated blood through the veins, and of lymph taking impurities back to the heart. The venous and lymphatic systems are mainly driven by the movement of the muscles, and so tend to become sluggish, especially as we get older and less active. Your pressure should be firmer on the upward stroke toward the body, using a light touch on the return movements. Use the flat of your hands or fleshy pads of your finger, or thumbs, as appropriate. Keep your wrists flexible and your hands supple and flowing in a long continuous sequence. Maintain contact with your partner at all times.

Kneading

This is a deeper movement than effleurage so it is mainly used on fleshier areas. Your hands do not glide over the surface of the skin but press much deeper so you can feel the skin moving against the soft tissues beneath to detect and relax specific areas of tension.

The action is similar to kneading dough. Your hands should be relaxed and supple as you pick up the soft tissues, separate them from the underlying structures, compress them and then allow them to relax. The movement is slow and rhythmic with a deep but comfortable pressure. The fleshy pads of your fingers or thumbs move in a circular motion with an increase in pressure on the upward half of the circle and a decrease on the downward half.

FACT

Do not worry about feeling awkward at first. Instead of trying to get every stroke technically correct, concentrate on massaging with care and affection to make your partner feel relaxed, nurtured and secure. With practice, your massage will flow freely and smoothly.

tip Practise the different movements on yourself to feel the effect of varying the speed or pressure of the strokes.

Once the circle is complete, your hand moves smoothly to the next part so that contact and rhythm are maintained. Be careful not to pinch or work too long in one area as this may cause discomfort.

Kneading is very effective in reducing the pain, tension and stiffness often felt in hands and feet. It is a wonderful releasing movement for taut muscles and aching joints, and has a positive effect on stimulating blood and lymph circulation. The rhythmical compression and relaxation of your hands acts like a pump to boost the flow of blood back to the heart and speed the flow of lymph to the nearest set of lymph nodes to be cleansed and filtered. However, as it creates so much heat, do not knead over arthritic, painful, hot or inflamed joints.

Tapping

This is an invigorating movement that strengthens slack muscles, warms the area and stimulates sensory nerve endings. It can play an important part in an energizing, circulation-boosting routine but

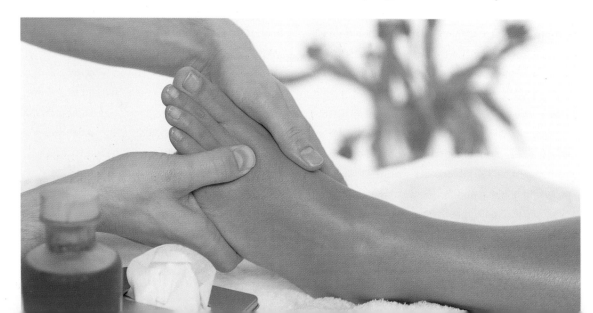

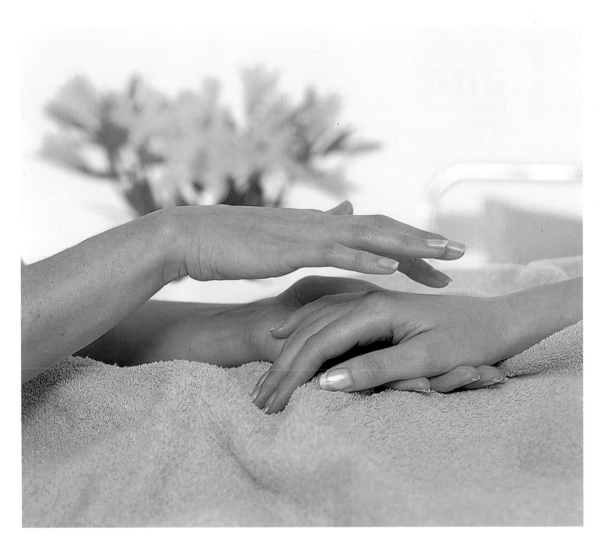

should not be used when massaging babies, children, elderly, arthritic or frail people as it may be too vigorous. Tapping involves striking the skin and then releasing in the same rapid, rhythmical way as a percussion instrument in an orchestra. Keep your wrists flexible and use your hands or fingers to tap the skin with a light, springy movement. Your hands or fingers bounce back up as soon as they land on the skin. It is best to start and finish each tapping sequence with a lighter pressure to avoid an abrupt shock. Do not use tapping movements until the area has been warmed and prepared with stroking or effleurage movements. Use gentle strokes afterwards to soothe the sensory nerve endings and aid the flow of any excess blood or lymph back to the heart.

tip With any form of massage it is important to remember that you are working 'with' and not 'on' another person – hence the term 'massage partner' used throughout this book.

Hand
massages

Our hands work for us continually, day in, day out. The many repetitive movements we perform can put strain, wear and tear on the tendons, ligaments and muscles.

Massage helps ease any build-up of tension, so increasing suppleness and preventing stiffness in the joints. Using a cream or oil helps moisturize and soften the skin, bringing an almost instant improvement in the appearance of even the most weather-beaten hands.

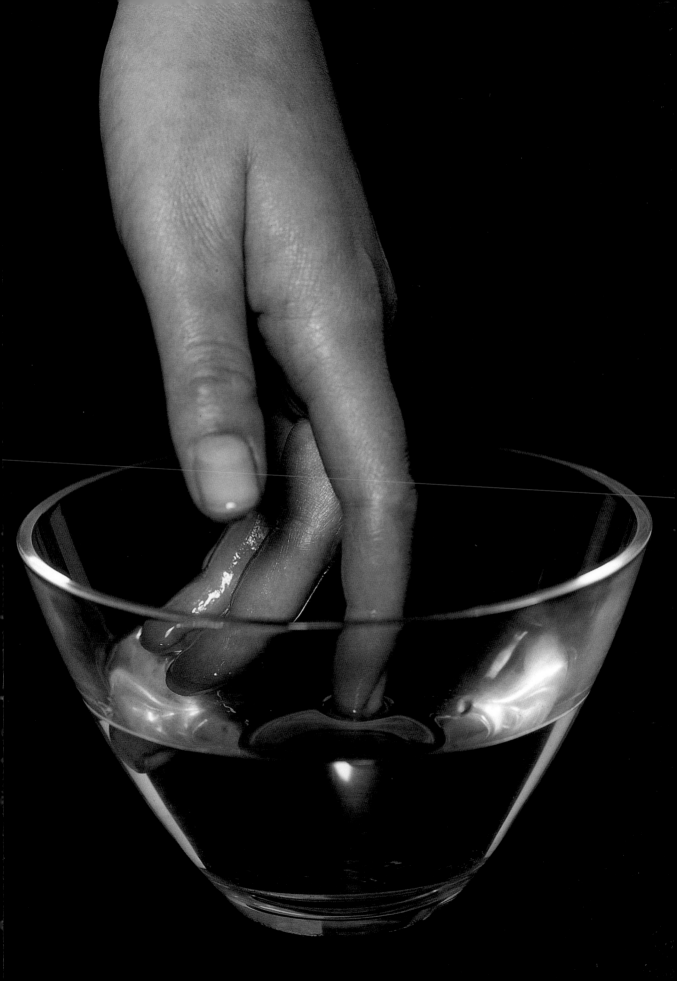

▶ Self-massage for tired and aching hands

This simple massage routine will help to reduce muscle fatigue, relieve everyday aches and pains, encourage joint mobility and increase the supplies of nourishing blood in order to improve the condition of the skin and nails. The use of oil or cream is optional, depending on when and where you massage your hands. If possible, sit on a chair and rest your elbows on a folded towel on a table or desk to offer extra support.

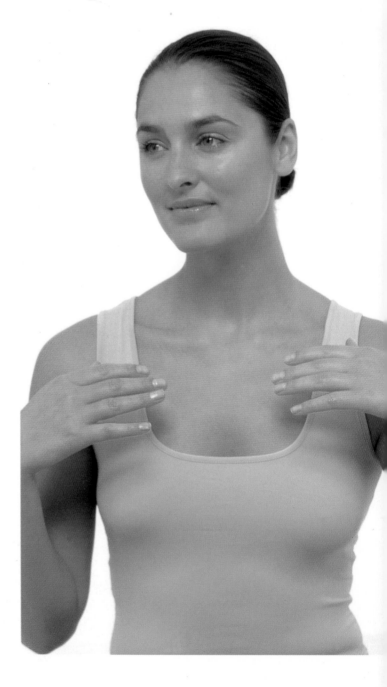

CHECKLIST
Preparation

- Go to the toilet
- Remove all jewellery on hands and wrists
- Roll sleeves up to the elbow
- Sit in a comfortable position
- Prepare a small amount of oil or cream (optional)
- Wash your hands

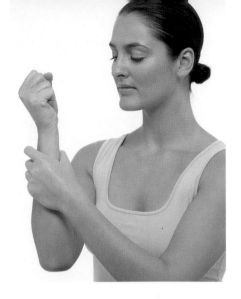

tip Practise the exercises on this page whenever you need some speedy relief from nagging aches or you want some natural warmth in the cold weather.

▲ Warm-up exercises

These simple exercises can help dissolve tension in tired hands and help boost circulation to cold fingers. Be cautious with these exercises if you have arthritis or another joint condition – seek the advice of your doctor or physiotherapist first.

1 Hold your hands at chest level and shake them from the wrist for a count of 10. Keep the movement loose and vigorous.

2 Interlock your fingers. Stretch your arms out in front at shoulder height and turn your hands so your palms face forward and thumbs down. Gently push the heels of your hands forward so that you feel a stretch from your wrist to fingertips. Hold for the count of five. Release and repeat.

3 Support one wrist by clasping it with the other hand. Make your free hand into a soft fist and gently rotate the wrist clockwise (see above). Keep your supporting hand still. Do not force the movement, stay within a comfortable range of movement. Repeat three to five times. Now rotate your hand in the opposite direction, three to five times.

▶ Hand rubbing

This sequence helps improve the flow of blood to the hands and fingers so bringing nourishment and generating warmth in the area.

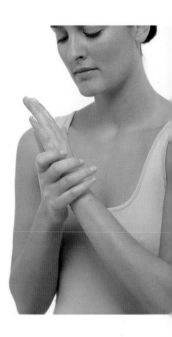

1 If you are using oil or cream, place a small amount in one of your hands. Now, rub your hands together so your palms and fingers are warm and well covered in lubricant. Massage your hands against each other – palm to palm, top of hand to palm and fingers to fingers. Really get them moving.

2 Place your palms together. Move them against each other for about 20 seconds in a circular motion with the heel of one hand exerting the pressure. Repeat, with the other hand leading the action.

tip These movements are useful for helping to spread oil or cream over your hands but they are also beneficial if you choose to do the massage dry – just pretend you are washing your hands with soap.

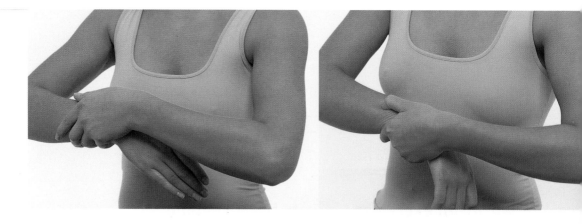

▲ Arm stroking

This sequence uses long, firm stroking movements to soothe the sensory nerve endings in your skin and warm your arms and hands.

1 With one forearm resting across your chest, or your elbow supported on a table or desk, use the palm and fingers of your other hand to stroke from the tips of your fingers to the elbow in a firm, smoothing action. When you reach the elbow, release the pressure and glide your hand back to the starting position. Continue until your forearm feels warm and relaxed, usually around 10 to 15 strokes.

2 Turn your forearm over and repeat the stroking action on the inner side of your arm.

• Keep your hand soft and relaxed so that it moulds naturally to the contours of your arm.

tip Keep focusing on your breathing as you massage your arms and hands. Try to let go of everyday stress for a few minutes – take some deep, calming breaths to help relieve any mental and physical tensions.

▲ Arm kneading

These strokes feel heavenly when massaging your own arms because you know exactly where to increase or decrease the pressure and speed of movement. Avoid the wrist if you have fragile bones or painful, swollen or arthritic wrists.

1 Rest one forearm across your chest, or support your elbow on a table. Grasp your forearm in the V between the thumb and forefinger of your free hand. The thumb is on top and fingers beneath. Make small, circular movements with the flat of your thumb and the inside of your hand, moving from wrist to elbow. Maintain skin contact at all times. Increase the pressure on the upward half of the circle and decrease on the downward half. The skin moving against the underlying tissues will reveal areas of tension. At the elbow, do a few circles around it, then glide back down to the wrist.

2 Repeat about six times to ensure the whole outer forearm is covered. Calm the area with some strokes as shown in 'Arm stroking'.

3 Turn your arm over and repeat on the inside of your forearm. Repeat six times and finish with 'Arm stroking'.

• Relax and feel the tensions of the day being released as you ease out the tension.

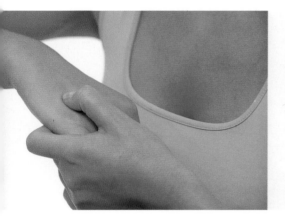

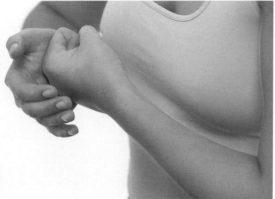

▲ Hand kneading

This sequence feels wonderful when your hands tend to ache through general tiredness.

1 Support your hand, palm downward, in the fingers of your other hand. Place your thumb between the knuckles at the base of your little finger and ring finger. Use the fleshy pad of your thumb to stroke deeply in a straight line between the tendons, toward the wrist. When your thumb reaches the wrist, release the pressure and glide back to the start. Repeat. Repeat along the other grooves on the top of your hand, finishing with the groove between the thumb and index finger.

2 With hands in the same position, use the pad of your thumb to make small circular kneading movements down the groove between the little finger and ring finger. Maintain skin contact. Be aware of increasing the pressure on the upward half of the circle and decreasing it on the downward half. Repeat twice. Repeat along the other grooves on the top of your hand, ending with the groove between the thumb and index finger.

3 Complete the sequence with some gentle stroking over the top of your hand.

• You may need to adjust your hand position to massage effectively.

▲ Palm kneading

Enjoy the wonderful sense of relief as you target taut and over-worked muscles – but be cautious when massaging the wrist as the bones are very delicate. Avoid working on the wrist if you have fragile bones or painful, swollen or arthritic wrists.

1 Turn your hand over to work the palm. With your fingers supporting the back of your hand, use the fleshy pad of your thumb to make deep, circular movements over the whole of the palm and inner wrist. Pay special attention to the muscular pad at the base of the thumb. Start gently and slowly increase the pressure to get it right for you. Continue until you have covered your whole palm.

2 Now make your massaging hand into a fist and use your knuckles to knead the palm of the other hand. Alternatively, use the heel of your hand.

• We all hold tension in different places in our arms and hands. So, once you have learnt the basic movements, vary the routine and moves to suit your own personal needs. Experiment to find the most effective movements. You will know when you hit the spot.

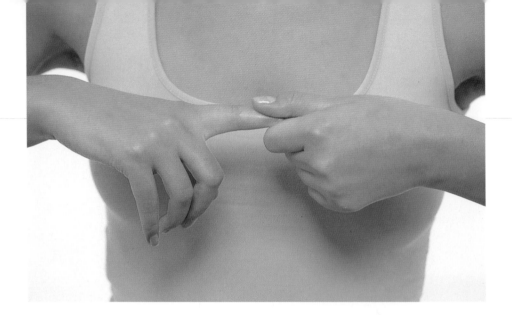

▲ Finger stretch

Avoid this sequence if you have painful, swollen or arthritic fingers.

1 Hold the little finger of your right hand between the thumb and forefinger of your left hand. Curl your left hand around the little finger. Now gently squeeze and massage along the finger with a circular pressure. Move from the base of the finger to the tip.

2 When your hand reaches the tip of the finger, glide back down to the starting point. Now gently pull to give the whole finger a glorious stretch.

3 Release your grip and slide your hand to the top of the finger in one long, continuous movement. Allow your fingers to float away from the tip.

4 Repeat this sequence, working on each of your other fingers and thumb in turn.

• Try this exercise to warm cold hands in the winter.

▼ Finger tapping

These soft tapping movements have an energizing effect throughout the body.

1 Rest your right hand on a table or your knees, palm downward. Use the flat of your fingers on your left hand to tap the back of the hand and fingers with light, rapid movements. Allow your fingers to bounce back as they land on the skin.

2 Turn your hand over and continue.

3 Complete the sequence with some gentle stroking to calm the sensory nerve endings.

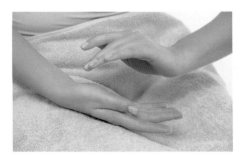

Final flourish

Complete your hand massage by repeating 'Arm stroking'. On the return stroke, make the movement progressively lighter and slower, with your fingertips floating from the end of your fingers. Enjoy the soothing sense of release.

Soothing
hand massage

Now that you have practised on yourself, you may wish to share the benefits of massage with others. The following simple hand-massage routine will help relax and calm your massage partner. Start with the right hand and then repeat the sequence on the left hand.

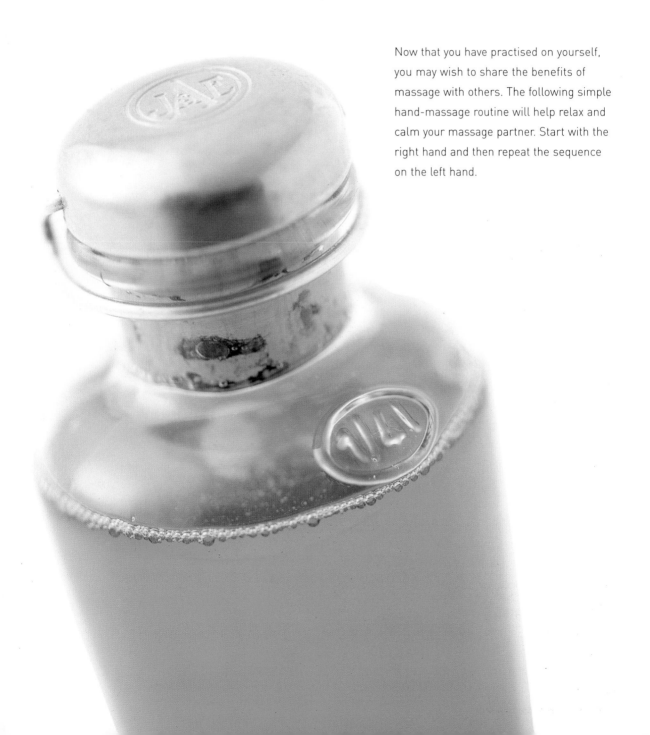

CHECKLIST
Things you will need

- Small pillow or cushion.
- Small table (optional).
- Two chairs.
- Suitable oil or hand cream in a small container
- Wooden or plastic spatula for cream.
- Two small towels.
- Paper towels to wipe your hands and absorb any spillage.
- Soft background music (optional).
- Blanket (optional).
- Clock (optional).
- Cologne (optional).
- Cotton wool (optional).

CHECKLIST
Advise your massage partner to

- Go to the toilet.
- Remove any rings, wristwatches or bracelets
- Roll sleeves up to the elbow.
- Wash hands. Alternatively, clean them with wipes or cotton wool with a few drops of cologne.
- Tell you about any medical conditions that may affect your massage. Ask about allergies and offer a choice of oil or cream.
- Try different positions to ensure you are both comfortable.
- Join you in breathing slowly and deeply, concentrating your thoughts on the massage that you are about to receive and give.

CHECKLIST
Things to do

- Dress in comfortable, washable clothes
- Reduce the lighting.
- Check the room is warm and free from draughts.
- Arrange some privacy. Ensure that you will not be disturbed for the next 20 minutes or so. Switch on the answerphone or unplug the telephone.
- Wash your hands. Check that your nails are short, smooth and clean. Remove any jewellery that may interfere with the massage.
- Warm your hands by rubbing them briskly together. Do a few mobility exercises (see pages 194–5) to help release any tension.

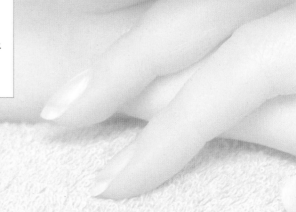

Getting prepared

Before you begin a massage, make sure those you massage know what to expect and are aware of the benefits. Give them the chance to ask any questions that may arise.

Talk it through

You may also like to ask whether they have had a hand massage before. If so, discuss any movements that they particularly liked or disliked. They may have some suggestions of their own. Use this time to discreetly assess, through looking and feeling, the condition of your massage partner's hand. Think about temperature, skin texture and colour (see page 126). Feel for any tension in the hand and check the condition of the nails. Check for any cuts, swollen joints or varicose veins.

NOTE

Hand massage brings you into close personal contact with your massage partner. You will be entering each other's personal space and this may feel a little uncomfortable at first. Be sensitive to your partner's reaction.

Get comfortable

Comfort is vital to relaxation. It is well worth spending a little time getting into a suitable position so you can massage without stretching or straining. You should both be able to move freely so that you can maintain a good posture during the massage. Depending on circumstances you may choose from the following:

Hand position one

You can sit facing each other. Cover a cushion with a towel and place it on a small table between you, or on your lap. Rest your massage partner's hand on the cushion for the massage. Your feet, and those of your massage partner, should be placed firmly on the floor or small stool, ankles uncrossed. This is a good position for maintaining eye contact, but do be prepared to have your movements closely watched.

Hand position two

You can sit side by side. Your massage partner may choose to sit in a chair with one hand resting on a pillow on their lap or the armrest. Check the angle so you can work in comfort. Alternatively, if your massage partner is bedridden, you can easily massage the hands while they rest on a pillow on the side of the bed. This position is especially useful when massaging elderly or ill people. The disadvantage is that you will have to move your chair so you can massage each hand in comfort.

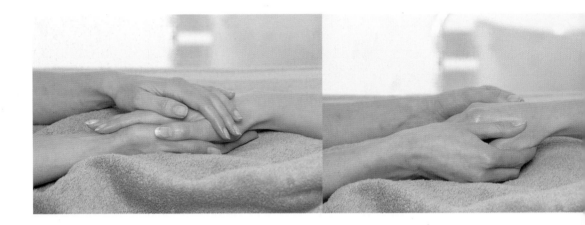

▲ Holding the hand

Holding your partner's hand in a caring way provides reassurance at the start of the massage. It offers a moment of peace and stillness that helps establish a bond and allows you both to let go of tension and relax into the experience. It is important not to rush this preliminary hold.

1 Begin with your massage partner's hand facing palm downward. Place one of your hands beneath and the other on top, so that the hand is cradled in the warmth and security of your palms. Maintain optimum contact by using the whole surface area of palms and fingers.

2 Hold for a minute. At this stage you may like to ask your massage partner to close her eyes and take some deep breaths to encourage relaxation. Remind your partner to try to 'let go' of her everyday hassles and enjoy being pampered.

3 Release your hold very gradually by sliding your hands toward the fingertips, and gently and slowly drawing away.

 tip Look out for areas of dry skin. Massage the cream or oil into these patches to moisturize and soften the hands.

▲ Gentle stretch

This stretching movement is wonderfully soothing, especially for tired, aching hands.

1 Place some oil or cream in the palm of one hand. If you use too much you may find your hands slipping and sliding over the skin. You can easily top it up during the massage if your hands are large or your massage partner's skin is very dry. Rub your hands together so that the palms and fingers are warm and well covered in oil or cream.

2 With your partner's hand facing palm downward, place a hand on either side with fingers curled underneath and your thumbs on top. Cup the sides of your massage partner's hand in your hands. Now draw your thumbs firmly out to the sides to achieve a pleasant rolling and stretching action over the back of her hand. Use the whole length of your thumbs to gain maximum benefit.

3 When your thumbs reach the sides of the hand, hold for a count of three, then release and repeat twice more.

• Work on the top of the hand, avoid pressing on your partner's fingers.

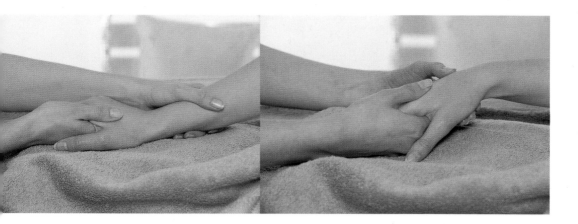

▲ Warming up

This sequence uses sweeping movements to relax your massage partner and stimulate blood circulation. Use these strokes as a way of becoming more familiar with the feel of your partner's skin beneath your hands.

1 With your partner's palm facing downward, place one hand beneath – in a loose 'shaking hands' position. Sweep your other hand firmly up from the finger tips along the upper side of the arm toward the elbow in a steady stroke. Work with your whole hand and keep it relaxed so it moulds to the shape of her arm. Glide around the elbow and return with a lighter pressure to the fingers. Repeat six to ten times.

2 Turn your massage partner's arm slightly and change your working hand to perform these gliding strokes along the inside of the forearm. Sweep lightly into the elbow crease before returning to the wrist. Repeat six to ten times.

3 Complete the sequence by gently holding your partner's hand for a few seconds.

• Ensure that any dry skin is well lubricated with oil or cream.

▲ Stroking the back of the hand

These rhythmical strokes help warm and soften the hand so that it is well prepared for the subsequent movements. The bones of the hand are very delicate, so maintain a light pressure.

1 With the palm of your massage partner's hand facing downward, wrap your hands around it, thumbs on top and fingers beneath. Use the pads of your thumbs to make alternate strokes along the top of the hand, working from the fingers to the wrist. Your thumbs move one after the other in a wave-like flowing motion.

2 When your thumbs reach the wrist, lessen the pressure and, without losing contact, slide them back to the starting position. Repeat the sequence six times to cover the whole of the top of the hand.

• Spend longer on these movements if you sense that your massage partner needs soothing comfort.

 tip Synchronize your breathing with that of your massage partner. Focus on your partner. Thinking about other things may well convey a feeling of detachment.

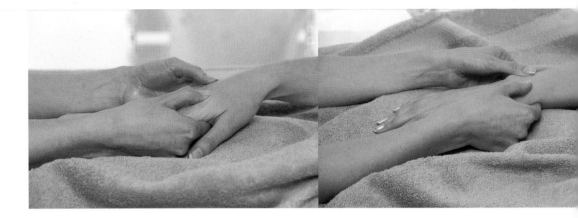

▲ Kneading the back of the hand

This sequence of movements is effective in releasing muscular tension and tiredness.

1 With the palm of your massage partner's hand facing downward, place your fingers beneath and thumbs on top as in the previous movement. Use the pads of your thumbs to make alternate strokes along the groove between the tendons of the little and third fingers. Work from the knuckles to the wrist. Begin with a firm but comfortable pressure and gradually release the pressure as your thumb reaches the wrist. Return with a light pressure, maintaining contact. Repeat. Repeat this stroking action along each of the grooves on the top of the hand, including between thumb and forefinger.

2 Return your hands to the starting position and use the pads of your thumbs to make alternate small circular movements along the groove between the little finger third fingers. Move toward the wrist. Repeat. Repeat the movement working along each of the grooves on the top of the hand.

3 Finish with some soothing stokes over the top of the hand working toward the wrist.

• You will need to change working hands to perform this effectively.

▲ Wrist release

Avoid this movement if a massage partner has fragile bones or painful, swollen or arthritic wrists.

1 Start with your hands on either side of your massage partner's hand. Place your fingers beneath her inner wrist and your thumbs on top. Now make small, alternating circles with the pads of both thumbs over the back of the wrist. The movement should be fairly slow and rhythmical with a comfortably firm pressure. Make around 15 to 20 small circles.

2 Now change the movement to a gentle fanning action, using both thumbs to stroke upward from the wrist in an arc. Your thumbs come gently off the skin at the sides of the arm about 5 cm (2 in) above the wrist. Repeat around six times.

• Do not press too firmly as the bones in the wrist are very delicate.

tip Keep your massage as fluid and rhythmical as possible, flowing smoothly between movements. Try not to stop and start.

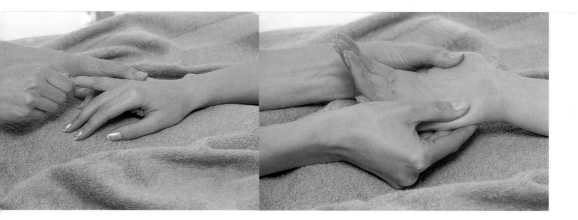

▲ Finger work

Avoid this sequence of movements if the person has painful, swollen or arthritic joints.

1 Clasp the hand, palm downward, with one hand. With your other hand, hold your massage partner's little finger between your thumb and forefinger. The finger should be well supported from the base. Rotate the whole finger three times clockwise, and then three times anti-clockwise. Ask your massage partner not to help with the rotation but to 'let go'.

2 Now place the little finger between your thumb and forefinger so that it is supported in the turn of your fingers. Use the pad of your thumb to make gentle circular movements along the finger, working from base to tip.

3 When your thumb reaches the tip of your massage partner's finger, push your thumb and fingers downward in a firm stroking movement. Hold, so that the finger is enclosed in your hand. Release the pressure slightly and draw your hand in the opposite direction, allowing it to slide off the tip of the finger in a gentle pulling, stretching action. Repeat.

4 Repeat the same sequence of movements on each finger in turn, finishing with the thumb.

▲ Palm stretch

This sequence helps stretch and soften constricted muscle fibres in the palm, so making the palm more relaxed and pliant.

1 Sandwich your massage partner's hand between your two palms and turn it over so that the palm faces upward. Make the movement definite so that you are in control.

2 Now rest the back of your massage partner's hand on your fingers and place your thumbs on the palm, pointing toward the wrist. Push your thumbs gently outward to the sides to spread and stretch the palm. Use your thumbs to hold the stretch for a count of five, then release and repeat twice.

tip Be aware of your massage partner's body language. Around 70 per cent of all communication is by means of non-verbal massages and gestures. Take note of any flinching or stiffening, which may indicate discomfort or unease. Similarly look for signs of pleasure such as relaxed breathing. Adapt your massage accordingly.

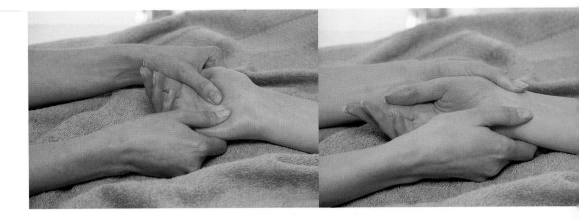

▲ Palm stroking and kneading

These movements ease tension in taut muscles in the palm. Some people call this 'walking in the palm'.

1 With your massage partner's palm facing upward, wrap your hands around the sides of the hand, fingers underneath and thumbs in the palm. Use your thumbs to make stroking movements covering the whole palm. Work from fingers toward wrist and glide over the surface of the skin.

2 Start kneading the palm. Make alternate, circular movements with your thumbs, increasing the pressure on the upward half of the circle and decrease on the downward half. Keep movements slow, firm and rhythmical, with one thumb working after the other. Cover all the palm, paying attention to the pad at the base of the thumb.

3 Follow this with firm sliding strokes. Use the pads of your thumbs to make a fanning movement from the base of the fingers toward the wrist. Your thumbs move at the same time. Repeat about 10 times.

4 Finish the sequence by repeating Step 1.

• The fleshy pad of the palm usually responds well to deep massage but check your pressure is comfortable as some areas may be tender.

▲ Inner wrist stroking

Avoid this if the person has fragile bones or painful, swollen or arthritic wrists.

1 With your massage partner's hand palm upward, rest your fingers on the back of the wrist and your thumbs on the inner wrist. Use the pads of your thumbs to make alternate, light circular movements. Cover the whole of the inner wrist.

2 Change the movement to a gentle fanning action, using both thumbs to stroke upward from the wrist in an arc. Your thumbs come off the skin at the sides of the arm about 5 cm (2 in) about the wrist. Repeat six times.

• Maintain a good support and keep your pressure very light in order to avoid causing pain or discomfort around the delicate bones of the wrist.

tip During a hand massage make every effort to ensure that your partner feels nurtured, cossetted and secure. Try not to rush any of the movements. Gentle, unhurried, rhythmical strokes are soothing and relaxing.

▼ Wrist rotations

This helps to mobilize wrist joints and prevent the problems of stiffness and swelling. Make movements firm and controlled but do not force the action. Be cautious if your partner has arthritis, or a previous wrist injury.

1 For this movement your massage partner's forearm is slightly raised. Use one hand to gently support the lower arm – avoid gripping tightly. Interlock the fingers of your free hand with those of your massage partner to ensure a firm, supportive hold. Alternately, clasp your hands as though shaking each other's hands.

2 Now slowly rotate the wrist. Repeat three times in a clockwise direction and three times in an anti-clockwise direction.

3 Gently lay down the arm and hand and slowly release your fingers.

tip Feel the range of movement in your partner's wrist and always remain within her own personal limits. You may find that your partner tries to help with the movement. If this happens, ask her to look away or close her eyes so that you can control the action.

▼ Finishing touch

Complete the hand massage with a series of soothing strokes that are designed to relax mind, body and spirit.

1 With your massage partner's palm facing downward, place one hand beneath it to offer warmth and reassurance. Repeat the same soothing strokes used at the beginning of the massage in the 'warming up' sequence to massage the hand and arm. Allow the strokes to become progressively lighter and slower.

2 Now use the tips of the fingers on your free hand to stroke the top of your massage partner's hand with a feather-like touch as though stroking a cat. Work from wrist to fingertips, allowing your fingers to float from the end of your massage partner's fingertips.

3 Place your free hand on top of your massage partner's hand to enclose it securely in the warmth of your palms for around 10 seconds, or longer if you wish. Release your hold and slowly draw your hands away.

• Cover your massage partner's hand with a towel and repeat the routine on the other hand.

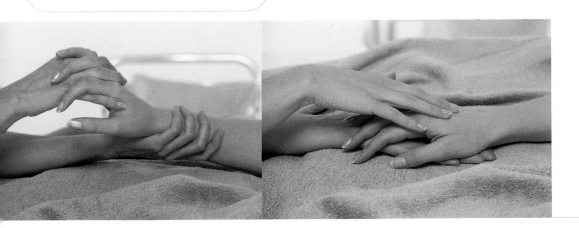

Foot
massages

Feet contain thousands of tiny sensory nerve endings, making them among the most sensitive areas of the whole body. Your massage can be adapted to stimulate or soothe these nerve endings and thus energize or relax yourself and your massage partner.

A brisk massage can help to boost energy levels and restore a sense of well-being. A slower massage can be extremely relaxing and offer comfort and reassurance during a stressful or difficult time.

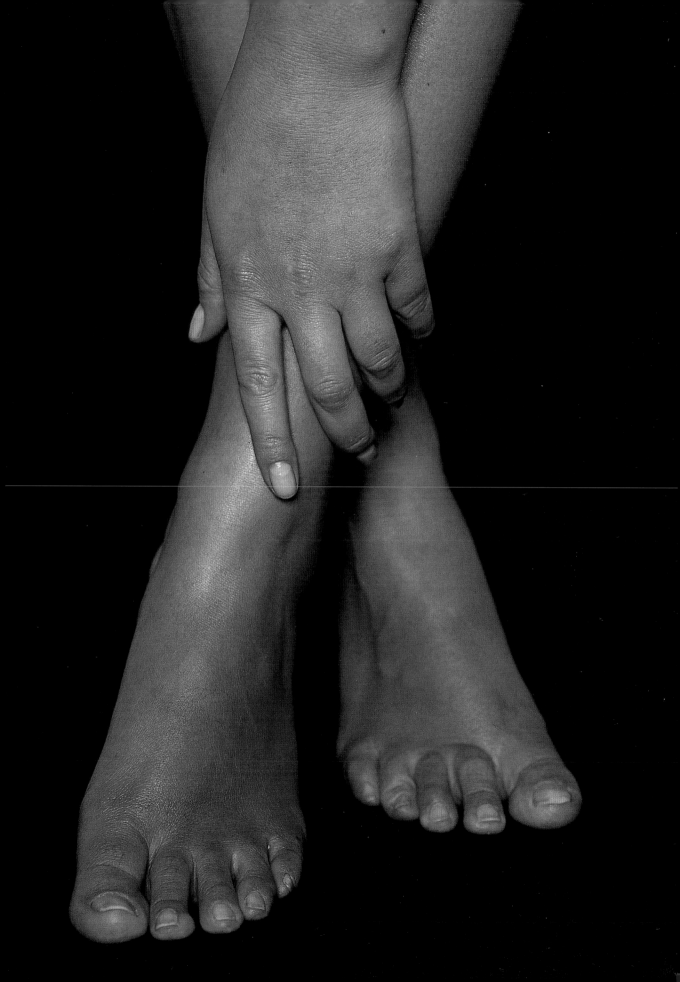

Self foot-massage
for boosting circulation

If you suffer the miseries of cold feet, then try this quick and effective self-help routine. It can be done wherever you are – at home or at work. You may choose to use a nourishing oil or cream, but many of the strokes are just as effective performed dry without even removing your socks or tights. You need to be able to reach your foot comfortably, either sitting on the floor, a chair or a bed. Experiment to find the most suitable position for you.

CHECKLIST
Preparation

- Remove all jewellery on hands, feet, wrists and ankles.
- Remove shoes.
- Sit in a comfortable position.
- Prepare a small amount of oil or cream (optional).
- Go to the toilet.
- Wash your hands in warm water – they need to be warm before you begin.

◀ Warming start

Give your circulation a kick-start with these smooth, sweeping strokes. A firm, confident pressure will improve poor blood and lymph circulation in the feet and lower legs.

1 If you are using oil or cream, roll up your trouser legs and remove socks or tights. (This is best done at the start when your hands are dry.) Place a little oil or cream in the palm of one of your hands. Rub your hands together so that they are warm and well covered in the lubricant.

2 With your knee bent, stroke both hands up your leg moving from the ankle toward the knee in a slow, rhythmical, flowing action. Keep your hands open and soft, maintaining as much contact with the palms and fingers as possible. Imagine your hands are plasticine or playdough and mould them to the contours of your legs.

3 Gradually increase the pressure using long, even and confident strokes on the upward movement toward the knee. Lessen the pressure at the knee and glide back down the sides of the leg to the starting position.

4 Work the back and front of the lower leg until it feels warm and relaxed.

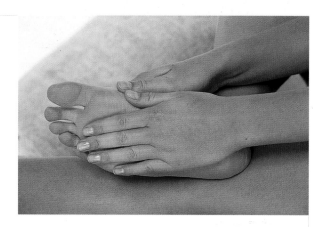

▲ Foot stroking

Rest the ankle of one foot on a towel across the thigh of the other leg. Alternatively, you may prefer to rest on a cushion.

1 Sandwich your foot between your hands and, with both hands moving at once, stroke from the toes to the heel in one long continuous movement. Repeat three times.

2 With hands held in the same position, start moving the flat of your hands in large circles, one on top and one beneath, rather like the wheels of a train.

3 Finish the sequence by holding your foot between the palms of your hands, fingers facing toward the toes. Draw your hands down your foot and slide very lightly right off the end of your toes. Repeat three times.

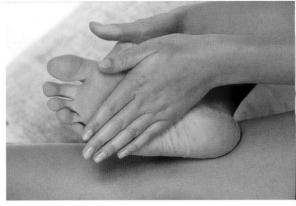 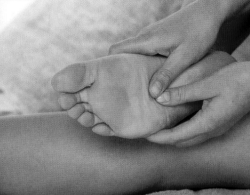

▲ Foot rub

Rubbing your feet is a natural response when we feel chilly as it helps to generate warmth – and feels wonderful. The pressure should be fairly firm to stimulate the local blood circulation and warm and invigorate your whole body.

1 With your foot sandwiched between the palms of your hands, rub briskly over the surface of the skin using short, stimulating movements back and forth in any direction. You will find that one hand naturally moves forward as the other moves backward. Your wrists stay flexible, fingers held quite straight. Cover your whole foot, including your toes, heel and ankle.

2 Finish with some soothing strokes over the whole foot.

3 Keep your hands moving so you do not stay in the same spot for too long.

▲ Sole fanning

This movement feels best when the pressure is comfortably firm. Relax and enjoy the sensation.

1 Support your foot in both hands, fingers on top of the foot and thumbs meeting on the arch of the foot. Now press with the pads of your thumbs and, with one long, sweeping fan-like movement, push them upward to the base of your toes and out to the sides of the foot. Your thumbs should stay fairly stiff and in contact with the skin as you sweep them up to form a curved T-shape.

2 Maintain an even pressure on the upward movement and then skim over the skin to return to the starting position. Repeat four times.

> ## NOTE
>
> The sole of the foot is very sensitive to touch. Notice how gentle strokes soothe the whole body while brisker strokes have a more stimulating effect.

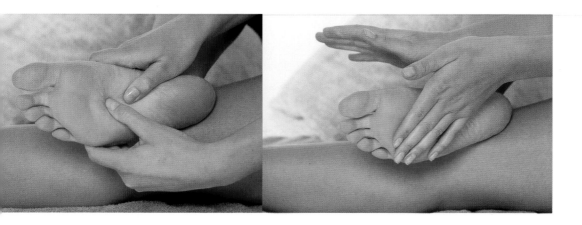

▲ Sole searching

Use these kneading movements to target the tension hot-spots in the sole of your foot. You will know exactly where to work for the best results. These techniques help to loosen muscles, ease aches and pains, and improve poor circulation.

1 With hands held in the same position as above, use the pads of your thumbs to make small circular movements over the whole of the sole of your foot and around your heel. Your thumbs work simultaneously, exerting a deep but comfortable pressure – feel the sense of relief as you knead this area.
2 Now support the top of the foot with one hand and make a loose fist with your free hand. Firmly rotate your fist over the sole of the foot using your knuckles to make small circular tension-releasing movements.
3 Complete the sequence by soothing any slight discomfort caused by deep kneading with some gentle stroking around the foot.

▲ Foot tapping

This is an energizing, uplifting movement that stimulates the blood circulation to your feet and makes you feel good all over. Avoid this action over inflamed areas or corns.

1 Lightly tap your toes with the flat of your hands, one hand moving after the other in the same rapid, rhythmical way as playing a percussion instrument. Keep your wrists loose and allow your fingers to bounce back as soon as they land on the skin. Begin slowly and then gradually increase your speed so the movement is energetic and springy.
2 Repeat this light striking action over the top and sole of the foot.
3 Follow this invigorating movement with some gentle stroking to soothe the area.
4 Try using the back or side of your hand to tap the sole of the foot.

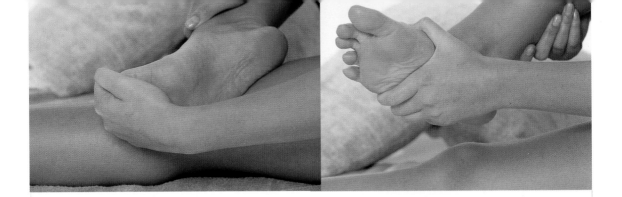

▲ Toe stretching and circling

If your toes tend to feel the cold, then practise this sequence regularly to help loosen joints and maintain good circulation to the extremities. If you have painful, swollen or arthritic joints in your toes, consult your doctor or physiotherapist before doing this exercise.

1 Supporting your foot in one hand, hold all five toes in your other hand. Clasp the toes firmly with the palm of your hand on the ball of the foot, fingers curled over the toes and pointing along the top of the foot toward the ankle. Gently push against your toes to bend them toward your leg. Hold for a count of six. Release. Repeat four times, keeping the movement slow and controlled.

2 With hands held in the same position, grasp your toes firmly and gently rotate all five toes at once. Begin by moving them in a clockwise direction. Repeat six times. Now reverse the movement so they are circled in the other direction. Repeat six times.

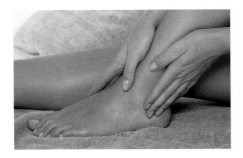

▲ Ankle circling

This simple movement helps maintain flexibility and prevents stiffness and is also a most effective circulation-boosting exercise. If you have painful, swollen or arthritic ankles, consult your doctor.

1 Support your leg with one hand placed just above the ankle. Clasp the foot with the other hand. Maintaining a firm hold, use your hand to rotate your ankle in a clockwise direction. Keep the movement definite and controlled, aiming to achieve your full range of movement – but do not force the movement. Repeat five times.

2 Circle the ankle in the other direction five times.

• Make ankle circling part of your daily routine. You will find that your ankle mobility gradually starts to increase.

◀ Final strokes

To complete your massage, soothe the nerve endings with some slow stroking.

1 Stroke your hands from your toes to your ankles. Continue the stroke up to your knee, if you wish.

2 Cover your whole foot and lower leg with light, calming strokes using the tips of your fingers.

3 Hold your foot between your palms. Stay still and feel the warmth of your hands against your foot. Slowly release the hold and draw your hands away.

• Cover your foot with a towel to keep warm and repeat the sequence on the other foot.

Reviving
foot massage

A foot massage can also help to refresh tired feet, get rid of aches, keep joints flexible and boost blood circulation. Try this sequence on a massage partner, varying the depth and speed of strokes as appropriate to the mood and occasion. Begin with the right foot and then repeat the sequence of movements on the left foot.

CHECKLIST

Things you will need

- Small pillow or cushion.
- Two chairs, small table and/or cushions depending on position.
- Suitable oil or cream in a small container.
- Wooden or plastic spatula (for cream).
- Two small towels.
- Paper towels to wipe your hands and absorb any spillage.
- Soft background music (optional).
- Blanket (optional).
- Clock (optional).
- Cologne (optional).
- Cotton wool (optional).
- Mirror (optional).
- Shoehorn (optional).

CHECKLIST

Things to do

- Dress in comfortable, washable clothes.
- Reduce the lighting.
- Check the room is warm and free from draughts.
- Arrange to have privacy. Make sure that you will not be disturbed for the next half hour or so. Switch on the answerphone.
- Remove any jewellery that may interfere with the massage.
- Wash your hands.
- Check your nails are short, smooth and clean. Cover any cuts or abrasions with sticking plaster.
- Warm your hands by rubbing them briskly together. Do a few mobility exercises (see pages 194–5) to help release any tension.

CHECKLIST

Advise your massage partner to

- Wear loose, comfortable clothing. Trousers are rolled up for lower leg massage.
- Remove any foot rings or ankle chains.
- Tell you about any conditions that may affect your massage. (Ask your massage partner about allergies and offer a choice of oils or creams.)
- Go to the toilet.
- Try different positions to ensure maximum comfort for you both.
- Join you in breathing deeply and slowly, allowing your thoughts to centre on the massage time you are about to share.

Getting prepared

Some people feel strange having their feet massaged. They may be concerned that their feet are ugly or smelly, or that your touch will tickle. So, before starting your massage, explain exactly what is going to happen and outline briefly some of the benefits. Give your massage partner the chance to ask any questions and reassure him or her that you will stop if any movements are painful or uncomfortable.

Be comfortable

There is a temptation to launch straight into a massage without thinking about your position. It is often only half way through that you realize your back is aching and your partner is still unable to relax. So spend a little time and effort making sure that you are both comfortable, well supported and at the right angle for massage. Ideally, your back should be straight with your partner's feet at chest height to avoid muscle tension in your arms. You should be able to move freely and breathe easily.

Foot position one

Your massage partner lies on a bed or reclining chair with her feet at the foot. You sit on a lower chair so that you face your massage partner and have easy access to the soles of the feet. Place a small cushion or rolled up towel beneath her knees. Make sure your massage partner feels comfortable and that her neck and back are supported. Use extra pillows to prop her up if she chooses to sit in a semi-reclining position.

Foot position two

Your massage partner sits on a chair with her legs resting on a stool or small table. Or she rests her feet on your lap. Place her feet on a cushion covered in a towel, knees slightly bent. You sit facing your massage partner on a chair, stool or cushion but do check your height and position so that you maintain a good posture. One drawback of this position is privacy – your massage partner may prefer to wear trousers or rest a towel over her lap.

Foot position three

Your partner rests against a pile of cushions on the floor. You kneel or sit cross-legged on the floor with your back against a wall or piece of furniture. Your massage partner's feet rest on a cushion on your lap.

Cleaning up

It is natural to feel concerned you may have smelly feet, even if you have just walked out of the shower. So put your massage partner at ease by cleansing her feet. Use antiseptic or baby wipes or cotton wool with some cologne. Use separate pieces for each foot to avoid cross infection. While cleaning the feet, handle them with tenderness and care as though saying a gentle 'hello' to them. Use the opportunity to assess temperature, texture, colour and tension. Look for any cuts, swollen joints, varicose veins or fungal infections.

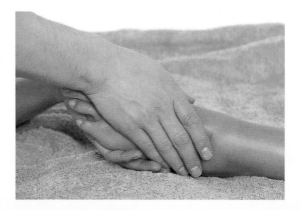

▲ Greeting the feet

First impressions matter – and your first contact with your massage partner's feet sets the tone for the whole massage. Be confident and reassuring. Feel how the person's feet gradually soften and become more receptive to your touch.

1 Gently cradle your massage partner's right foot in both hands. Hold the foot securely with maximum skin-to-skin contact, so encouraging the foot to relax within the warmth and comfort of your palms.
2 Hold for a minute or two. You may like to ask your massage partner to take some deep breaths to help her relax and gain the optimum benefits from your massage. You can join in too. It is surprising how effective deep breathing can be in allowing you to let go of everyday tensions.
3 Release your hold by slowly drawing your hands away.
• Do not be tempted to rush this initial hold. It helps inspire a feeling of trust from your partner.

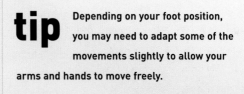

tip **Depending on your foot position, you may need to adapt some of the movements slightly to allow your arms and hands to move freely.**

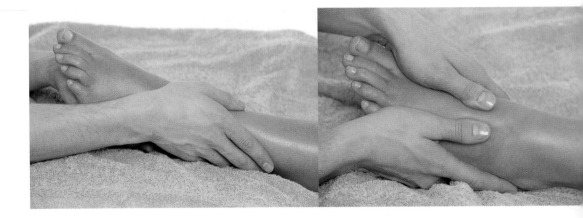

▲ Warming strokes

These flowing strokes smoothes in the cream or oil, and warms and prepares the foot for massage.

1 Place some oil or cream on your palms. Add more if the skin on your massage partner's feet is dry but be careful not to overdo it or your hands will slide. Rub your hands together so your palms and fingers are warm and covered in lubricant.

2 Sandwich the right foot between your palms – one hand covering the top of the foot, the other on the sole. Place your hands in a prayer position so you obtain maximum skin-to-skin contact.

3 Slide your hands gently but firmly from the tips of the toes up toward the body. When your hands reach the ankle, glide back with a lighter pressure down toward the toes, maintaining contact throughout. It is a smooth, rhythmical, sweeping action, following the contours of the foot. Your hands should be aiming to mould themselves to the foot.

4 If you choose, sweep the strokes right up to the knee, keeping a firmer pressure on the upward movement and gliding back down to the ankle.

5 Repeat several times until the foot feels warm.

• Cover your partner's other foot to keep it warm.

▲ Opening the foot

This is a wonderful stretching and releasing movement for tired feet. Try it on yourself when you have been on your feet all day.

1 Position your hands either side of the foot – fingers on the sole and thumbs on the top. Now exert a slight pressure with your thumbs to stretch out the top of the foot and bring the sides toward you. As your thumbs move outward, feel the foot gently arching. Hold for a count of five and gently release.

2 Repeat three times, moving a little further down the foot each time.

• Keep the pressure on the top of the foot, be careful not to press on your partner's toes.

> ## NOTE
>
> Your massage partner's feet deserve some care and respect. After all, it has been estimated that during an average lifespan most of us walk the equivalent of four times the circumference of the Earth. Every time we take a step we put around one and a quarter times our body weight on each foot. For most people this amounts to a total force of over one million pounds every day.

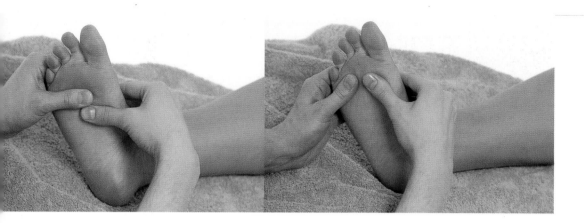

▲ Sole criss-cross

Firm massage movements on the sole of the foot can be really pleasurable. This deep stroking movement helps to ease tension and warm the sole of the foot. Try to maintain a slow, steady rhythm with even pressure throughout the movements.

1 Clasp the foot with both hands, positioning your thumbs on the heel and fingers overlapping on top of the foot. Now, slide one thumb above the other in a criss-cross action toward either side of the foot. Your thumbs move with a firm pressure toward and past each other, moving simultaneously in opposite directions. Without losing contact with the skin, use this alternate back-and-forth action to move your hands up the foot so that the whole sole is covered.

2 Continue the criss-cross action moving down to the heel.

3 Repeat three times.

• Try using different speeds. A slow action is very soothing while a brisker movement has more of an invigorating effect.

▲ Thumb circles

This sequence works a little deeper, helping to stimulate blood circulation to the sole of the foot. This not only generates warmth, it also encourages flexibility.

1 With your hands in the same position as the start of the previous movement, use the fleshy pads of your thumbs to make small circular movements over the sole of the foot. Your thumbs work simultaneously to rotate the skin against the underlying tissues. It is a rhythmical, kneading movement – press, lift, squeeze and release the flesh.

2 Work upward from the heel to the base of the toes in a smooth, flowing, continuous movement. Make sure that your thumbs do not leave the skin. Repeat these thumb circles so that the entire sole is covered.

• Keep checking the pressure with your partner as some areas of the foot may be a little tender.

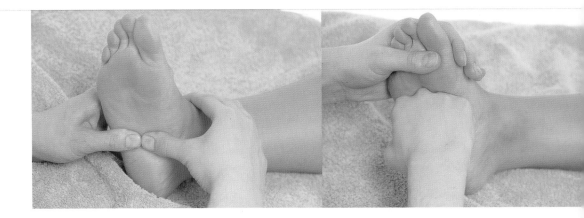

▲ Thumb stroking

This deep, stroking sequence of movements feels blissful after the previous kneading movement. You must be in a position where you can lean slightly backward and keep your back straight.

1 Hold the foot with both hands, fingers overlapping on top and thumbs on the ball of the foot. Mould your fingers to the foot so that it rests securely in your hand. Now make short, sweeping, downward movements with your thumbs. One thumb strokes after the other, in a rhythmical, wave-like movement.
2 Follow this action down to the heel, so that the whole sole is covered.
3 When your thumbs reach the heel, release the pressure and glide both thumbs up the sides of the foot simultaneously. Then, with thumbs touching at the tips, draw them down the foot with a firm, confident stroke to the heel.
4 Glide your thumbs back to the starting position and repeat the sequence four times.
• Encourage your massage partner to enjoy the tingling sensation in their foot as the blood circulation improves.

▲ Sole stretch

This is a stretching and releasing movement that complements perfectly the previous movements on the sole, and helps to loosen and soften the foot.

1 Rest the flat of one hand on the top of your massage partner's foot. Make a loose fist with your free hand and place your knuckles just under the ball of the foot. Stroke your fist firmly down the sole of the foot toward the heel so that the backs of your fingers, not your knuckles, press into the skin. This creates a deep and very satisfying stretch. Repeat three times.
2 Now use the heel of your free hand to make a firm, circular movement around the arch of the foot. Make a generous circle maintaining as much contact as possible. Keep your hand soft and relaxed with your palm flat against the skin. Repeat three times.

▼ Stroking the top of the foot

This is a light stroking movement that can be either refreshing or very calming, depending on the speed of the stroke used. For the best effect, you should be in a position where you can lean slightly backward. Keep your back straight and bring your elbows out to the sides.

1 Hold your massage partner's foot with both hands, your thumbs resting underneath and the tips of all fingers placed in a line on the top of the toes. Lift your elbows to the sides to stroke all eight fingers lightly down the top of the foot to the ankle.
2 Stroke your fingers around the ankle bone – your right hand on the right side, and left hand on the left side – in a circular movement.
3 Now lean back and, at the same time, bring your fingers back up to the toes with an even lighter pressure than before.
4 Repeat this sequence of movements a total of four times.
• Be careful not to press too hard on the bones on the top of the foot – check with your massage partner that the pressure you are using is comfortable.

▼ Toe tonic

This series of movements has a surprisingly relaxing effect. You may need to move your elbows out to the sides in order to do it more effectively.

1 Hold the foot in both hands, fingers overlapping on the sole of the foot and thumbs on top. Place your thumbs on the base line of the toes between the big toe and second toe. Now stroke the pad of one thumb downward with a fairly firm pressure for about 2.5 cm (1 in). Your thumb follows the groove between the tendons on the top of the foot. As one thumb completes a stroke, the other follows the same path in a rhythmical way.
2 Repeat this wave-like movement, one thumb flowing after the other, for around 10 strokes.
3 Move your hands to repeat this movement along the other groves on the top of the foot, finishing with the little toe.

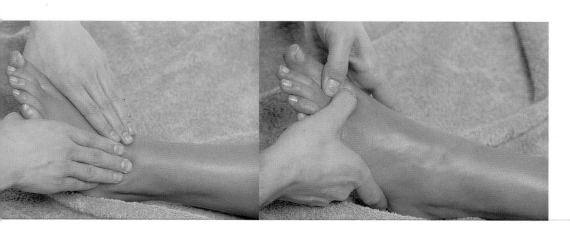

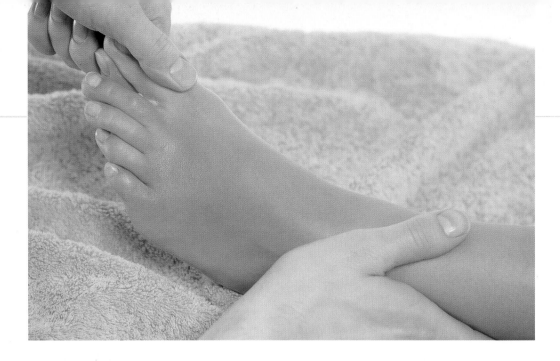

▼ ▲ Toe squeezing and stretching

This sequence is refreshing and reviving for tired feet. It helps mobilize stiff joints, strengthens muscles and stimulates the blood circulation, bringing warmth, nourishment and relaxation. Do not try to reshape malformed toes – work around them. Avoid this movement if your partner has

painful, swollen or arthritic joints. Move your position and change working hands as necessary as it can be rather fiddly with small toes.

1 Hold the foot with one hand. Use the other hand to grasp your massage partner's big toe between your thumb and index finger. Hold the toe at the base, not the tip, ensuring it is well supported. Now rotate the toe slowly and deliberately in a clockwise direction three times. Then rotate it in the other direction three times. Keep the movement smooth and continuous but always work within your partner's range of movement. Do not force the action.

2 With your thumb and index finger held in the same position, gently roll and squeeze the toe as you move your hand toward the tip.

3 Glide your thumb and index finger back to the starting position and then gently pull them toward you so they slide along the length of the toe to achieve a pleasant, stretching sensation. Gradually allow them to float off the end of the toes. To create a really relaxing effect, continue the movement as though pulling a piece of string from the tips of the toes.

4 Repeat this sequence of movements on each toe in turn finishing with the little toe.

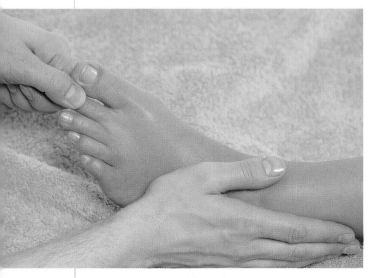

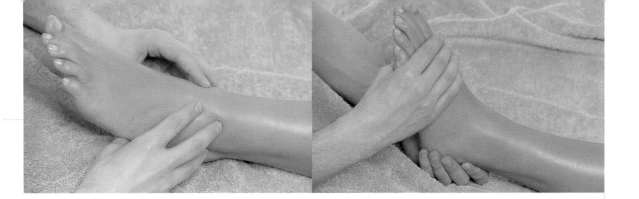

▲ Ankle kneading

This movement helps to refresh and relax stiff, tired and puffy ankles by squeezing out waste products and excess fluid.

1 Cup the heel in both hands. Place your fingers around the ankle bone and thumbs on the arch (don't press with the thumbs). Use the pads of two or more fingers to make circular kneading movements around the two prominences either side of the ankle. Massage both sides of the ankle simultaneously. Repeat three times.

2 Cup the heel of the foot in the palm of one hand. With your hand still held in this cupped position, use the palm and fingers to gently massage your partner's heel with a firm circular action.

3 Release your cupped hand and massage the Achilles tendon at the back of the heel, between your thumb and fingers. Use a circular motion working up both sides of the tendon toward the back of the calf. Keep the pressure light.

• Use your free hand to offer support to the foot.

▲ Ankle rotating

This rotation movement helps ease the tendons and ligaments around the ankle joints and stretches and relaxes the Achilles tendon. If your massage partner has painful, swollen or arthritic ankles, check with her doctor that this movement is appropriate. Work within your massage partner's range of movement.

1 Place one hand in a cupped position to support the heel of the foot. Use the other hand to gently hold the foot at the base of the toes and then rotate it from the ankle in a clockwise direction three times. Repeat the movement rotating the foot in the other direction.

2 With hands in the same position, stretch the top of the foot toward you. Hold and release. Then push it away from you in a slow, controlled and rhythmical movement. Hold and release. Repeat around five times.

• When practised regularly ankle rotations can make a real difference to flexibility and circulation.

Final touch

Complete your foot massage with some gentle strokes to soothe the sensory nerve endings.

1 Use both hands to make soft strokes with the tips of your fingers over the whole of the foot. Make the movement slow but definite. Work from the ankle to the toes. Repeat three times.

2 Gradually decrease the pressure so that your fingers hardly touch the skin in a feather-like movement. Allow your hands to slide very slowly off the end of the toes. Repeat three times.

3 Hold the foot securely between your palms for a few seconds.

Massage
for all ages

Everyone can benefit from hand and foot massage – from the very young to the very old – not only physically but emotionally too. And those benefits are even greater when the massage is given with love and tenderness by a family member or close friend.

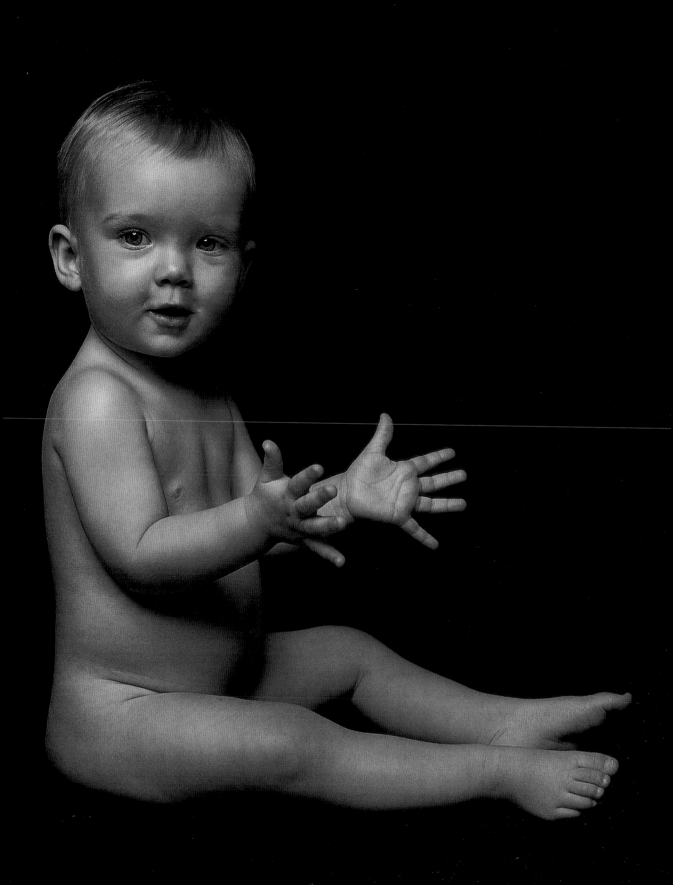

Massage during pregnancy

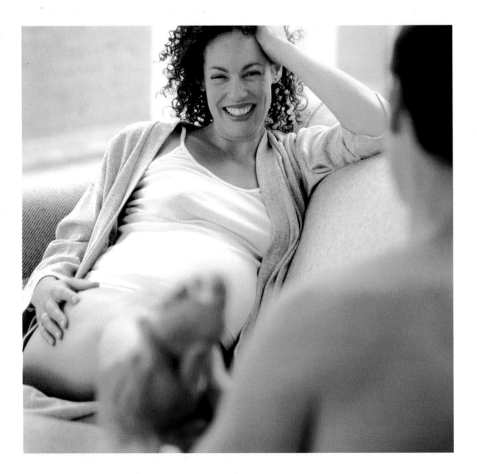

The benefits of massage during pregnancy and childbirth are now so well recognized that many nurses and midwives are learning the techniques and actively encouraging partners to develop their own massage skills. Pregnancy brings increased demands on mind, body and spirit and many women find themselves riding a roller-coaster of emotional and physical ups and downs. A gentle hand or foot massage, or indeed, a manicure or pedicure, can help during this exciting but stressful time.

Follow the routines on previous pages using plenty of light, calming massage strokes. Avoid any deep or vigorous movements during pregnancy. Choose a good quality nourishing cream or oil but do not add any essential oils without the advice of a qualified clinical aromatherapist.

Benefits for mothers-to-be

- Simple hand or foot massage techniques can ease ante-natal anxieties and help to encourage deep relaxation in preparation for a more positive childbirth experience.
- Massage allows time for you to relax, unwind and recharge, thus increasing energy levels and making it easier to cope with the exhausting physical stresses of pregnancy.
- Nourishing creams and oils help moisturize skin and cuticles, which often become extremely dry during pregnancy.
- Foot massage can release tension in tired feet and so help to prevent swollen ankles, which are so often associated with pregnancy.
- Massage releases chemicals known as endorphins in the brain, which are the body's natural painkillers, and sends them racing around the body to help boost well-being and alleviate general aches and pains.
- Manicure and pedicure help to boost your confidence and make you feel better about your general appearance. And when you cannot reach to cut your toenails, you can rely on someone to clip them for you.
- Massage from a birth partner can be wonderfully reassuring and comforting during labour and childbirth. Although many women do not like having their bodies touched during contractions, a hand massage can help relieve tension and pain.

FACT

In India and Japan, massage is regarded as an essential part of a midwife's skill. Women are traditionally given a regular massage during pregnancy and, then for forty days after the birth, new mothers and their babies receive a daily massage to help them recover from the physical and emotional strain of childbirth.

NOTE
A few cautions

- If you have any doubts, do not give a massage during pregnancy. Seek the advice of your massage partner's doctor or midwife if she is suffering any long-term medical condition.
- Check your massage partner has not developed a new medical condition such as high blood pressure or gestational diabetes, both are relatively common in pregnancy.
- Do not use essential oils during pregnancy, unless advised by a qualified clinical aromatherapist. Pure essential oils can have a very powerful effect and should be treated with extreme caution.
- Avoid massaging deeply around the heel, ankle bones and Achilles tendon as reflexologists believe these areas are related to the uterus and firm massage in the area may stimulate contractions. (Never massage the abdomen during pregnancy.)

tip Partners get very stressed, tired and anxious too! So set time aside to share a loving massage – and show each other just how much you are valued and cared for. Make an effort to keep massaging each other after your baby is born.

Enjoying massage with your children

Babies and children love to be held, cuddled and massaged – and not only is it a comforting, loving experience but a caring touch brings positive health benefits for both parent and child. In the animal kingdom, the young are snuggled and cuddled by their mother at every opportunity. And nature obviously knows best. Studies now reveal that babies who receive the warmth and security of close physical contact in their early days tend to cry less, have fewer tantrums and sleep more soundly. Similarly, parents can benefit from nurturing their children with touch. Research among new mothers shows that giving regular massage to their babies helps boost confidence, promote well-being and ease the baby-blues.

Sharing the caring

Expressing love and affection through touch is a basic parental instinct. Most parents naturally enjoy playing games of 'Round and Round the Garden' or 'This Little Piggy' with their child's tiny hands and feet. And as children get older, it is instinctive for parents to rub a sore spot to ease aches and pains, or offer comforting strokes to soothe and reassure. The physical and emotional benefits of the therapeutic power of touch can be extended still further by giving your child a regular hand and foot massage – whatever her age – whenever you feel she needs some extra love and attention.

Children enjoy giving massage, too. Young people have fewer inhibitions about touch and find it perfectly natural to communicate love for parents, siblings and friends through their hands. Indeed, you may well find that your child has a wonderfully firm and caring touch that brings almost instant benefits of relaxation and well-being – to both giver and receiver. Hand and foot massage can also be beneficial during those stormy teenage years when many parents and adolescents seem to be at loggerheads. Current studies show that the 'warring sides' still hold a great affection for each other – they just do not always know how to show it. A caring hand or foot massage can go some way toward keeping open the channels of communication.

Giving and receiving

As hands and feet are so accessible, you can massage them anywhere, at anytime. And there is no need to undress, which appeals to many children, teenagers and adults. There is no need to make it a formal session or follow the steps rigidly, just take

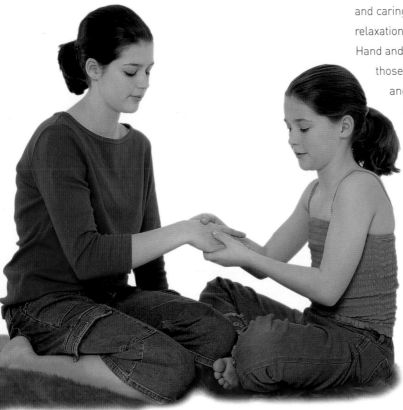

advantage of any opportunity when you are both in the mood for massage. All children are different and you will soon start to discover their particular likes and dislikes, skills and preferences. Indeed, getting to know your child's character and changing moods is one of the pleasures of sharing a massage with each other. Do not force your child either to give or receive a massage; judge the right time. And stop as soon as either of you becomes bored or grumpy. Try again another time.

The following routine provides a few suggestions for a quick and simple hand and foot massage to share with your child. You can follow the whole sequence or massage hands and feet at different times. Chances are that once you have massaged your child a few times, she will be keen to return the favour and also to massage friends and siblings. However, it may be best that she does not use oil, as you could both get rather messy.

Massaging your child safely

- Choose your massage oil with care as a child's skin is very sensitive – make sure it is suitable. Avoid nut oils and all pure essential oils unless advised by a qualified clinical aromatherapist.
- Do not use oil on young children's hands in case they rub it in their eyes.
- Always get the go-ahead from the midwife or health visitor before massaging a baby.
- Do not massage if the child is unwell, particularly if he or she has a fever or is being given medication. Wait at least one week after immunization.
- Work carefully around any areas of broken skin – but avoid massage if your child has a rash or skin infection.
- Massage movements should be light and gentle using soft, flowing strokes that glide over the surface of the skin.

Get cosy

Position yourself so you have close contact with your child . You both need to be comfortable and well-supported so you can move freely and breathe easily. Check that you do not need to twist or stretch.

- A baby will love the security and warmth of your lap. Sit on a cushion with your back supported, if possible, against a wall or heavy piece of furniture. Try cushions of different sizes to find the most comfortable one for you. Place the baby on your lap, with your legs crossed or together and knees bent. Rest her on a changing mat, cushion or pillow covered in a towel.
- If you suffer from back pain, try resting the baby on a table or changing unit that is the correct height. Never leave a baby unattended.
- For a young child, try sitting with your legs stretched out in front of you in a V shape with the baby lying on the floor between your legs.

CHECKLIST
Things you will need

- Pillow, cushion or changing mat. Cover with a clean, soft, warm towel.
- Good-quality oil or cream suitable for a baby or child's delicate skin (only needed for foot massage). Ask your pharmacist for advice.
- Wooden or plastic spatula for cream.
- Spare towel and baby wipes.

Things to do

- Ensure the room is warm and free from draughts.
- Remove jewellery that may scratch the child's skin.
- Check that your nails are short, smooth and clean.
- Wash your hands in warm water.
- Check that you are both in a comfortable position.

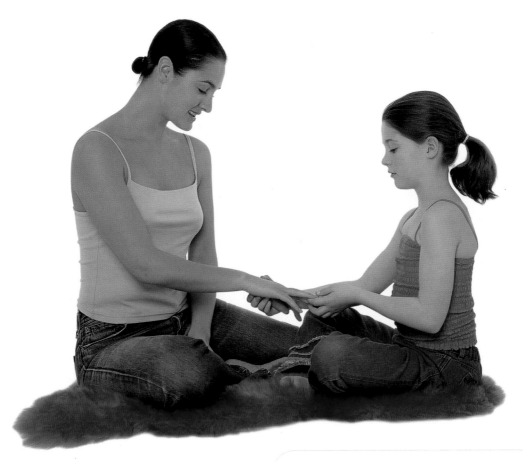

- An older child or adolescent may enjoy being massaged in a favourite chair, sofa or bed or while sitting on the floor. Rest hands or feet on a towel-covered pillow so they can be reached comfortably while maintaining eye-to-eye contact.

Foot massage

Place a tiny drop of a suitable oil or cream in the palm of one hand. Rub your hands together briskly so that they are warm.

Saying hello

Hold the child's feet securely, one in each hand, with fingers on top and thumbs beneath. Enjoy the softness of the child's skin against your skin. Keep the touch gentle but confident. Hold for a minute or so to help him or her feel reassured in your presence. Slowly remove your hands in a stroking action from ankle to toe.

- Repeat these soothing strokes if children appear fractious to help them relax and prevent the movements causing tickles.

Sole strokes

With hands cradling the baby's feet, gently massage the soles of the feet with the fleshy pads of your thumbs. Move your thumbs in circles using a very light, even pressure so that they glide over the top of the skin. Mould your hands to the shape of the baby's delicate feet.

- If feet feel ticklish, try making the movements just a little deeper.

Foot rub

Sandwich your child's right foot between your palms. Keeping your hands soft, move the flat of your hands gently backward and forward across the top and bottom of the foot. Repeat on the left foot.

• This is a lovely way to warm cold feet.

Toe squeeze

Cup your right hand under the heel of the child's right foot to offer support. Using the thumb and forefinger of your free hand, softly squeeze and then pull the big toe very gently, allowing your hand to float from the tip in a gentle, stretching action. Do not tug the toe. Repeat on each toe in turn, finishing with the little toe. Repeat the sequence on the left foot.

NOTE

If you have enjoyed sharing hand and foot massage with your baby, why not attend a parent and baby massage class in your area? Here you will meet other parents and learn how to give your child a full body massage, with an expert on hand to guide you.

NOTE

As you massage your baby's feet, let the infant's hands explore your body too. However, since tiny hands tend to enjoy stroking your face and rearranging your hair, do take off your glasses first.

Foot hold

Complete the foot massage sequence by holding your child's feet in the warmth of your hands. Hold for a minute or so as you breathe deeply and evenly.

• Cover your child's feet with a towel so that they remain warm while you are massaging the child's hands.

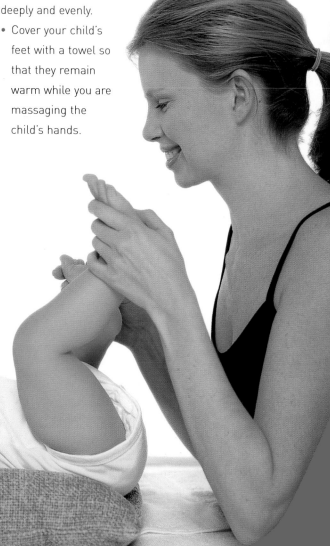

Hand massage

Greeting the hands

Remove any oil or cream on your hands and avoid the risk of babies rubbing their eyes with oily hands. Hold your child's hands gently in yours for a minute or so. A child will enjoy the reassuring sound of your voice so softly talk, hum or sing.

Palm circles

Hold your child's right hand, palm facing upward, with one hand on either side. Your fingers rest on the back of the hand and thumbs in the palm. Gently uncurl her hand, and using the fleshy pads of your thumbs, make small circles round the palm and up the backs of her fingers and thumb. Keep the pressure very light and even so the strokes skim over her skin. Repeat on her left hand.

Finger circles

Hold and support your child's right wrist in one hand. Using the index finger and thumb of your free hand, gently squeeze and rotate the thumb on her right hand. Repeat on each finger, finishing with the little finger. Repeat the sequence on the left hand.

Finger stroking

With your child's right hand supported at the wrist, use the fleshy pads of the fingertips on your free hand to gently stroke along the top of the hand from the wrist to the finger tips. Your touch should be feather-like as your fingers float slowly off the end of her fingertips. Do around 10 of these light strokes. Repeat on the left hand.

Signalling the end

Conclude by holding your child's hands in the same way as the start of the massage. This brings the massage to an end in a calm and balanced way.

Massage and the older generation

Human touch through massage can be valuable for older people. Massage is a way of showing respect and affection for older relatives and friends in a way that words cannot express. Increasingly, nurses are realizing the physical and psychological benefits of 'professional love' and are learning massage skills to support medical practice. Gentle hand and foot massage is very beneficial for less mobile elderly people as there is no need to change position.

Easing aches and pains

On a physical level, receiving a regular hand or foot massage combined with hand and foot mobility exercises can help strengthen muscles and keep joints flexible and mobile. This is important as we get older as it enables us to enjoy a better quality of life and continue participating in favourite activities or pastimes. Massage also boosts blood and lymph circulation and keeps skin soft and supple, thus helping to prevent many of the hand and foot problems associated with ageing. It also gives a caring friend or relative the chance to check the health and conditions of elderly hands or feet. Everyone in their later years should be encouraged to examine their own feet regularly using a mirror.

Boosting self-esteem

Many older people can find themselves alone at the end of their lives when they may have spent a life giving love to others. There may no longer be people there to hug or kiss them goodbye and hello. Receiving a massage can bring a caring touch back into an older person's life and go some way toward alleviating any feelings of isolation and loneliness. The tenderness of someone else's touch can boost self-esteem and promote optimism and well-being.

tip Massage can be a wonderful way of strengthening the bond between family members of different generations. In many cultures, grandparents ask their grandchildren to massage away their aches and pains – and enjoy using the time together to exchange stories and memories.

Growing older brings a whole new set of fears and worries – research shows that a simple five-minute hand or foot massage can reduce anxiety levels and relieve emotional stress. A gentle massage aids relaxation and brings an inner calm, which can help make it a little easier to cope with difficult situations.

Massage with care

Most older people will gain pleasure from a hand or foot massage. However, it important to be sensitive to your partner's emotional and physical state of health. Always ask permission and stop if she shows any signs of tiredness or distress. You should be aware that your touch may trigger an expression of sorrow or sadness. Be prepared to listen. Do not expect to be able to answer difficult questions, but just by paying attention you are providing emotional comfort.

Ensure your massage partner is in a comfortable position and can move and breathe freely during the massage. Keep the massage light and short, and modify your movements to suit her particular needs. Use plenty of soothing, feathering strokes and reassuring holds. Simply holding your massage partner's hand or foot for a few minutes can increase circulation and reduce stiffness.

As we age our joints tend to get stiff, painful and swollen. Massage can be very soothing but should always be performed with great care around affected joints.

Never work on a swollen or inflamed joint as massage creates heat that can aggravate the condition. Apply gentle massage above and below the joint to improve blood circulation and remove excess waste products and fluid from the area. Stroke from the toes up to the ankles, and from the fingers to the wrists, but never force the movement.

With age the skin often becomes thin, dry or fragile and is easily damaged. Ensure your nails are short and remove any rings or jewellery that could scratch. Another condition associated with ageing is osteoporosis, which causes bones to lose their density and become weak and brittle. Avoid strong pressure on delicate bones as this could cause a fracture. Be very careful of the fragile bones in the wrists. Keep your touch light, gentle and comforting.

FACT

Research among older people attending massage classes shows that the psychological benefits of sharing a loving touch can actually be even greater when you are the giver.

tip If you suffer from stiff joints or an arthritic condition, book in for a professional manicure with paraffin wax treatment. The wax generates a steady level of heat which alleviates pain and leaves your hands warm and relaxed.

Manicures
and pedicures

Manicure and pedicure treatments are not simply cosmetic luxuries – they are valuable conditioning therapies for hands and feet. A good manicure or pedicure includes a relaxing massage, which can stimulate local blood circulation, strengthen nails, improve skin condition and offer protection from daily wear and tear.

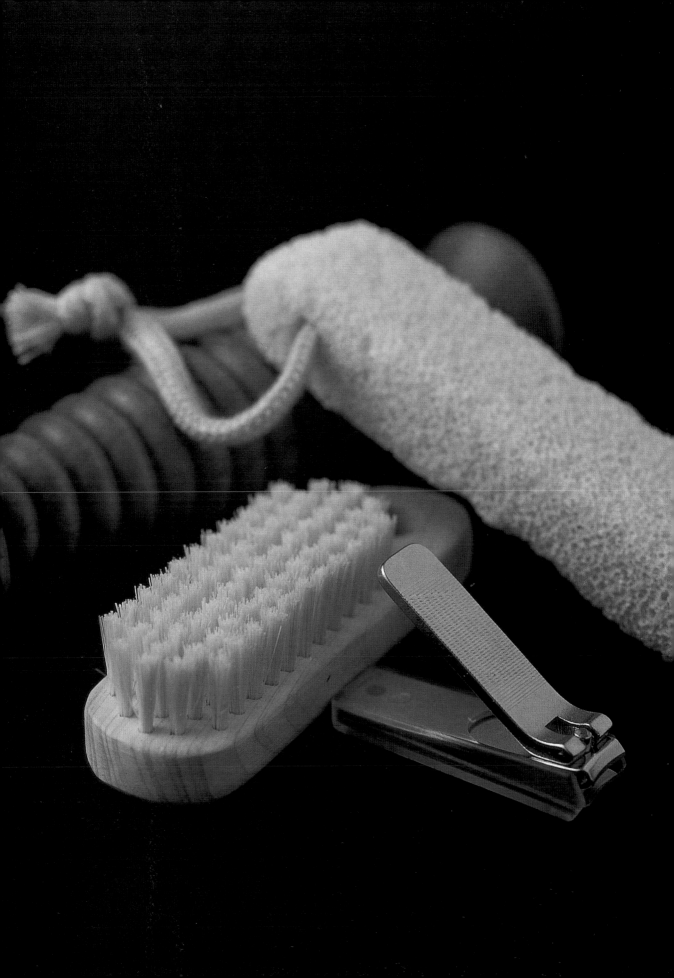

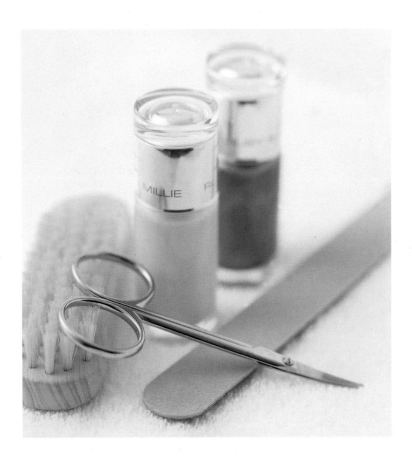

Giving a manicure

Set half an hour aside and treat a friend or relative to a quick and easy manicure or pedicure. The following steps can easily be adapted for a do-it-yourself treatment, too. Taking time and trouble to care for your hands is a great morale-booster.

It is no coincidence that patients in hospital report a greater sense of relaxation and well-being when they have had their hands manicured by a volunteer. You will find hands respond quickly to some care and attention.

CHECKLIST
Things to do

- Three small towels – for drying hands and placing over the table.
- Paper towels – to absorb any spillage and catch nail clippings or filings.
- Cotton wool balls – for removing polish and placing on tips of orange sticks. Choose natural cotton wool as it is better at absorbing polish and less likely to stick to nails.
- Cologne (optional) – for cleaning hands.
- Nail enamel remover – for removing old polish. Use sparingly and choose a good-quality acetone-free moisturizing remover as this will not cause brittleness and dryness.
- Nail scissors (optional) – for cutting long nails.
- Emery board – for filing nails. Avoid metal nail files as they can tear or split your nails. Emery boards usually have different textures on each side. The coarser side is used to take off excess length and the smoother, while the finer side is for shaping the nail and removing any rough edges or snags. If the nails are weak, only use the finer side.
- Hand soak – fill a small bowl half full with warm water. Add a small drop of mild shampoo as it is less drying than most soaps or washing up liquids. Alternatively, add some sweet almond oil or three drops of pure essential oil.
- Cuticle softener or sweet almond oil – for loosening tough cuticles.
- Natural bristle nail brush – for scrubbing nails.
- Hoof stick, or orange stick tipped with cotton wool, for gently pushing back the cuticles and cleaning under the nails. Do not use anything metal and steer clear of cuticle knives or trimmers, which take skill to use properly. It is important not to cut the cuticle as it offers protection and prevents foreign bodies getting beneath the skin – if the skin is damaged this could lead to a nail infection.
- Suitable cream or oil – for massaging into the skin. Take a look at page 18 to help make a selection.
- Wooden or plastic spatula – for applying cream.
- Nail buffer – for boosting blood circulation and polishing nails to a natural shine.
- Buffing paste (optional) – for adding an extra shine to nails.
- Basecoat and nail enamel (optional) – always use a clear basecoat to give a smoother surface and prevent enamel discolouring nails.

CHECKLIST
Things to do

- Lay out your tools on a towel or the tabletop so that everything is to hand.
- Remove any jewellery from yourself and the recipient of the treatment. (Keep it nearby so it does not get left behind.)
- Wash and warm your hands. Cover any cuts or abrasions with sticking plaster.
- Ask your partner to:
  – wear old clothes (or offer an apron or similar to cover her clothing and protect from any accidental spillage) and roll sleeves up to the elbow;
  – wash or cleanse hands with wipes or cotton wool soaked in cologne.

Working in comfort

You should both be sitting at the correct height and close enough so you do not need to lean forward. One of the most practical positions is to sit facing each other across a small table. Spread a towel over the table, then fold another towel into a pad as a support for your partner's elbow. Put a paper towel in place to collect any nail filings for quick and easy disposal. Keep the third towel by your side to use as necessary. An alternative position is to sit opposite each other with a towel-covered pillow on your lap.

Plan your manicure

Before you begin, examine your partner's hands thoroughly to get a feel for them. Check that she is not suffering from an infectious nail or skin disease as it would be unwise to continue with a manicure, or that she has any conditions where special care should be taken with the massage step. You also need to find out if she has any allergies to creams, oils or nail cosmetics. If she is allergic to nail enamel, then leave out the final step of the manicure. Ask about personal preferences too, such as nail shape and enamel colour.

tip Take the opportunity to look at the general condition of your partner's nails and skin – you may like to offer some of the advice on hand care outlined on pages 188–97.

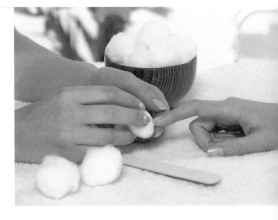

▲ Remove old enamel

This step ensures that all traces of old polish are removed so allowing you to begin afresh.

Soak a cotton pad or ball with nail enamel remover and press on the nail for a moment, then wipe off slowly. A quick swipe is not enough to dissolve polish, especially glittery textures. If necessary, use a tipped orange stick soaked in nail enamel remover to clean up the cuticle and free edge of the nail.

tip Treat yourself to a professional manicure to keep your hands or nails in good condition. Watch the expert at work and learn. Do not worry if your nails are bitten or battered – the manicurist has seen plenty of similar hands and will have helpful advice to offer. And once you see how much better your nails look after a manicure, you will feel more inclined to look after them.

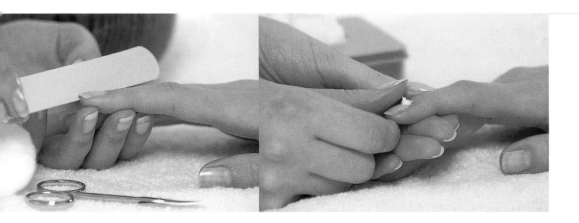

▲ File the nails

Now shape the nails. Your partner may have a strong view on this. If not, file the tips to the same shape as the base of the nail. Begin by doing this step and the next step on the right hand first.

Shape each nail in turn with the emery board. A good guide to correct filing technique is to hold the emery board as though about to shake hands with it. Tilt the emery board at a 45° angle so that you concentrate on the underside of the nail. Use the finer, smoother side of the emery board to file the free edge, working from the side to the centre to form a gentle curve. Work in one direction only with long, rhythmical strokes. Avoid a sawing action on one spot, which can cause the nail layers to split. Be careful not to file deep into the nail corners as this weakens the edge and the nail is more likely to split.

- If the nails are very long it is quicker to trim them to the approximate length with nail scissors first. Cut from one side to the centre, and then repeat this process on the other side.

▲ Softening the cuticles

This step helps soften and loosen cuticles (the dead skin around the edge of the nails) so they can be more easily pushed back.

Using the tip of your index finger, massage a small amount of cuticle cream or almond oil into each nail base and the surrounding skin on the fingers.

- If cuticles are very dry, soak fingernails in a small bowl of warm almond oil for five minutes first.

▼ Soak the nails

This step helps to loosen any stubborn dirt from around the nails and helps soften cuticles.

Place the right hand into a hand soak. Leave for three to five minutes. While the right hand is soaking, repeat the previous two steps on the left hand. Then place the left hand in the soak (see page 179).

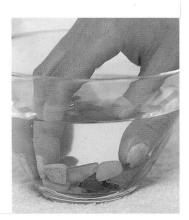

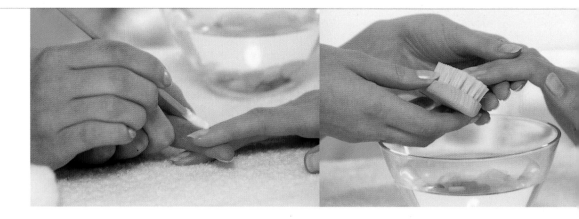

▲ Push back the cuticles

This helps improve the appearance of cuticles
and prevents them attaching to the nail plate.

1 Take the right hand from the water and pat
   each nail and finger dry with a towel. Apply
   a little cuticle cream to the nail base of the
   fingers and massage it in gently.
2 The cuticles should now be soft enough for you
   to gently ease them back using a hoof stick or
   orange stick tipped with cotton wool. Hold the
   stick like a pen and do not apply too much
   pressure. Repeat on the left hand.
• Alternatively, wrap a soft towel around your
   fingertip and use this gently to push back the
   cuticles. You can do this on your own cuticles.

▲ Wash the hands

This step helps remove any excess cuticle
cream, which is caustic and could dry or
burn the skin.

Dip both hands in the warm hand soak to
wash off any remaining cuticle remover. Then
take hands from the bowl and pat dry. If your
partner's hands or nails are a little dirty, use
a soft, natural bristle nail-brush to scrub away
any dirt or stains. The light, rubbing action
helps increase blood circulation to the nails
so encouraging healthy growth.

◀ Massage hands and arms

This helps boost circulation, improve joint
mobility and nourish dry skin.

Apply a rich moisturizing cream or oil, rub them
together and follow the steps shown in the
routine on pages 134–49 You could also dip
your partner's fingertips in the warm water and
scrub the nails gently with a nail brush. Any
stubborn dirt can be removed with an orange
stick – but do not dig too deep.

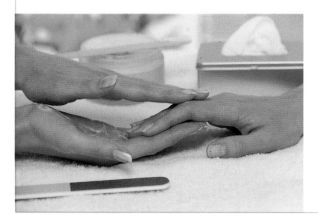

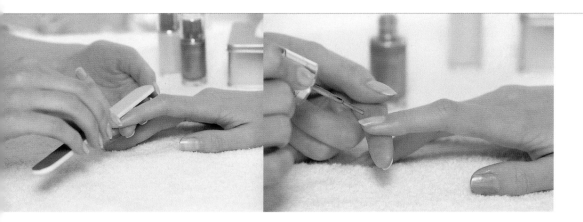

▲ Buff the nails

Buffing is a simple way to give the nail plate a healthy shine and it helps smooth out ridges. It also stimulates blood supply, so promoting healthier, stronger nails. Buffing is also useful for removing yellowish tints on nails caused by nicotine or sunlight.

With the buffer held loosely in your hand, work on each nail plate in turn. Buff in one direction only from the base of the nail to the free edge. Use firm, smooth strokes. Around six strokes for each nail is usually sufficient – do not overdo it. Tidy up nails with an emery board to give a smooth finish.

• If not using nail enamel, apply a little buffing paste to achieve extra shine.

tip Men benefit from manicures too – and usually thoroughly enjoy the pampering. The only real differences are that most men prefer to have nails cut straight across and not shaped at the sides and that their nails may take a bit more effort to scrub clean. It is unlikely that a man would want nail enamel but buffing can give his nails a healthy sheen.

▲ Apply nail enamel

This is very much a personal choice. Offer your partner a selection of coloured or clear enamels before commencing.

1 First, make sure that the nail is free from any grease or cream, as this will cause the enamel to bubble or go streaky. Apply a clear base coat and leave it to dry for 15 minutes. Avoid waving your hands about to dry them as this may create an uneven texture.

2 When the base coat is completely dry, apply varnish in three straight strokes – one down the middle, and one on each side. Remove any enamel on surrounding skin with an orange stick tipped with cotton wool. Allow it to dry and harden thoroughly before using your hands to avoid chipping.

• Before using nail polish, roll the bottle in the palms of your hands. Avoid shaking it as this creates air bubbles, which can lead to chipping.

Giving a pedicure

Regular foot care including a pedicure and foot massage not only helps make feet look more attractive but also reduces hard skin, odours and sweat, relaxes tired, aching feet and helps prevent many common problems from developing.

Check your position

It is worth spending a little time and effort making sure that you are both comfortable and at the correct height. One of the most practical positions is sitting facing each other. Place a small table between you with a towel-covered cushion to support your partner's leg and foot. Ensure that the knee is slightly bent so the foot is relaxed. The foot bowl can be placed on a towel on the floor. Keep a towel handy for drying your partner's feet, and another for wrapping them to keep warm.

CHECKLIST
Things to do

- Check your partner has no infectious or contagious skin or nail diseases that would make it unwise to continue with the pedicure, and that she does not have any conditions where special care should be taken with the massage step. Ask about allergies to creams or oils. Choose colour of nail enamel.
- Lay out everything you need so that it is all to hand.
- Ask your partner to wear loose clothing and remove shoes, tights and socks. Trousers should be rolled up to the knees.
- Remove your jewellery and your partner's toe rings or anklets.
- Wash your hands. Cover any cuts or abrasions with a medical dressing.

CHECKLIST
Things you will need

- Three towels – used for drying and warming feet.
- Cotton wool balls – used to remove polish and place on top of orange sticks. Choose natural cotton wool as it is better at absorbing polish and is less likely to stick to the nails.
- Paper towels – used to absorb any spillage and catch nail clippings.
- Nail enamel remover – used for taking off old polish. Use sparingly and choose a good-quality moisturizing remover that is free from acetone, which can cause brittleness and dryness.
- Nail clippers – for cutting nails to the right length.
- Emery board – for filing nails. Do not use metal files as these can damage nails.
- Foot soak – use a large bowl half full of comfortably warm water. The bowl should be deep enough to immerse the feet to the ankles. A washing-up bowl is ideal. Add a few drops of mild shampoo or bath lotion as it is less drying than soap or washing-up liquids (detergent). Alternatively, add some sweet almond oil or three drops of pure essential oil.
- Cuticle softener or sweet almond oil – for loosening tough cuticles.
- Natural bristle nail brush – for scrubbing nails.
- Hoof stick, or orange stick tipped with cotton wool, for gently pushing back the cuticles and cleaning under nails. Do not use anything metal for this job, and never use cuticle knives, which can be dangerous in untrained hands.
- Pumice stone or exfoliating cream – for removing rough skin.
- Suitable cream or oil – for massaging into the skin.
- Wooden or plastic spatula – for applying cream.
- Basecoat and nail enamel (optional).

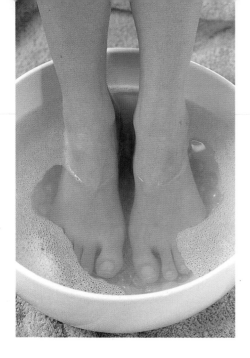

▲ Cleanse the feet

At the start of the pedicure your partner may feel concerned that her feet are smelly or dirty and otherwise unpleasant. Put her at ease by soaking her feet in a relaxing, cleansing foot soak before starting.

1. Ask your partner to put both feet in the foot soak. Leave the feet in the bowl for three to five minutes. While her feet are soaking, encourage your partner to relax and unwind. She may like to close her eyes and enjoy the pleasing sensation of warmth on her feet.

2. Remove feet from the soak and dry thoroughly. Be extra vigilant about drying between the toes as bacteria and fungi thrive in moist, dark conditions and can cause skin disorders.

3. Soak a cotton pad with nail enamel remover and press against each nail for a few seconds, then wipe off slowly. If necessary, use a tipped orange stick soaked in nail enamel remover to clean up the cuticle and free edge of the nail.

- Use this opportunity to assess the general condition of your partner's feet and, if appropriate, offer self-care advice.

▼ Clip and file the nails

Toe nails should be kept straight, allowing only a gentle curve at the sides, as this prevents the nail cutting into the skin and so protects against ingrowing nail. Place a tissue to collect any clippings or filings for easy disposal.

Use clippers to cut a straight line across the nail. Do not use scissors as they can cause the nail to split. Trim the nails of the left foot in turn. Using the coarse side of the emery board, file the nails to remove any sharp corners or rough edges. Do not try to shape them or file into the corners.

- Hold the emery board so that it is slightly angled beneath the free edge of the nail. Using long strokes, file each side of the nail toward the centre.

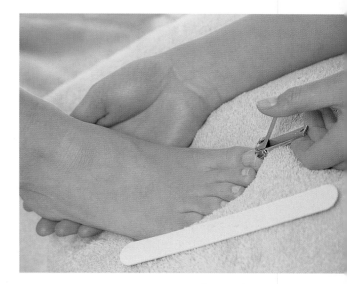

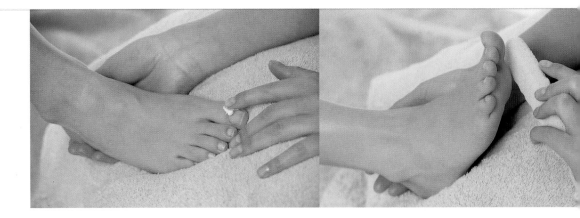

▲ Easing back the cuticles

This step is a must if you wish your feet to look pretty in open-toe sandals. It is also important for your nail health as it keeps the cuticles in good condition.

Apply a small dab of cuticle cream or almond oil into each nail base and massage in gently with your forefinger. Now place both feet back into the warm water. Allow to soak for a minute or so. Remove and dry thoroughly. Massage a little more cuticle cream into each nail base. Ease the cuticles back very gently using a hoof stick, or orange stick tipped with cotton wool. Try using circular movements to ease the cuticle down and away from the nail. Wipe off any excess cuticle remover with cotton wool.
- Be careful not to damage the cuticle as it acts as a protective barrier against fungi and bacteria.

tip At last people are waking up to the need to respect our hard-working feet. There is now a wide selection of good-quality natural foot care products and treatments on the market – enjoy browsing to find those that appeal to you.

▲ Removing hard skin

During a pedicure, excess hard skin can be removed to improve the appearance of your partner's feet.

If there is only a mild build-up of hard skin, massage the feet with some exfoliating cream. Use a deep, circular movement, working with your fingers. On very rough areas around the heels and balls of the feet, use a pumice stone, friction pad or chiropody block. Never use metal files or attempt to cut or shave hard skin. Avoid sawing back and forth with the pumice stone, which can be quite painful, and be careful not to overdo it as this can cause irritation.
- If hard skin is causing pain or discomfort seek the advice of a state registered chiropodist or podiatrist.

NOTES

Regular pedicures are especially important if you usually wear synthetic shoes and socks, or if you suffer from poor circulation or diabetes as it is vital to keep your feet in good condition to prevent further problems.

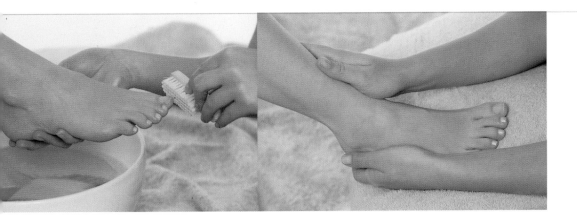

▲ Brushing the nails

This step helps remove any loosened dirt and all traces of cuticle remover.

Place both feet in warm water. Use a natural bristle nail brush to scrub around the nails. Clean under the free edges of the nails with a cotton-tipped orange stick soaked in water. Take both feet from the water. Remove the bowl to prevent it being knocked over.

▲ Massage the feet and legs

A moisturizing massage helps to relieve tension in hard-working muscles and tendons and promotes general relaxation.

Rub rich, moisturizing cream into your hands. Now follow the steps in the foot massage routine on pages 150–65.
• Ensure that all the cream or oil has been massaged in or remove any excess with tissue.

◀ Apply nail enamel

Offer your partner a choice of colours. Before applying, check the nails are free from grease.

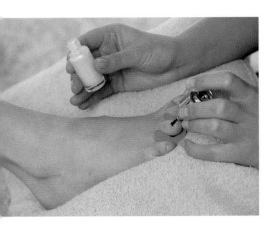

To prevent smudging, use a specially designed toe separator or divide toes with a tissue, folded length-wise and threaded between the toes. Apply a clear base coat and leave to dry for five minutes. When the base coat is completely dry, apply varnish in three straight stokes – one down the middle, and one on each side. Clean any smudge marks with a cotton-tipped orange stick dipped in polish remover.
• Leave for 10 to 15 minutes to dry before removing toe separators. Wait at least an hour before putting on tights or shoes.

Caring for
hands and feet

Once your massage partner starts to enjoy the benefits of regular hand or foot massage, it is helpful to offer some general tips and advice to help keep skin and nails in good condition. Do not forget to follow your own advice!

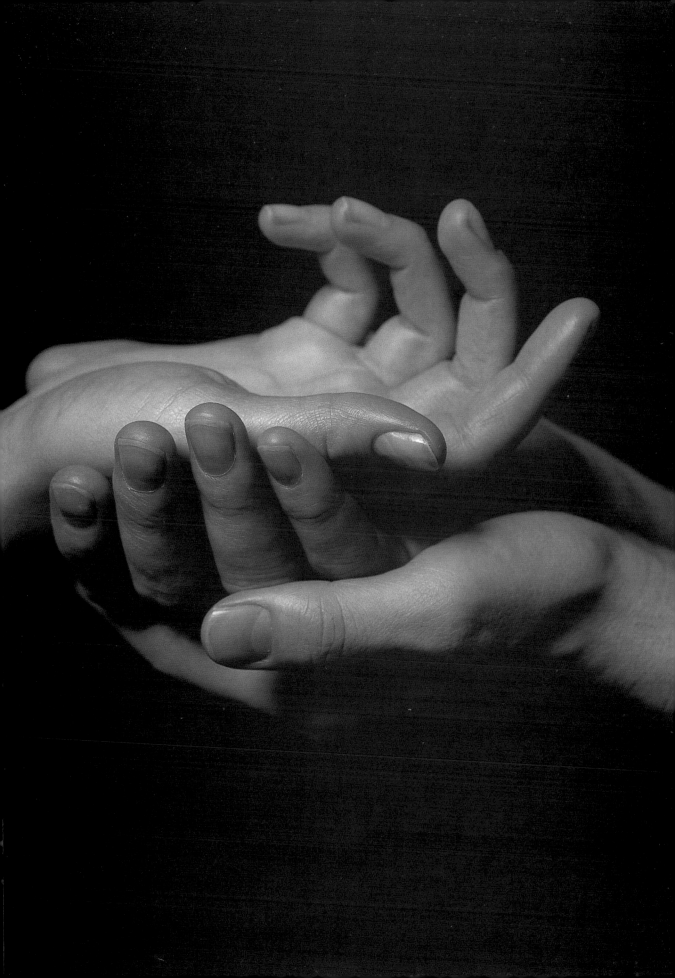

Looking after hands and feet

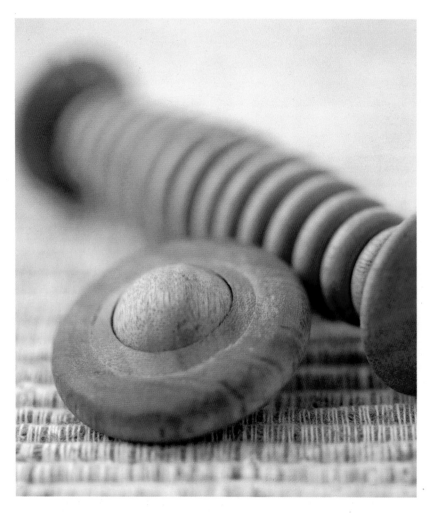

Sensible hygiene and care can enhance the benefits of massage and help prevent many common problems developing. These simple self-help measures are easy to follow and will make a noticeable difference to keeping skin and nails healthy and attractive. It is well worth spending a little time on caring for hands and feet – when they look and feel good, then you feel good too!

Clean and fresh

Wash your hands and feet every day with a gentle, soap-free cleanser. The water should be warm but not hot, which can cause drying and tightening of the skin. If you have a loss of sensation in your hands or feet, because of diabetes or other condition, check the temperature with your elbow. Rinse and dry thoroughly, especially between the toes, as bacteria and fungi thrive in warm, moist conditions. The area between the fourth and fifth toe on each foot is the most common site of infection. It is important not to share towels and flannels if a member of the family has warts, nail infection or other contagious

> **tip** Try massaging and rubbing one foot against the other to boost the circulation. It is amazing how dexterous your toes can be. Use the heel and sides of your feet to work into all the curves and bends to ease out all the tension and get blood flowing to the feet.

conditions as they can be so easily passed to others. Choose shoes and socks made from natural fibres, which allow cool air to circulate. It is best not to wear the same shoes two days running; so allow shoes time to dry before wearing them again.

Soft and supple

Hands and feet will benefit from a relaxing soak in a bowl half full of warm water – but do not soak them for longer than five minutes as this can upset the natural balance of protective oils. A handful of Dead Sea salts added to the water can help improve circulation, soften the skin and fight infection.

Hard skin should be treated with care – gently rub away with a pumice stone every day to keep it under control. Attempting to remove it all in one go could lead to very sore feet. If you have a build-up of hard skin, ask the advice of a registered chiropodist or podiatrist. Regular massage with a rich moisturizer

will keep the skin and nails on the feet and hands supple and prevent chapping or cracking. Rub in well but avoid the area between the toes as this should be kept fairly dry to avoid infection. A useful tip is to keep pots of moisturizer in different places all over the house to jog your memory. Try this skin-softening routine: once a week, just before going to bed, apply a generous amount of moisturizing cream to your hands and feet. Now put on a pair of white cotton gloves and socks and allow your skin and nails to reap the benefits while you sleep.

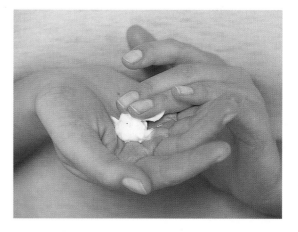

Protecting your skin

During the day it is wise to get into the habit of wearing gloves whenever your hands are immersed in water for some time – if you do not like rubber gloves then lightweight surgical gloves are suitable. Limit the amount of detergent used in washing up or cleaning. Detergent left on the skin may cause uncomfortable dryness and rashes. Always rinse your hands with fresh water after contact with detergent, especially between the fingers and under rings. Wear protective gloves for dirty, dry work such as gardening and do not forget to shield your hands from the elements: warm gloves help maintain blood circulation to the hands and nails during cold weather.

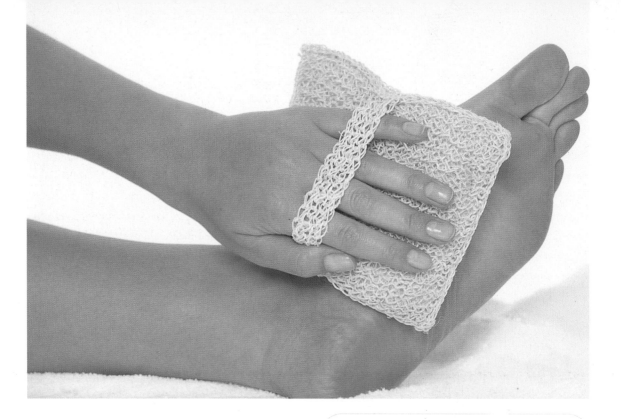

Hands also need protection from the sun's ultra-violet rays. Use a sunscreen lotion or moisturizing cream that filters out harmful rays to protect your health, and prevent dehydration and age spots – do not forget to massage sunscreen into your nails, too. Never use your nails to prize open lids or do similar jobs; find the right tool for the task or you could end up with split nails.

Early warning

It is good advice to get into the habit of inspecting your hands and feet every day – especially if you have a medical condition such as diabetes that can lead to foot disorders. Look for redness, cuts, swelling or cracks in your skin, or any changes in colour or temperature. If you find it difficult to view your feet, use a mirror or ask a friend to look for you. If you have doubts, see your doctor. The earlier problems are reported, the quicker they can be treated. Cover any breaks in the skin with a plaster to guard against infection. Keep your nails trimmed – toenails should be cut straight across. Do not pick or tear finger and toenails. They are often easier to cut after a bath.

tip If you are elderly or diabetic, your eyesight is poor or you have difficulty cutting your nails, seek the advice of a state registered chiropodist or podiatrist.

Boost circulation

A sluggish blood circulation can cause misery – not only do hands and feet feel cold and uncomfortable but poor circulation is at the root of many disorders that affect the extremities. Following a few simple guidelines can help improve blood circulation but if you are concerned then see your doctor as poor circulation may be associated with a medical condition.

To boost sluggish circulation in the morning, sit on a chair or the side of a bed and move your legs briskly up and down, one after the other. The movement comes from your knees with your ankles staying soft and flexible. Then take a warm bath to pep up your circulation and raise your body temperature. Brush palms and soles with a soft body brush using firm, circular strokes. Dry thoroughly with a rough towel. Rub a moisturizing cream or oil into areas that are likely to become chilled. After your bath, do some hand and foot mobility exercises (see page 194–7) and repeat them at regular intervals.

If possible, eat breakfast and have a hot meal and plenty of hot drinks during the day to maintain body heat. Cut back on smoking as this constricts the blood vessels and makes the problem even worse. It also discolours skin and nails, and robs the body of vital nutrients. Exercise is vital to a healthy blood circulation. Walking, especially up hills, is particularly good exercise for the feet as it strengthens muscles, ligaments and tendons. Try to take a brisk walk every day, wearing correct footwear. When you get a chance to sit down – put your feet up above the level of your hips to encourage the flow of blood back to the heart.

If it is chilly outside, wrap up warm as the cold hinders blood circulation to the extremities. Wear several layers of thin, loose clothing to trap body heat and put on gloves, thick socks, a scarf and hat. Avoid clothing that restricts blood circulation – a red ring on your lower leg is a sure sign that the elastic in your socks is too tight. Choose shoes or boots with warm, inner soles. Wear bed socks at night.

Choosing footwear

Poorly fitting shoes are the cause of many uncomfortable or painful foot problems. Shoes that are too narrow, for example, or too tight, long, high or wide not only make feet tired and aching, but

tip If your hands or feet get very cold then warm them gradually. Be wary of heating them on radiators, hot water bottles or near a fire as the sudden change in temperature can lead to further problems.

they can also speed up the onset of problems or aggravate any existing ones.

Correct shoe fitting is not just for children. Every time you buy new shoes you should ask to have your feet measured for size and width by a trained shoe fitter. Shoe size is only a guide. Shoes that are the same size can have a different fit, depending on the style and manufacturer. The best time to buy shoes is in the afternoon as your feet tend to swell during the day. Put on both shoes and stand up and walk around. The shoe should be about 1 cm (½ in) longer than your foot with room for your toes to move. It

tip Alternate your style of footwear and heel height regularly. This helps tone up your calf muscles and reduces strain on the feet and ankles.

should fit snugly at the heel and instep and be wide enough to prevent friction, squashing or rubbing when you walk. Never buy shoes in the hope that they will stretch. Check that there are no holes or rough edges in socks, tights or shoes.

For best support and comfort, choose a shoe with a heel no higher than 4 cm (1½ in) and a rounded toe. Shoes with laces, straps or a buckle are preferable. Always choose the most suitable shoe for the occasion. Keep high heels for special occasions as constant wear can cause muscular imbalances in the lower leg, leading to aches and cramps. In high-heeled shoes your toes are crushed forward and the tendons on the top of the foot are stretched, while the Achilles tendon at the back of the heel is shortened.

Hand exercises

Hand and finger exercises can help boost blood circulation, ease aches and pains and maintain strength and flexibility in your hands and wrists. Repeat these exercises several times a day, and perform them as a warm-up routine just before giving a massage. It is best to remove all jewellery from your hands and wrists. You may find it more comfortable to rest your elbows on a folded towel on a table or desk for some of the exercises.

NOTE

Hand and foot mobility exercises can be beneficial if you have arthritis, Raynaud's disease or repetitive strain injury – but if you suffer from these conditions, or any other medical condition, consult your doctor or physiotherapist before doing hand or foot exercises. It is important that all movements are tailored to your particular needs.

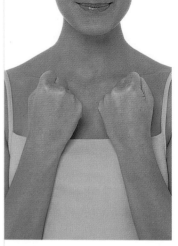

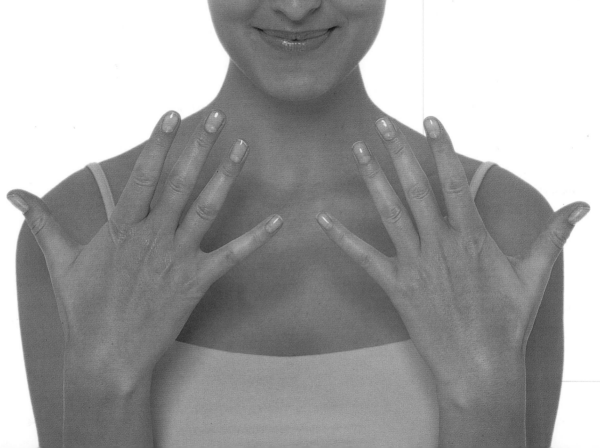

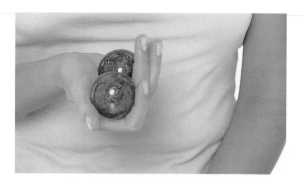

1 Make soft fists with both hands. Then quickly separate your fingers and thumbs and stretch them out as far as you can reach (see left). Hold for a count of 10. Feel the tension in your fingers. Slowly release and return to the soft fists. Repeat three times.

2 Put your hands on a flat surface with the palms facing downward. First, lift your thumbs, then each finger in turn, as though playing a piano. Return to the starting position by placing your little fingers on the surface, followed by each individual finger. Repeat three times.

3 Place the palms of your hands together in the 'prayer' position. Press one hand firmly against the other and hold for a count of five. Release and then repeat. With your hands in the same position, keep your wrists, thumbs and fingertips in contact while pushing out your knuckle joints to form a diamond shape with your hands (see below right). Hold for a count of five. Return to the starting position and then repeat three times.

4 Try this exercise if you suffer from poor circulation in your hands. Stand with your hands by your sides. Now raise your arms in front of you as high as you can comfortably reach. Turn your wrists so that your palms face downward and then lower your arms to your sides in a swinging action. Repeat three times. Rest and repeat the sequence another three times, allowing yourself to get into a steady rhythm.

5 Hold a small soft, rubber ball (buy one specially designed for 'stressbusting') or some playdough or plasticine in your hand. Squeeze and mould it in your hands to work the muscles, but without straining them. Repeat, this time holding the ball in the other hand.

6 Take a tip from the East and invest in some Chinese hand balls for a fun way to keep your hands and fingers supple (see above). These small balls, which are available in oriental craft shops and health food stores, work by stimulating acupuncture points on the hands to increase the flow of vital energy through the body. Hold two balls in the palm of one hand, and circle them around each other in your palm and fingers. Some even come with musical accompaniment to help soothe your nerves.

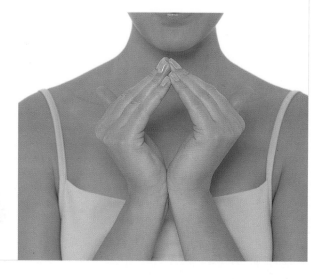

Foot exercises

Feet and toes need to be kept on the move. Without sufficient exercise, the muscles in your feet slacken, arches weaken, joints stiffen and blood circulation slows down. These simple exercises will strengthen and relax muscles, tendons and ligaments, thus helping prevent foot problems and keep your feet healthy, flexible and warm. Remove your shoes and allow your feet the chance to exercise freely – set aside a few minutes every day and you will soon notice the improvement.

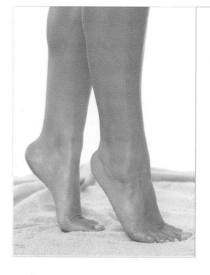

NOTE

Walking barefoot – especially going up and down stairs – is good for stimulating circulation and strengthening the muscles in your feet. Whenever it is safe and practical, take off your shoes and socks to allow the bones in your feet some welcome freedom from the pressure of tight shoes, tights and socks. Avoid walking barefoot if you have diabetes as there is a slight risk of injury.

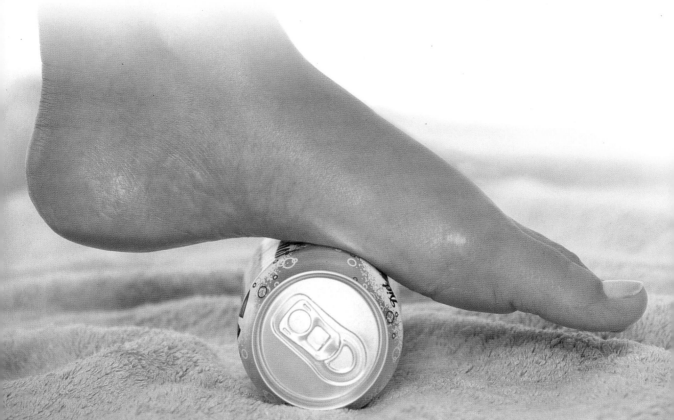

1 Stand straight, feet about 20 cm (8 in) apart, toes pointing ahead. Now raise yourself up slowly on your toes, hold for a count of five, lower. Repeat five times. Try walking on tip toes for a few paces (see left).

2 Place a soft ball, orange or can of drink (try it cold from the fridge) under the ball of your foot and roll it backward and forward for one minute to improve circulation and relieve any aches in the arch. Repeat with the other foot. Alternatively, use a specially designed foot massager (see below far left).

3 Sit on a chair with your feet flat on the ground. Press the toes of your left foot into the floor and raise the toes of your right foot firmly upward. Hold this position for a count of three and then release slowly. Repeat with the opposite foot. This may take some practice to do properly, but do persevere. Try raising the toes individually.

4 Sitting in the same position as above, grasp a pencil with your toes. Hold for a count of five, release. Repeat. To add an extra dimension to this exercise, place a sheet of paper on the floor and try writing or drawing with the pencil.

5 Sit on the floor with your legs pointing straight ahead. Point your toes down and away from you (see below left). Hold for a count of 10. Release and repeat. Now, flex your feet so that your toes are pointing toward your nose (see below right). Hold for a count of 10. Release and repeat. Point your toes inward toward the middle of the body. Hold for a count of 10. Release and repeat. Finally move your feet out toward the side of your body. Hold for a count of 10. Release and repeat.

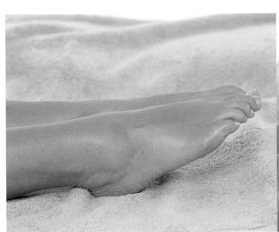
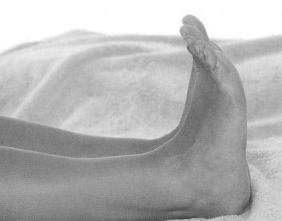

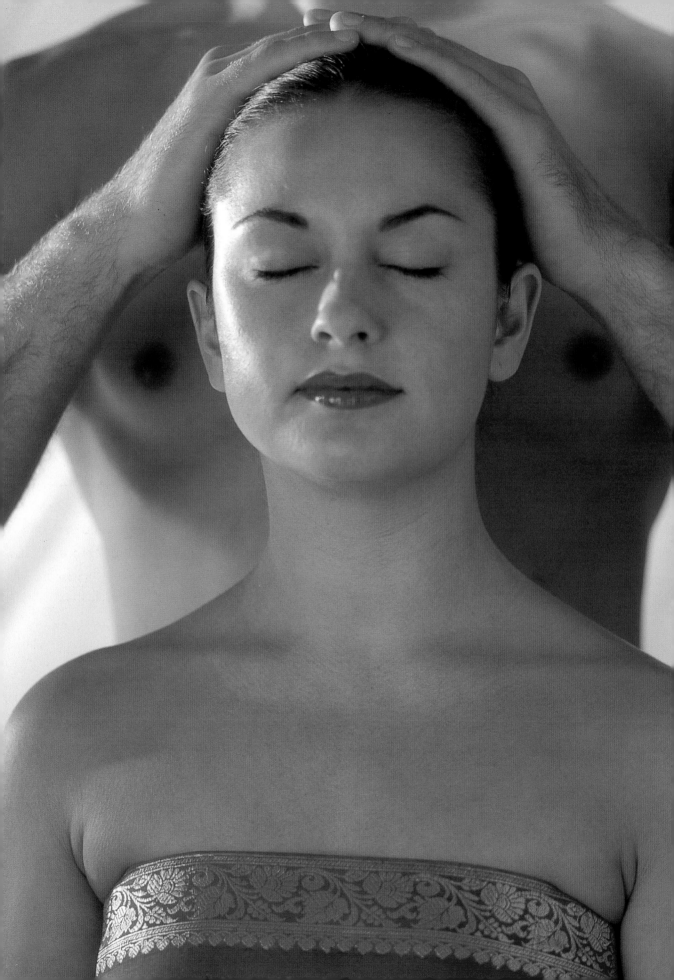

3 Indian head
massage

As you begin to practise the techniques, you should find this ancient art to be calming, revitalizing, uplifting and incredibly rewarding. Much of the joy lies in its simplicity, effectiveness and accessibility – no special equipment is needed and it takes less than half an hour to complete. With a few basic strokes, you can relax and soothe or invigorate and stimulate. It is a wonderful way of pacifying a troubled child to sleep, refreshing a jaded computer-user or pampering your loved ones with some tender loving care. You can also continue a long tradition followed by Indian women, men and children and enjoy head massage to give hair a healthy, lustrous shine. Indian head massage not only works on the scalp, but also on the face, shoulders, upper back and arms. The movements can help to relax taut muscles, ease stiffness, stimulate blood circulation and drain away excess toxins, so helping to relieve headaches and eye strain and increase joint mobility. It also encourages deeper breathing and helps boost the flow of freshly oxygenated blood to the brain, resulting in more focused thought, greater concentration and better memory.

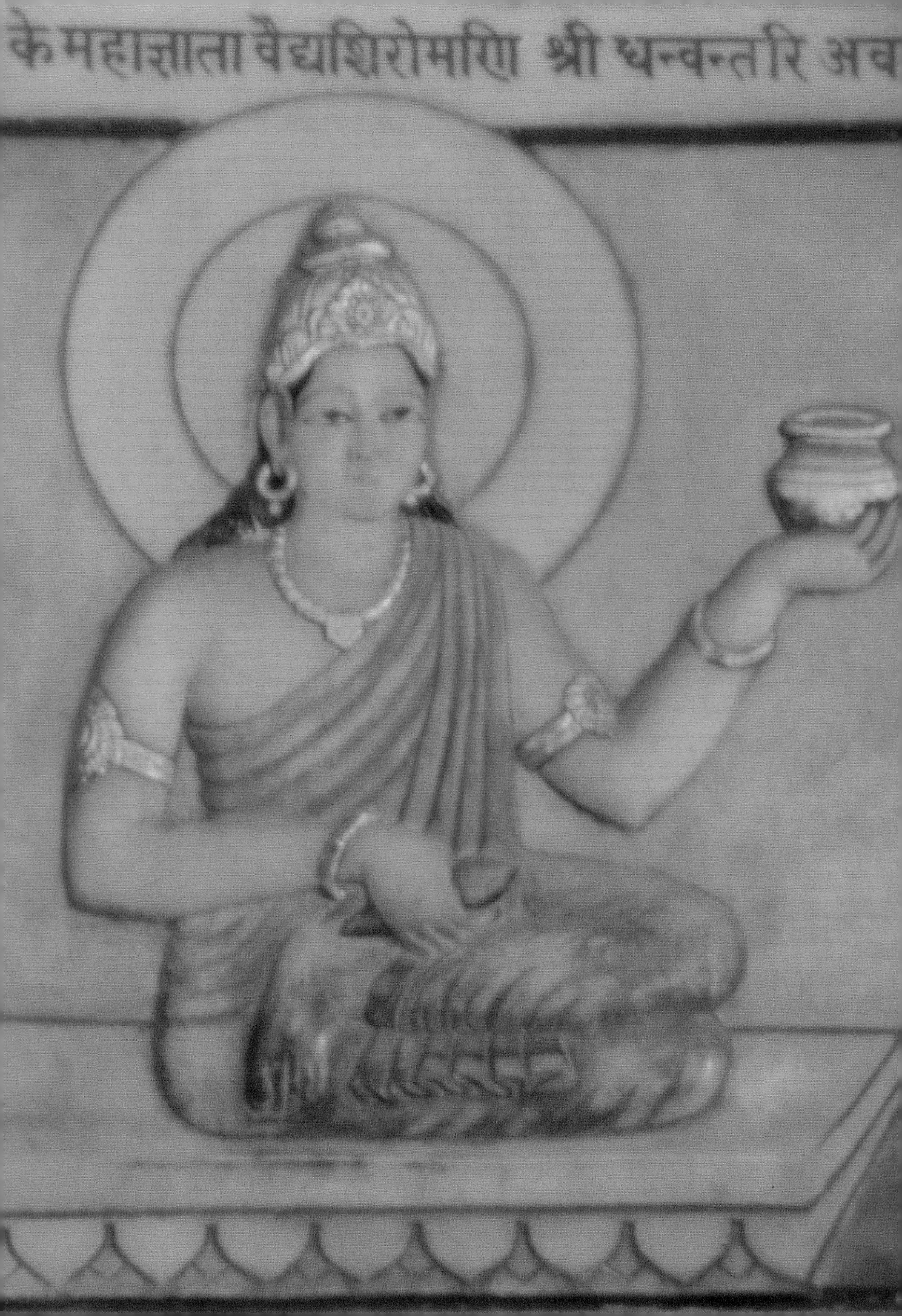
के महाज्ञाता वैद्यशिरोमणि श्री धन्वन्तरि अव

An ancient art
in a modern world

Indian head massage has a long and colourful history. It is
based on a traditional system of medicine known as Ayurveda,
which has been practised in India for over three thousand years
and is becoming increasingly popular in the West. The word
'Ayurveda' comes from Sanskrit, the ancient language of India,
and means 'science of life' or 'knowledge of life'. Ayurveda is a
complete healing system, possibly the oldest in the world, which
teaches a truly holistic approach, concentrating on achieving a
balance of mind, body and spirit to promote physical, emotional
and spiritual health and well-being.

The origins of Indian head massage

According to the Ayurvedic system, there are five fundamental elements in all living things – air, fire, water, earth and ether – that are forever changing and interacting with each other. These are represented in the human body by three vital energies, or forces, known as 'doshas', which are individually called vata, pitta and kapha. The level of these doshas within the body is influenced by certain foods, varying temperatures, times of the day, levels of stress and many other factors. In their normal balanced state, the doshas provide strength and govern the normal functioning of all bodily systems, while an imbalance of the doshas leads to disease, illness and unhappiness.

Ayurveda works on the philosophy that each person is a unique entity with her own balance and combination of doshas. A trained practitioner asks many detailed questions and performs various tests, such as taking the pulse and examining the tongue. The practitioner seeks to establish the patient's particular doshic constitution and find any imbalances before prescribing medication or other treatments. However, most of us have one or two dominant doshas that can be readily identified.

In general terms, vatas tend to be slightly built with dry skin and hair, fluctuating moods, a creative mind and a tendency toward insomnia and vivid dreams. Pittas are of medium build, with fair or medium colouring and fine, straight hair that has a tendency to go grey prematurely. They are usually efficient and ambitious and have a good memory. Kaphas usually have smooth, oily skin, thick hair and find it hard to lose weight. They tend to have a large build, are strong and are rather lethargic with a caring and patient temperament.

A tailored lifestyle programme

An ideal lifestyle programme to maintain good health and prevent ill health is specified for each doshic constitution. What is good for one person may not be right for another. All aspects of health and well-being are covered by Ayurveda, including diet, yoga, exercise, meditation, personal hygiene, internal cleansing, herbal remedies and massage. Although few modern families adhere to all the rituals and rules of a strictly authentic Ayurvedic way of life, the basic principles are followed in many homes and it remains the dominant health-care system in the Indian subcontinent.

The value of massage

Massage has long been an integral part of everyday life in India. According to Ayurvedic custom, a weekly massage is recommended for men and women to maintain a healthy balance of doshas and promote soft skin and strong, shiny hair. Before a wedding, the bride and groom are massaged with special oils to promote health, beauty and fertility. Women are massaged to help them cope with the physical and emotional strain of labour and, for forty days after the birth, new mothers and their babies receive a daily recuperative massage.

For Indian mothers, massage is regarded as an essential skill and an important means of communicating and bonding with their children. From the age of three or four, children receive a daily or weekly head massage, given with a selection of pungent oils, in the belief that this will help prevent scalp disorders, make their hair grow strong and also boost brain power. It is a custom that still holds fast, despite the fact that many youngsters, especially boys, rebel against being made to go out and play while they have oil on their heads.

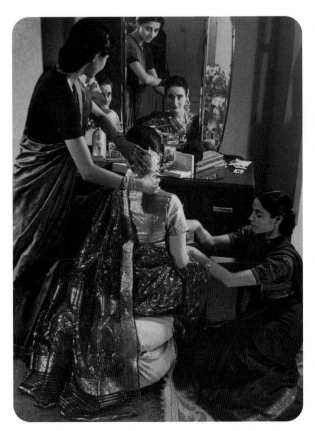

ABOVE **Indian wedding preparations. A head massage is often given prior to the big event to promote health, beauty and fertility.**

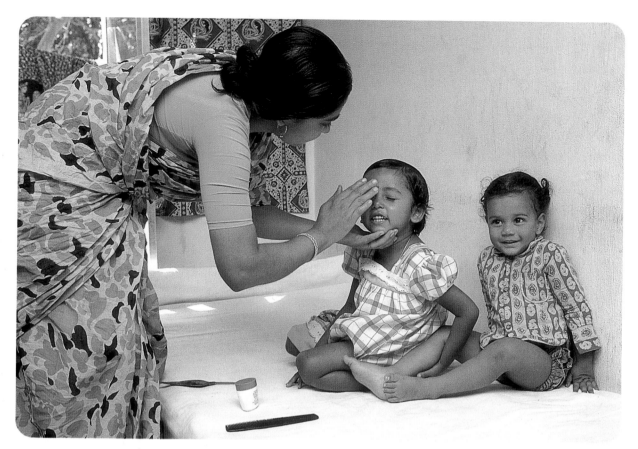

ABOVE **A woman from Calcutta moisturizes her daughter's face.**

In the West, we tend to view the scalp as independent from the rest of the body and treat it in a different way. In India, however, the scalp is regarded as an extension of the body skin and lavished with the same care and attention. Most Indian women continue to massage their heads with nourishing oils and are rewarded with the long, vibrant, glossy hair that is much admired in Indian society. Mothers share suggestions for hair care and beauty routines with their daughters who, in turn, hand them down to their own offspring. There is no formal structure or set routine but, rather like a recipe that has been passed down through the generations, head massage has been developed and refined, with each region and family adding their own special touches to suit the climate, personalities and particular occasions.

Oils and herbs

In India, a head massage is not complete without the use of ghee (clarified butter) or warm organic vegetable oils, chosen according to the season and availability within the region. These oils are often mixed with a selection of herbs, spices or fruits, such as amla (Indian gooseberry). Another popular ingredient is henna, a pale green powder from the dried shoots and leaves of the Lawsonia alba plant, which is used to dye and condition hair. Oils may be blended to a special family recipe or to alleviate a certain condition – perhaps to ease anxiety or moisturize a dry scalp. In Ayurvedic health centres, blends of oils and medicinal herbs are recommended to suit the dominant dosha. Vatas, for example, are generally advised to use a 'warming' oil, such as sesame or mustard, as a base, whereas kaphas should choose a 'cooling' oil, such as coconut or sunflower, mixed with herbal extracts. In some parts of India, women like to leave the oil on their heads for 24 hours or more, while others shampoo it off after a few hours.

Head massage has not remained an entirely female practice. Over the years, it has become incorporated into treatments offered to men by barbers and masseurs. There are even stories that these masseurs sometimes acted as spies who were able to draw out secrets while their clients were in the soporific state that can be induced by massage. Today, head massage is still included in any treatment provided by a barber, and many men claim that it helps prevent early balding and greying.

Powerful touch

The massage generally performed in Ayurvedic health centres in India and usually offered to visitors tends to be extremely brisk and powerful. Although Indian masseurs may look very frail, their fingers can feel like rods of iron against your scalp. The massage is often too rough and vigorous for Westerners, who prefer a gentler touch. Many have vivid memories and claim 'I thought my eyes were going to pop out of my head' or 'It felt like my head was a spin drier' and 'I was worried his fingers would go straight through my scalp'. However, it must be added that these same people nearly always go on to extol the many benefits they derived from it, including deep relaxation, freedom from aches and pains, more restful sleep and better concentration.

A Western dimension

The concept of Indian head massage as a complementary therapy was first introduced into the United Kingdom by Dr Narendra Mehta, who arrived from India in the early 1970s to train as a physiotherapist. Like many Indian people away from their home country, he began to miss the benefits of a regular head massage and so decided it was time to develop it in the West. He returned to India to study different family and regional techniques and extended his particular style of scalp massage to include the neck, shoulders, upper back, upper arms and face. Balancing the flow of the body's subtle life energy – or 'prana', as it is known in India – is an important part of Ayurveda and many other Eastern medical philosophies. Dr Mehta's form of Indian head massage, which he calls 'champissage', also involves balancing the flow of energy by working on the body's energy centres – or 'chakras'.

A chakra is believed to be a whirling vortex that draws energy into the body, allowing it to flow freely through the network of energy centres. 'Chakra' also comes from the ancient Sanskrit language and literally means 'circle of movement'. There are seven main chakras located at different levels, running from the master chakra on the crown of the head to the lowest one at the base of the spine. Therapists work with the chakras to release stagnant energy within the body and restore a balance that brings a feeling of inner harmony.

Indian head massage has become so popular that it is now widely taught at colleges. The massage has also been adapted so that it can be performed without oil, therefore clients do not need to disrobe and so the working day is not interrupted for long. As such, it has become firmly established as the ultimate antidote to the demands of modern life and is taken into offices, schools, nursing homes and even airports.

OPPOSITE **An Indian head massage is now becoming a popular way to release tension and promote well-being in the work place.**

CASE STUDY

HEALTHY HAIR

Saradha, 23, a trainee shop manager, moved from India when she was six. She follows her mother's and grandmother's example by giving herself a head massage every week to keep her long hair strong and shiny. Sometimes her mother gives her a massage. 'It is a lovely feeling when my mother tends my hair,' she says. 'She knows instinctively what mood I'm in and does a different kind of massage depending on how I'm feeling. When I'm tired and stressed, it is just so relaxing. I have tried using all sorts of different oils on my hair but I find that coconut is very light and easy to apply. It doesn't have much smell, which is good as I like to sleep with the oil on my head. Some of the oils my mother prefers have such strong aromas that I would wake up with a migraine!

'While she massages my head, my mother tells me all about my early life in India. I love hearing the old stories about how children have their head massaged by their mothers and grandmothers. I haven't got any children yet but I would like to follow the tradition. My sisters massage their children's heads using the same kind of movements as my mother. But they don't sit still for long – just enough to get the oil into the hair and scalp!'

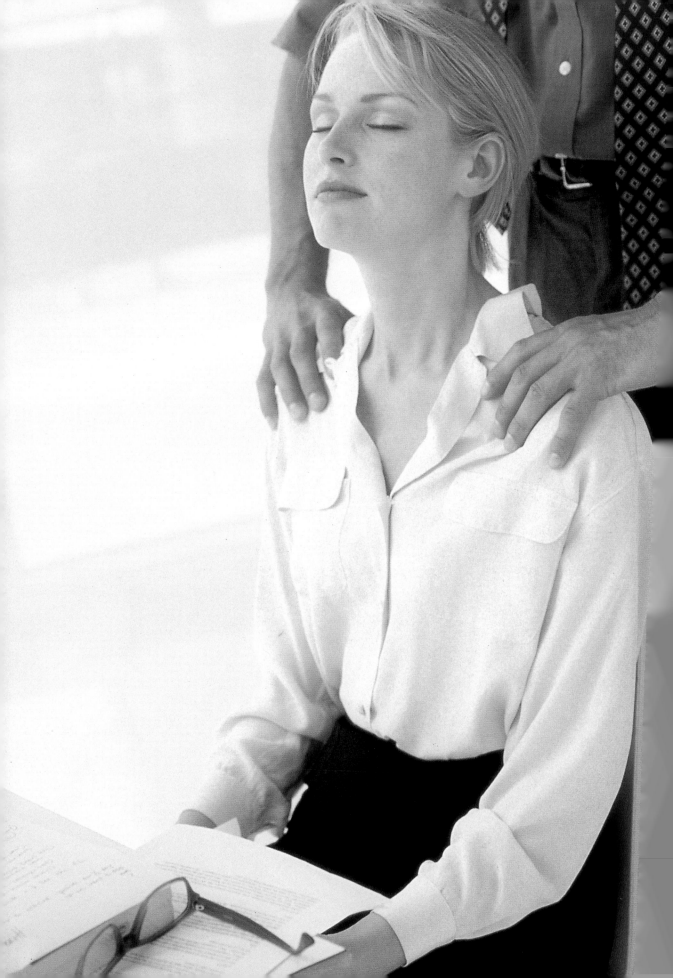

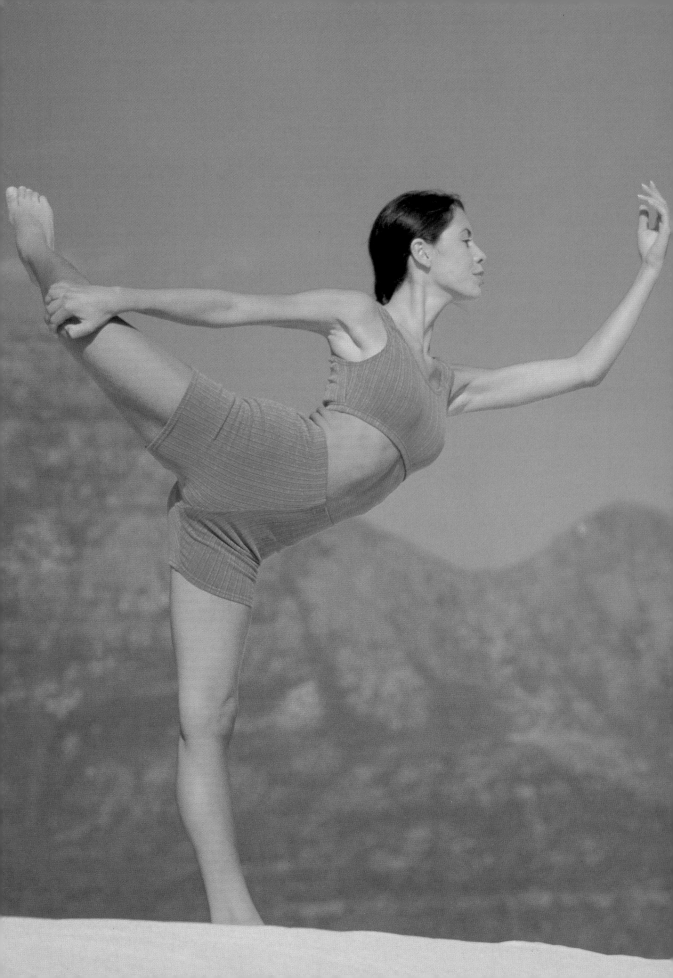

Healthy body,
healthy mind

A basic knowledge of how Indian head massage affects some
of the main structures and systems of the body can help you to
appreciate the benefits of the therapy and enable you to give a more
effective and personal massage. As you start to realize the amazing
intricacies of the miraculous body machine, you will develop a
greater understanding of the impact of the various different
techniques and learn how to adapt your sequence of movements
to meet the individual needs of your massage partner.

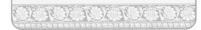

CHECKLIST

BENEFITS OF INDIAN HEAD MASSAGE

The therapeutic effects of Indian head massage last long after the treatment is over. The short- and long-term benefits are individual, varied and cumulative and include the following.

- Relief from pain and stiffness in the muscles of the face, scalp, neck, upper back and shoulders.
- Increased mobility of the joints in the neck and shoulder area.
- Relief from tension headaches, eye strain, nasal congestion, jaw-ache and hangovers.
- Increased energy levels.
- Alleviation of stress, anxiety, lethargy and mild depression.
- Greater creativity, clarity of thought and concentration.
- A sense of tranquillity, calmness and positive well-being.
- More restful, refreshing sleep.
- Deeper, calmer breathing.
- Strengthened immune system.
- Improved skin condition and colour.
- Strong, healthy, shiny hair.
- Increased self-esteem and self-worth.
- Greater self-awareness, which often brings the additional benefit of a change to a healthier lifestyle.

Qualified Indian head massage practitioners have the skills and experience to help relieve the symptoms of a number of disorders, such as sinusitis, tinnitus and migraines, but these advanced techniques do require hands-on training. Without formal training, it is important that you do not attempt to treat any medical conditions.

Therapeutic effects

This chapter looks at the blood and lymph circulation, the musculoskeletal system, skin and hair, and the effect of stress on our lives. When studying aspects of anatomy and physiology, however, it is important not to regard any mental or physical system in total isolation. Everything within the mind and body is interlinked and interacts so that an imbalance in one system can have a profound effect on your overall health and well-being.

Life-giving blood

Blood is the body's main transport system. It distributes vital supplies of oxygen and nutrients to the billions of living cells within the body and removes their waste products. Cells are the basic building blocks of life – varying in size, shape and function. Groups of cells form body tissues, such as skin and muscle, or make up organs, such as the brain and heart. Cells require a constant supply of oxygen and nutrients to produce the energy needed to fuel the thousands of different chemical activities within the body. During the process of creating energy, known as cell metabolism, various waste products, such as carbon dioxide and water, are released into the spaces between the cells. If the blood circulation is poor, the cells are starved of oxygen and nutrients, and toxins begin to accumulate in the tissues.

The healthy circulation of blood is essential to the health and vitality of all the bodily systems. When the blood circulation to the cells is sluggish or impaired, energy levels plummet, muscles may feel stiff, painful and tired, the brain starts to suffer lapses in concentration and memory, hair looks lacklustre, skin takes on a dull appearance and spots may develop. Indian head massage can boost the flow of blood through the cells in the brain, scalp, face, neck and shoulders, helping to keep the mind alert and the body active and promoting fresh, clear skin and healthy, vibrant hair.

Continuous circuit

Blood is pumped around the body by the heart, a hollow muscular bag that forces the blood through a continuous figure-of-eight circuit, travelling between the lungs, the heart and the tissues of the body. It carries unwanted carbon dioxide from the cells to the lungs to be

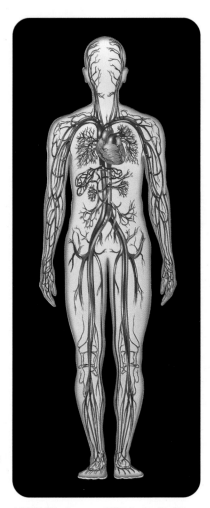

ABOVE **The organs and blood vessels of the human body that work together to enable the circulation of blood.**

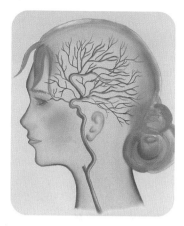

ABOVE **The red (oxygenated) and blue (deoxygenated) blood to and from the head.**

exhaled and then collects the freshly inhaled oxygen and distributes it around the body. Blood picks up nutrients, such as glucose, vitamins and minerals, from the digestive tract and delivers them to the cells. Toxic wastes are dropped off at the lungs and sweat glands to be eliminated, or taken to the liver to be prepared for excretion by the kidneys. Blood also carries heat around the body and takes hormones from the endocrine glands, where they are produced, to the target organs.

Transporting supplies

Blood that is rich in fresh oxygen is known as oxygenated blood. This oxygen-rich blood surges from the heart under pressure into a network of blood vessels called arteries. Blood is travelling under such pressure that if you cut an artery it would bleed profusely. When the heart contracts and pumps out blood, the thick, elastic walls of the arteries expand slightly and then return to their normal shape as the heart relaxes. The wave of pressure that causes this temporary change in shape in the artery wall is felt as the pulse.

- Press very gently on the carotid artery at the side of your neck and you will feel your pulse. If you have difficulty locating it, trace a line down from your earlobe to the hollow under your jaw. The number of pulses that occur in a minute is known as the pulse rate. This is the same as the number of times the heart beats in a minute. The normal pulse rate for an adult at rest varies between 60 and 80 beats a minute. This increases with activity, stress and strong emotions.

Blood pressure

When the heart contracts, blood is pumped into the arteries. When it relaxes, blood flows into the heart from the veins. The force with which the heart pumps blood through the arteries is known as blood pressure. This is usually based on two measurements. The force exerted when the heart contracts is known as the systolic blood pressure; the reduction in force when the heart relaxes is known as diastolic pressure. Blood pressure often changes, rising with exercise and strong emotions. Fluctuations in blood pressure are normal but a permanently raised level can be detrimental to health and is a contributory factor in strokes and heart disease.

If the blood was not under pressure it would naturally gravitate to the lower parts of the body. Blood pressure ensures that some blood is forced upward through the aorta, the largest artery in the body. The aorta branches into the carotid arteries on either side of the neck, which divide and sub-divide into smaller arteries to supply the tissues of the brain, face and scalp. Most arteries lie deep within the body, where they are protected by bones and muscles, but the carotid arteries are near the surface of the neck. When massaging this area, it is important not to press too heavily as you could interrupt the flow of blood to the brain, possibly causing unconsciousness.

Fair exchange

Arteries continually branch into smaller and smaller arteries until they become tiny arterioles, which divide into a network of blood capillaries. Capillaries are only one cell thick, which allows blood plasma (the liquid base of blood, holding nutrients and other substances in solution) to seep through the thin capillary walls, where it becomes known as tissue fluid. This fluid acts as a medium for the exchange of nourishing oxygen and nutrients with the unwanted carbon dioxide and waste products. The cells absorb the nourishment from the tissue fluid and, at the same time, eliminate their waste products through diffusion into the tissue fluid and then through the thin capillary walls back into the bloodstream.

Deoxygenated blood, which contains very little oxygen, is carried back to the heart via the venous (vein) system. These blood vessels begin as tiny venules that gradually increase in size to become a network of veins. This blood is under much less pressure than blood in the arterial system and so many veins have non-return valves to prevent a back-flow of blood. In general, veins are closer to the surface of the skin than arteries. Blood drains from the head, largely by the force of gravity, via the jugular veins, which join the two main veins – the superior and inferior vena cava – leading directly to the heart. Once the deoxygenated blood arrives back at the heart, it is ready to begin its journey to the lungs and around the body again.

Monitoring the flow

The amount of oxygenated blood delivered to the cells is determined by the arterioles. The walls of these tiny blood vessels can expand and contract considerably to control their output and ensure that cells are supplied with exactly the right quantity of blood for their needs. If any area needs extra energy, such as the muscles when exercising, oxygenated blood is diverted from other parts of the body to satisfy the demand. This is known as blood shunting. As the blood vessels in the working area dilate to allow extra blood to enter, there is a reddening, known as erythema, that gives the skin a radiant glow.

Heat transfer

Blood also carries heat, so the increased flow through the cells will automatically warm the tissues. The production of energy in the cells generates a huge amount of heat. This is carried in the blood where it is evenly distributed around the body to maintain a constant temperature of around 37°C (98.6°F). If too much heat is produced, the 'superficial' blood vessels – near the surface of the skin – dilate so that excess heat can be carried to the surface and dissipated into the atmosphere. If the temperature outside the body is cold, the superficial blood vessels constrict to conserve heat and the skin takes on a more sallow appearance.

Blood composition

Blood contains 55 per cent plasma and 45 per cent blood cells, such as erythrocytes, leucocytes and platelets.

- Plasma is a straw-coloured liquid. It is 91 per cent water and holds sugar, amino acids, mineral salts, enzymes and other substances in solution.
- Erythrocytes, or red blood cells, contain haemoglobin, a protein that absorbs oxygen from the lungs and releases it to the body cells. The erythrocytes appear dark red when haemoglobin is carrying oxygen, but the colour changes to a paler red once the oxygen has been released.
- Leucocytes, or white blood cells, play a vital part in the immune system by attacking and destroying infectious

micro-organisms, such as bacteria, and producing antibodies to guard against future infection.
- Platelets, or thrombocytes, are capable of sticking together to form a clot or mass, especially when blood is exposed to the air, as a result of a cut, for example. This binding action seals the wound to prevent bleeding, fluid loss and infection.
- It is important to remember that Indian head massage is designed to complement – and not replace – orthodox medical treatment. Therefore, it should not be seen in any way as an alternative to your own doctor's diagnosis and treatment.

CHECKLIST

INDIAN HEAD MASSAGE AND BLOOD CIRCULATION

- Indian head massage works with the circulatory system.
- The various massage manipulations can help improve the flow of deoxygenated blood back to the heart and speed the flow of freshly oxygenated blood to the superficial and deeper tissues of the neck, shoulders and head.
- A more efficient flow of arterial blood enables more oxygen and nutrients to be brought to the cells, so aiding their proper functioning and stimulating cell growth, division, renewal and healing.
- A speedier flow of venous blood back to the heart helps remove carbon dioxide and metabolic waste products at a quicker rate. This helps muscles function more efficiently, prevents muscle stiffness and pain and improves the condition of hair and skin.
- The increased supply of blood produces warmth, which promotes general relaxation (the same effect as lying in a warm bath) and encourages small amounts of oil to be absorbed through the skin.
- Massage causes dilation of the superficial blood vessels, which gives a healthy glow to the skin. The generally relaxing effect of massage can help to lower a permanently raised blood pressure.

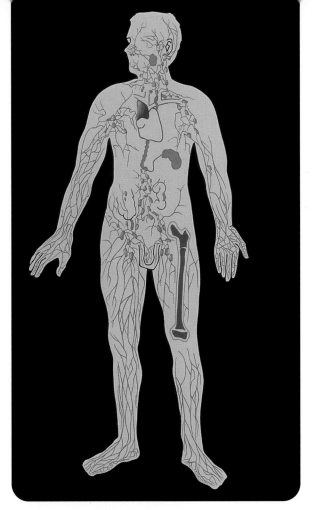

ABOVE **The human lymphatic system.**

Lymphatic system

We are bombarded by toxins that can enter the body in many ways – including through food and drink, pollution in the air and the invasion of bacteria and viruses. Toxic waste matter is also created internally as a by-product of normal metabolic processes. The body has a highly efficient self-cleansing system to eliminate these potentially harmful substances from the body through the skin, the kidneys, the colon, the immune system and the lymphatic system. When these systems slow down, toxins are able to accumulate and circulate around the body. This can give rise to a number of symptoms, including tiredness, nasal and sinus congestion, susceptibility to coughs and colds, frequent headaches, puffiness, disturbed sleep and dull skin and hair.

Indian head massage can help discourage the build up of toxic matter in the head, neck and shoulders by boosting the efficiency of the lymphatic system. This system is an intricate network of glands, vessels and tubes that extends throughout the body, removing viruses, bacteria and other foreign materials and draining excess fluid from tissue

spaces. The lymphatic system is integrally linked with the circulation of blood. However, it has several differences. It does not have a muscular pump equivalent to the heart and it does not form a complete circuit around the body. It is a one-way system of tubes that takes fluid from the body tissues to the heart but does not collect fluid from the heart.

The flow of lymph

The fluid that travels through the lymphatic system is known as lymph. This straw-coloured liquid is derived from the tissue fluid that bathes the body's cells. Tissue fluid contains both unwanted waste matter, which has been eliminated by the cells, and oxygen and nutrients, which have been delivered by the arterial bloodstream to nourish the cells. Once the cells have absorbed what they need for maintenance, growth and repair, most of the fluid and waste materials are returned to the bloodstream through the thin walls of the blood capillaries. The remaining fluid and foreign matter becomes lymph and seeps through the walls of the lymph capillaries to enter the lymphatic system.

Unlike blood capillaries, lymph vessels are blind-ended tubes. The walls of lymph vessels are more permeable than those of blood capillaries, allowing them to absorb larger particles of foreign material, cell debris, bacteria and viruses in the tissue fluid. They also drain any excess fluid that has built up as a result of infection, tissue damage or the presence of a foreign body. If drainage is sluggish, it can lead to water retention. Lymph vessels in the small intestine absorb fat, which is slowly emptied into the bloodstream.

Lymph vessels join together to form a network of tubes that carry lymph to the heart. Lymph is forced through the vessels by the rhythmic relaxation and contraction of nearby muscles during breathing and other body movements. Regular exercise has been shown to have a beneficial impact on lymph drainage. To ensure the lymph travels in the right direction, some lymphatic vessels have non-return valves that prevent back-flow. Lymphatic vessels get progressively larger until they eventually empty into two ducts: the right lymphatic duct and the thoracic duct. These two ducts drain the lymph into the subclavian veins at the base of the neck and finally into the vena cava, where it mixes with venous blood and is carried to the heart.

- The skin complements the lymphatic system by playing a major role in eliminating toxins from the body. These waste products are released in the sweat that seeps through the pores. A buildup of dirt, grime and dead skin cells can block pores. Use a loofah or body brush on your body as this helps purge the body of toxins by stimulating the lymphatic system and sloughing off dead cells .

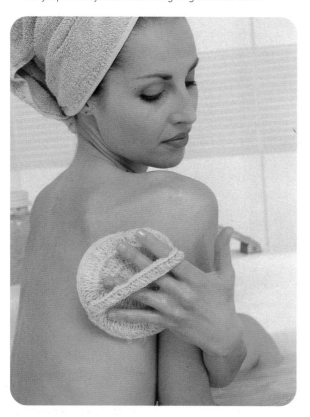

ABOVE **Aid your body in eliminating toxins by using a loofah to stimulate a sluggish lymphatic system.**

Cleansing and defending

All lymphatic vessels drain through lymph nodes, or 'glands', which are placed in strategic positions along the network. Lymph nodes are small, oval-shaped structures that act as filters to cleanse the lymph and remove any potentially harmful micro-organisms before they are allowed to enter the bloodstream and travel from one part of the body to another. Cancer cells may also be spread along the lymph vessels. There are around a hundred lymph nodes in the body and these vary greatly in size – some are as small as the head of a pin while others are as large as an almond. They are grouped into clusters that can lie near the surface or deeper in the body and drain a particular area. Lymph passes through several lymph nodes on its journey to the heart.

Lymph nodes store two types of leucocyte, or white blood cell – phagocytes and lymphocytes – that are part of the cleansing and filtering process. Phagocytes trap, engulf

and digest unwanted matter, such as dirt, dead cells and destroyed bacteria. Lymphocytes produce antibodies to combat viruses and bacteria. The lymphatic system also comprises organs such as the spleen, thymus gland and tonsils that play a major role in protecting and defending the body from infection and disease.

Whenever there is a threat of invasion by disease organisms, the lymph nodes in the area produce extra lymphocytes to repel the invaders. It is the accumulation of soldier cells and dead germs that causes the lymph nodes to become hard, swollen, inflamed and tender whenever the body is fighting a major disease. We have all experienced swollen lymph 'glands' in our neck when suffering a throat infection. Disease organisms and white blood cells travel along the lymph vessels until they reach the nearest set of nodes. An infected hand, for example, may result in swollen lymph nodes in the armpit. It is important not to massage over swollen lymph nodes.

- Manual lymph drainage is a specific form of massage therapy that uses a gentle, pumping action to stimulate the lymphatic system and drain the buildup of fluids and toxins. Massage strokes are always performed in the direction of the lymphatic pathways – toward the heart.

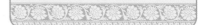

CHECKLIST

INDIAN HEAD MASSAGE AND THE LYMPHATIC SYSTEM

- Indian massage techniques can have many beneficial effects on the lymphatic system.

- They can help squeeze out any excess lymph from the tissue spaces and direct it to the nearest group of lymph nodes.

- The improved flow of lymph flushes out the toxins and drains any excess fluid from tissues in the massage area that can contribute to headaches, dull skin and general lethargy.

- The body's defence mechanisms are stimulated to increase resistance to 'the bug that is doing the rounds' and ensure that infections do not linger.

Muscles and bones

Indian head massage works on the muscles in the face, scalp, upper back, neck and shoulders. When these are tense, the flow of blood and lymph through the tissues is restricted, leading to reduced supplies of oxygen and nutrients and a buildup of stagnant wastes. This leads to stiffness, aches and pains, eye strain and feelings of anxiety and may contribute to greying and early hair loss. Massage helps relax tense muscles, thus stimulating the flow of blood and lymph through the area and easing tension headaches, aiding joint mobility, increasing concentration levels, encouraging healthy hair growth and promoting a general sense of well-being.

Muscle control

There are three different types of muscle. Indian head massage is applied to the voluntary muscles, which, as the name implies, are the muscles over which we have conscious control to bring about movement. Voluntary muscles are also known as skeletal muscles because they move and support the skeleton. Most of these muscles are attached to bones that pivot around joints. Different types of joints allow a varying range of movement. The bones of the skull, for example, are locked tightly together to form a protective casing for the brain, whereas the shoulder joints are designed to allow for greater freedom of movement.

- There are around 650 voluntary muscles, which make up around 40–50 per cent of body weight. Some are large and powerful, allowing movements such as climbing and running; others help perform very accurate and precise movements.

Voluntary muscles are attached to the bones on either side of a joint by fibres of connective tissue, known as tendons. Muscles exert a pull on the tendon, which moves the bone and any weight it is carrying. This action enables an arm to be raised, for example, or the head to be turned. Muscles work in pairs. When one contracts to raise a bone, the other will relax to facilitate movement. You can see this process in action by moving your lower arm up and down. As your biceps muscle contracts to raise your lower arm, your triceps muscle relaxes – and vice versa.

Muscle fibres

Muscles are made up of a collection of many long cells, or fibres, which are enclosed in a tough sheet of connective tissue, known as a muscle sheath. Each fibre is made up of bundles of even thinner strands, called myofibrils. These myofibrils comprise even finer strands, called filaments. When a muscle contracts, the filaments slide over each other and the muscle becomes shorter and fatter. When a muscle relaxes, the filaments slide back and the muscle returns to its original length. Voluntary muscles are usually stimulated to contract or relax by messages sent from the brain to the motor nerve cells controlling the muscle fibres.

Muscles have their own supply of blood and lymphatic vessels. As muscles relax, oxygenated blood flows in to nourish the tissues; as muscles contract, deoxygenated blood is forced out, carrying away waste products. The energy muscles need comes from oxygen, combined with its stores of a simple sugar called glycogen. This sets off a chemical process that releases energy and heat. If supplies of oxygen are limited, or muscles are working so vigorously that oxygen is used up quicker than the body can deliver it, a waste product, called lactic acid, is produced. This reduces the efficiency of muscles.

Muscular aches and pains

Some muscle fibres are always partially contracted. This partial contraction, known as muscle tone, is essential for maintaining posture. Without muscle tone we would collapse under the force of gravity. Muscle tone also adds definition and shape to the body. However, if muscles are held in an abnormal state of contraction for long periods – for example, when sitting hunched over a steering wheel or computer screen – the normal contraction/relaxation sequence does not occur and the flow of blood and lymph through the fibres is impeded.

Under these adverse conditions, the muscle is slowly starved of oxygen and nutrients and toxic waste products begin to accumulate and stagnate, making the situation even worse. Over time, the muscle tissue gradually begins to change in structure. The connective tissue may start to thicken and fibres stick together so they can no longer slide over each other so easily. Some tense muscles can be felt as hard lumps or nodules beneath the skin, a condition known as fibrositis, which is often most apparent in the muscles of the shoulder and upper back. This situation means there is little space for the free flow of blood and lymph. Unfortunately, muscular tension tends to build up so slowly that we often do not realize what is happening until the sensory nerve receptors in the area register soreness, discomfort, aching and pain.

Bones of the head, neck and shoulders

It is important to have some idea of the position of the underlying structures so you know which areas to massage – and which to avoid. It is particularly important not to exert any pressure on the spine. This bony column protects the spinal cord and a vast number of individual nerves connecting the brain to the rest of the body.

Skull

The skull is at the top of the vertebral column. It is divided into two sets of bones forming the cranium and the face. The cranium is the part of the skull that surrounds and protects the brain. It consists of eight immovable bones. The following ones are of relevance to Indian head massage.

- One occipital bone forms the lower back of the cranium.
- Two parietal bones form the sides of the cranium and the roof of the head.
- Two temporal bones form the sides of the head around the ears.
- One frontal bone forms the forehead.

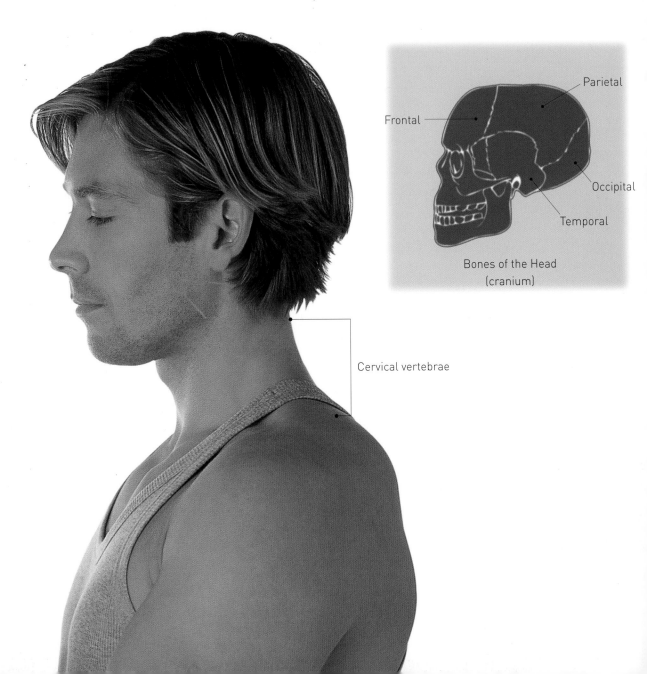

Frontal

Parietal

Occipital

Temporal

Bones of the Head (cranium)

Cervical vertebrae

Face

The face is formed from fourteen bones. The following ones are of particular relevance to Indian head massage.

- Two zygomatic bones form the cheekbones.
- Two maxilla bones form the upper jaw.
- One mandible bone forms the lower jaw.

Neck

The neck is made up of seven cervical vertebrae, which form the very top of the spinal column and the neck.

- First vertebra supports the head.
- Second vertebra allows rotation of the head.

Shoulders

The shoulders are formed by the following bones.

- Two scapulas (shoulder-blades). These triangular-shaped bones in the upper back are attached to muscles that move the arm.
- Two clavicles (collar-bones), one on either side of the sternum (breastbone). These form a joint with the sternum and scapulas, allowing shoulder movement.

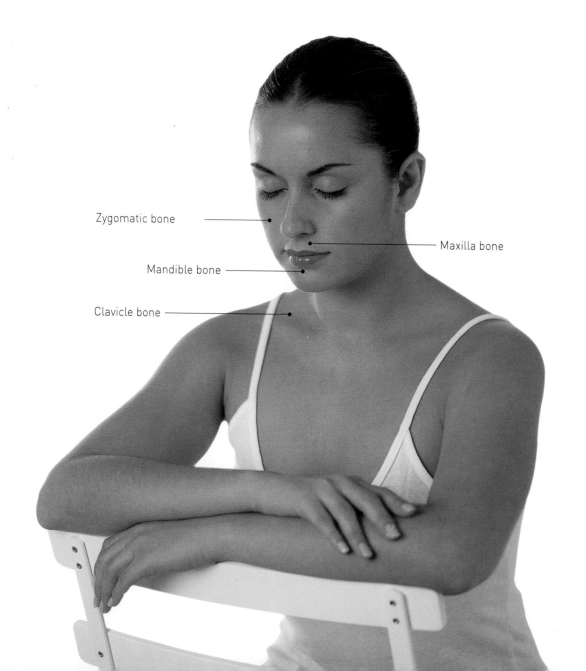

Zygomatic bone

Maxilla bone

Mandible bone

Clavicle bone

Muscles of the head, neck and shoulders

It is helpful to be able to locate the main muscles of the face, skull, neck, upper back and shoulders so that you can be sure that you are massaging in the right place for optimum benefits.

Muscles of the neck, shoulders and upper back

The following muscles are responsible for controlling the head, neck and shoulder area.

- Two sterno-cleido mastoid muscles work together to bend the head. Individually, they allow rotation of the head sideways toward the shoulder.
- One trapezius muscle draws the shoulders together and downward, pulls the head backward and allows movement of the shoulder.
- Two deltoid muscles raise the arm sideways away from the side of the body and help draw it backward and forward.

Muscles for chewing

The following muscles are responsible for chewing (or mastication).

- Masseter clenches the teeth and raises and closes the lower jaw tightly for chewing.
- Temporalis raises the lower jaw and presses it against the upper jaw to aid chewing.

Muscles of facial expression

These are mainly responsible for our facial expressions.

- Frontalis raises the eyebrows in surprise.
- Corrugator draws the eyebrows together in a frown.
- Orbicularis oculi closes the eyelid to wink.
- Risorius draws the corners of the mouth to grin.
- Buccinator compresses the cheeks to blow.
- Zygomaticus (major and minor) lifts the corners of the mouth upward and outward to smile.
- Orbicularis oris closes the mouth and purses the lips to kiss and whistle.
- Triangularis draws down the corners of the mouth to show sadness.
- Mentalis raises the lower lip, thereby wrinkling the chin, to indicate doubt.
- Platysma draws the corners of the mouth downward and backward to show horror.

The average adult head weighs 3–4 kilos (6½–9 lb), so the supporting muscles have to work hard to co-ordinate its movements. The head is designed to balance on the upper neck vertebrae, but most of us tend to push our heads forward during routine actions, and this imposes an enormous strain on the muscles of the shoulders, back and neck. This tension tends to spread to the tissues that cover the skull, impeding the flow of blood and lymph and leading to headaches, eye strain, stiffness and undernourished skin and hair roots.

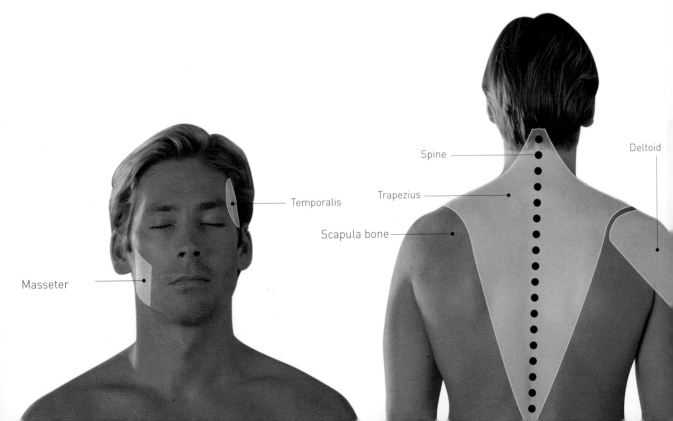

Temporalis

Masseter

Spine

Trapezius

Scapula bone

Deltoid

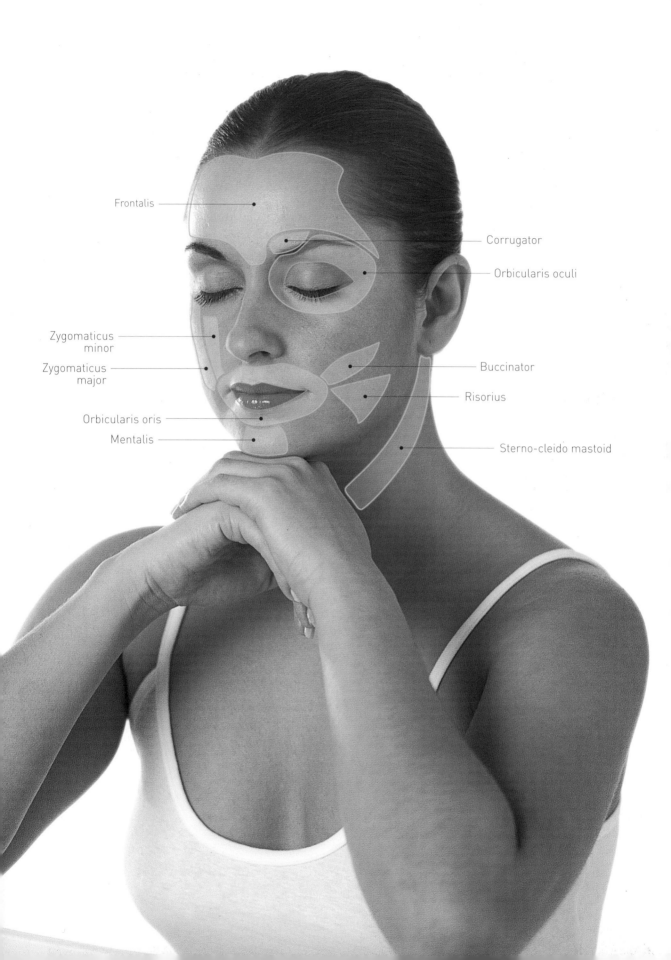

Frontalis

Corrugator

Orbicularis oculi

Zygomaticus minor

Zygomaticus major

Buccinator

Risorius

Orbicularis oris

Mentalis

Sterno-cleido mastoid

Muscles of expression

Many of the muscles in the face are tiny and very delicate. They are attached to the facial skin so that when they contract, they literally 'pull a face' – that is, they pull on the skin to create a facial expression. If these muscles become tense and taut through frowning, worry or pain they lose their flexibility and the face tends to look hard and set. It only takes 17 muscles to make you smile, but 43 for the average frown.

Indian head massage and muscle

The various massage techniques work on muscle tissue in different ways to help relax tense muscle fibres, tone slack fibres and increase blood and lymph flow through the tissues.

- The increased flow of oxygenated blood to the muscles brings fresh supplies of oxygen and nutrients to the muscle fibres.
- At the same time, a speedier venous flow and more efficient lymphatic drainage helps to prevent a buildup of waste products. This helps improve efficiency, aids repair and recovery and reduces pain, stiffness and muscle fatigue.
- The increased blood flow and frictional heat create warmth in the area. This encourages the muscles to relax so they are more receptive to the benefits of massage. The muscle fibres are stretched, broadened and separated, and any adhesions are broken down, enabling muscles to contract and relax more efficiently. The layer of tissue covering the skull is relaxed, which reduces headaches and eye strain and allows the hair follicles to be well supplied with nourishment, so encouraging healthy hair growth.
- Massage aids mobility of the neck and shoulder joints. Some facial muscles are encouraged to relax, which helps erase fine tension lines, while others are toned to give a younger, fresher appearance. Massage can also be an aid to greater awareness of the muscular tension that is being stored in the body by everyday activities.

Skin and hair

Massage with nourishing oils has long been used by Indian women as part of their beauty routine to promote strong, lustrous hair and keep their skin healthy, soft and supple. Scalp massage cannot reverse baldness or greying, which are often hereditary, but may help prevent excessive hair loss and will certainly make your hair soft, silky and shiny, with a natural bounce. Similarly, facial massage cannot remove wrinkles, which are largely due to smoking, pollution and excessive exposure to the damaging rays of the sun. However, by relaxing the underlying muscles, boosting the blood and lymph circulation and helping to shed dead skin cells, massage can give your face a younger, more attractive appearance.

The skin is one of nature's finest works of art. This complex organ, the largest in the body, provides a highly flexible protective covering to keep the body fluids in and to shield the internal structures and systems from injury and invasion by harmful micro-organisms. The skin contains thousands of sensory nerve endings that make it extremely sensitive to heat, cold, pain, light touch and deep pressure. The different sensory receptors respond to specific stimuli and send messages about these stimuli to the brain. The brain may respond by stimulating the motor nerves to carry out an appropriate action – such as tensing with pain or cold, or relaxing with the enjoyment of a pampering touch.

- There is a large number of sensory nerve receptors in the face and scalp so massage to these areas can be particularly effective in influencing moods. Massage movements may be adapted to create a soothing and calming effect or to stimulate and invigorate. Appropriate selection of massage techniques for the face and scalp area can have a profound effect on the mind and body.

Skin structure

The skin has three main layers, the epidermis, the dermis, and the subcutaneous, or 'below the skin', layer, each with a different composition and function.

Epidermis

The top skin layer is called the epidermis and is the one that can be seen and touched. It has no blood vessels and only a small number of nerve endings. This layer is where cell renewal takes place. The skin is made up of millions of cells that are constantly growing and replacing themselves. Over a period of around 27 days, cells push up through the epidermis, gradually changing in structure. Their nuclei (cell control centres) break down and the fluid within the cells is replaced by keratin, a tough and durable protein that makes the skin so hard-wearing. Skin cells have died by the time they reach the surface of the epidermis. As old cells are shed, fresh ones take their place and so the cycle continues. If these dead, scaly cells are allowed to accumulate, they give the skin a dull appearance.

- Dead skin cells are continually being rubbed off by the friction of everyday activities such as towel drying or wearing clothes. It is estimated that around 80 per cent of household dust is made up of dead skin cells and that we shed a complete surface layer every five days.

Some of the cells in the epidermis react with the sun's ultraviolet rays to produce a dark-brown pigment called melanin, which blocks some of the harmful effects of the sun. Melanin is mainly responsible for the normal colour of skin and hair – the more melanin there is, the darker the skin colour. Another function of the epidermis is to produce vitamin D – 'the sunshine vitamin'. When skin is exposed to the sun, its cells form vitamin D, which combines with calcium and phosphorus to

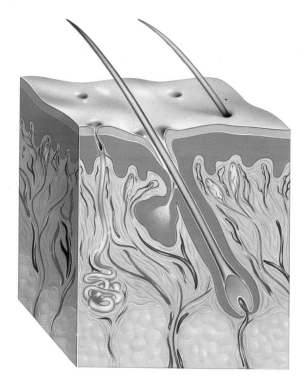

ABOVE **A cross-section of human skin. A hair pokes through the epidermis from the follicle, or pit, that holds it.**

develop and help maintain a healthy bone structure. A daily quota of sunlight is essential to health and well-being, but over-exposure can have a detrimental effect, not only on your health but also on your skin, leading to wrinkles, age-spots and a leathery appearance. This is why it is important to protect your skin during very sunny weather.

Dermis

The dermis lies directly underneath the epidermis and its main function is to support and nourish the epidermis. The dermis contains blood and lymph vessels, nerve endings, sweat and sebaceous glands and hair follicles. It is a much thicker layer than the epidermis and is made up of two types of protein fibres, collagen and elastin.

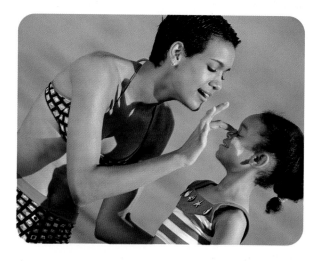

ABOVE **Protection from the sun, whether by using sunscreen or some form of shade, is important to protect our body's delicate skin.**

Collagen strengthens the skin and protects against over-stretching. Elastin, as the name suggests, gives the skin its elasticity and allows it to regain its shape after it has been stretched – following pregnancy, for example. These fibres weaken and become stretched with age, so the skin tends to become looser and more wrinkled over time.

The dermis has tiny projections, known as papillae, that extend into the epidermis. Papillae contain nerve endings and blood and lymph vessels to ensure a healthy flow of blood and lymph around the living cells of the top layer. The blood vessels in the dermis also help maintain a constant internal body temperature of 37°C (98.6°F). If the body gets too hot, the blood vessels leading to the skin dilate to allow more warm blood to come to the surface so that the excess heat is lost. If the body gets too cold, the blood vessels near the skin constrict to stop too much heat from escaping.

Removing heat and toxins

Sweating, or perspiration, is the body's other main reaction to raised temperature. The skin contains two to three million sweat glands, each consisting of a coiled section in the dermis, where sweat is produced, and a long tube that

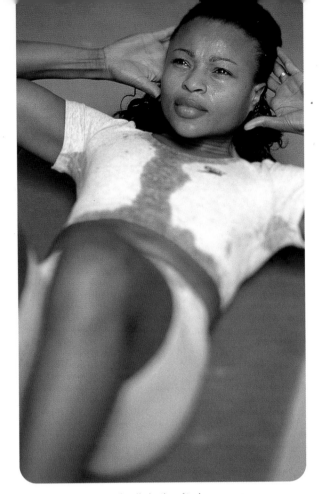

ABOVE **Sweat promotes the elimination of toxins.**

leads directly on to the surface of the skin through an opening called a pore. Sweat extracts heat from the blood flowing just beneath the surface and then oozes out through the pores. As the sweat evaporates, it removes heat from the skin. Some sweat glands respond to factors such as heat and exercise, others to emotional and hormonal changes. The sweat glands also play a major part in the body's excretory system and help eliminate toxic waste products through the pores. It is important to wash and rinse your skin thoroughly to prevent debris blocking the pores and hindering the flow of toxins from the body.

- The skin is used as a diagnostic tool in traditional Eastern medicine, as the colour and texture can indicate areas of ill-health within the body. As general health and well-being increases with regular Indian head massage, so the condition of the skin and hair will also improve.

Natural moisturizer

The dermis contains sebaceous glands that secrete an oily liquid known as sebum. Sebum is a natural moisturizer, helping to keep the skin and hair soft and supple. Sebaceous glands tend to be more active following puberty,

which accounts for the oiliness of the skin and hair during adolescence. When these glands are underactive, skin and hair tend to be very dry. Sebum helps keep the skin waterproof and combines with sweat to create an acidic coating, known as the acid mantle, to guard against the growth of bacteria and fungi. Harsh soaps and chemicals can upset the balance of this natural coating, so a mild cleanser suitable for your skin type is recommended.

- Skin varies in thickness over the body. The thinnest part is around the eyes, where it is only 0.5 mm thick. The thickest part is on the palms and soles of the feet, where it is around 6 mm thick.

Subcutaneous layer

The subcutaneous layer lies beneath the dermis and contains connective tissue, known as adipose tissue, where fat is stored. The subcutaneous layer helps to conserve body heat. Fat is a poor conductor of heat, thereby reducing heat loss through the skin.

Hair growth

Hair grows up through hollow spaces in the dermis known as hair follicles. Hair follicles are found all over the body except on the palms of the hands, soles of the feet, lips and the nipples. At the bottom of each hair follicle is an area known as the hair papilla where the living cells are nourished and drained of toxins by the blood and lymph vessels. Stress and illness can affect hair growth. This is because the body does not regard hair as being essential to life, so in times of crisis blood may be diverted away from the cells in the follicles toward more important areas that are in need of extra oxygen and nutrients. If the living cells continue to be deprived of essential nourishment, scalp problems may develop and the hair roots can start to weaken, leading to dull, brittle hair and even mild hair loss.

Cells in the hair papilla multiply to form the hair root and shape the hair bulb and then push up through the follicle in the same way that skin cells migrate up through the epidermis. As the cells move upward through the follicle, they change their structure, fill with the durable protein keratin and eventually die. There are around 120,000 hairs on the average head. Each hair grows at a rate of around 1 mm every three to four days. Over a period of between one and six years, an individual hair fibre grows, then stops, rests, degenerates and falls out. Around 50–100 hairs are lost from the head each day. Before a hair is shed, there is usually another one ready to replace it.

The visible strands of hair are all dead tissue. Each strand has an inner shaft, containing a pigment that gives the hair its colour, and an outer cuticle. The cuticle protects the interior of the hair shaft and is lubricated by sebum, the body's natural moisturizer, secreted from sebaceous glands at the base of the hair root. Sebum makes the hair soft to touch and reflects light to give a glossy sheen. If the cuticle is damaged by too vigorous brushing, chemical treatments or excessive exposure to the sun, the hair can become coarse and prone to tangling.

- The shape and size of the hair follicle determines the thickness and type of hair. Follicles with round openings produce straight hair, while follicles with oval openings produce curly or wavy hair.

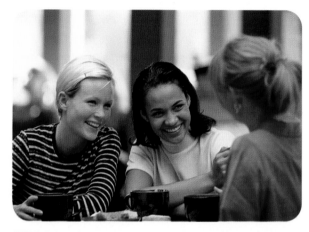

ABOVE **Hair varies not only in colour but also in thickness and type, resulting in straight or curly locks.**

There are thousands of hair follicles in the dermis, each one attached to a small muscle called an arrector pili, which is activated by a motor nerve. When a person feels cold or has a sudden fright, these muscles respond by making the strand of hair stand on end. Small bumps are formed over the skin, giving the appearance of a plucked goose – hence the term 'goose bumps'.

- Traditional treatments for preventing baldness include rubbing a fresh cut onion on the scalp or applying stinging nettles to stimulate the circulation of blood in that area. An Indian head massage, however, is a far more pleasant treatment.

Indian head massage and skin and hair

Massage has many beneficial effects on the condition of the skin and hair.

- The circulation of blood and lymph is stimulated, thereby delivering fresh supplies of nutrients and oxygen to the living cells and removing unwanted metabolic wastes and excess tissue fluid. This provides a healthy environment for cell growth, renewal, repair and division.
- Massage also aids desquamation, or the shedding of dead skin cells, as it stimulates cell division, so more cells move up toward the surface. The friction of the hands also helps rub off dead cells. Fresh new cells are exposed, which improves the skin's appearance.
- Massage leads to dilation of superficial blood capillaries, which gives a healthy glow to a sallow complexion. The sebaceous glands are stimulated to produce more sebum, which keeps the skin and hair soft and supple, and raises the temperature of the skin, which ensures optimum benefits from any oils used.
- Massage also has a cleansing effect by stimulating the sweat glands to produce more sweat, which assists the removal of metabolic wastes and helps prevent the pores getting clogged with dirt and dead skin cells.

Stress factor

Stress affects us all, whether adults or children, from the first jangle of the alarm clock in the morning to the final struggle with the duvet cover at night. It is the natural response to any kind of extra demand, pressure or change, pleasant or unpleasant, placed on the mind or body. Stress is often given a bad name, but without it we would soon become bored and lethargic. It can provide the motivation to finish tasks, give a competitive edge when playing sport and raise performance at meetings and in exams. Stress provides the tingle before an exciting event and the exhilaration of a high-risk leisure activity. It can increase your self-confidence and boost your energy.

Stress is only harmful when the extra burden becomes too great to handle and you lose your ability to cope in a calm and rational way. It is a very personal response. Perhaps other factors become involved, the demands get too severe or go on for too long, circumstances change for the worse, or your support network breaks down. We all have different stress thresholds and these can vary under different circumstances. What is invigorating for one person at a certain time may cause anxiety in another situation. And we all respond to stress in different ways. While some people react to even minor upsets by becoming aggressive and blaming everyone around them, others retreat into themselves. 'I can't cope' and 'It's all too much for me' are common cries when suffering from too many pressure.

Negative factors

Among the main causes of negative stress are major life crises or changes such as bereavement, divorce, moving house and starting a new job. In our fast-moving modern society, however, there are a very great number of potentially stressful situations – major or minor, at work and at home – that can build up over time and lead to mental, physical and emotional overload. The pressures may be external, such as a hostile boss, critical spouse, argumentative children, or even a constantly ringing telephone or the noise of road works in the street. They can also be internal, such as persistent worries about being made redundant, feelings of inadequacy or guilt about a relationship or event.

Physical tension and illness are also directly linked with mental and emotional health and well-being and can exacerbate the problem. We all know that when we are emotionally stressed or worried, our bodies respond with physical symptoms, and vice versa. Think how often anxieties about a family argument or a visit to the dentist have been transformed into a headache or stomach cramps, so making the situation even worse. When we are suffering from a headache or flu, we feel irritable and depressed, which, in turn, hinders our recovery. Our language is rich in sayings that reinforce the connection. We 'grit our teeth' and 'carry the weight of the world on our shoulders' and we complain that people 'get under our skin' or 'make us sick'.

Fight or flight

When you are faced with a stressful situation, whether real or perceived, physical, mental or emotional, internal 'alarm bells' sound and the body responds by secreting hormones such as adrenaline and cortisol to prepare for instant action. This 'fight or flight' response is a primitive survival tactic to cope with a purely physical threat, such as an attack from a wild animal.

Muscles contract for optimum performance, either in facing the attacker or making an instant getaway. The heart and lungs work extra hard to speed up the flow of blood and oxygen to the muscles and brain. Blood pressure and pulse rate rise. Breathing becomes quicker. Sugars and fats are released into the blood-stream. Blood is diverted from the skin (causing it to go white) and the stomach (leading to the sensation of 'butterflies') to provide the muscles and brain with extra supplies of energy. Hairs stand on end as protection against the attacker and to produce a more menacing look. Sweat glands produce more sweat to cool the body ready for the expected physical effort.

The fight or flight response was designed to prepare the body for rapid and efficient physical action in a crisis. In primitive days, normal functions were restored as soon as the threat was over and physical action, whether in fight or flight, had utilized the increased energy supplies circulating in the body. In modern times, however, although our stress is more often psychological, the body responds in the same way. As we have no physical outlet (except exercise which is very beneficial, or perhaps punching a pillow!), stress hormones build up and we live under a low level of 'threat' for days, months and even years.

BELOW **Stress levels are exacerbated by the constant demands made on you every day.**

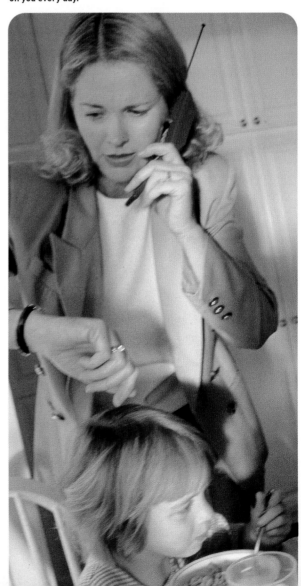

Effects of chronic stress

While short bursts of positive stress can be revitalizing, prolonged (chronic) negative stress keeps the mind and body in a constant state of mild 'overdrive' and saps mental and physical energy. These effects often creep up so slowly that many people do not notice the changes within themselves. All aspects of life can be affected. Minor hassles become major traumas and you may find yourself lying awake at night with your mind buzzing. You may find it hard to concentrate at work and doubt your ability, so your productivity can decline. You may then swing between bouts of weeping, with feelings of helplessness and hopelessness, to fits of aggression, when you pick fights with colleagues and neighbours. You may feel so down that you cannot face getting out of bed in the morning or find yourself turning to food or alcohol to lift your mood. You may start to get unexplained stomach upsets, headaches and feel a stiffness in your neck and shoulder muscles.

When the body is exposed to excessive stress for long periods of time, physical and mental health can become seriously affected, largely because the stress hormones interfere with the circulatory and immune systems. If allowed to continue, chronic stress can lead to raised blood pressure, digestive disorders, migraine, back pain, heart disease and skin and hair complaints. Stress hormones also depress the immune system, leading to greater susceptibility to diseases and allergies. Around 70 per cent of all illness is believed to be directly associated with physical, mental and emotional stress.

Indian head massage and stress

Indian head massage works simultaneously on a physical and psychological level, counteracting physical and mental tension or lethargy and encouraging well-being.

- On a physical level, massage relaxes tense and tight muscles, eases aches and pains, mobilizes the joints and regulates blood and lymph circulation, so restoring normal functioning. As the physical aches and pains are rubbed away, you will start to feel calmer and more able to cope with daily pressures in a relaxed and positive frame of mind.

- The deep physical and mental relaxation induced by massage has been proved effective in relieving the symptoms of stress, thus preventing serious health problems.

- On a psychological level, a massage gives you time to unwind so that nagging worries and problems can be viewed in a new light. The peace and quiet of massage allows the mind the time to relax and recharge. The caring, physical contact of massage helps boost self-esteem and encourages the release of 'feel good' endorphins, which counteract the stress hormones and boost the immune system, so helping to fight infection.

- Massage can facilitate the release of suppressed tension, which often brings a great sense of emotional relief. The relaxation effect encourages deep breathing, which relaxes the body and calms the mind.

- Massage can encourage an increased sense of self-awareness, which often leads to early recognition of stress signals and the realization of the need for mental and physical relaxation in everyday life.

CASE STUDY

TIME FOR MYSELF

On her 40th birthday, Janice, a full-time mother of four young children, was given a gift voucher for an Indian head massage. 'I was really touched,' she said. 'It was such a thoughtful present, especially as it came with an offer to look after my children too, so there were no excuses. My friends are always telling me that I get so bogged down with the children and house that I rarely spend any time or money on myself. This is true, but I feel so guilty when I do. However, I thought that this was something that I would really enjoy. It doesn't involve too much time or needing to show off all your lumps and bumps.

'I was converted after the first five minutes. It was just heaven. I really look forward to my weekly sessions – and notice if I have to miss for some reason. It is my time, my indulgence, my pleasure. No constant demands, no responsibilities, no expectations, no telephone – just peace and quiet. My therapist always makes me feel really well looked after. My weekly 'time out' has helped me to see things in a different way. I have stopped worrying about little things – and now enjoy life more. I'm much less of a nag with my husband and children.'

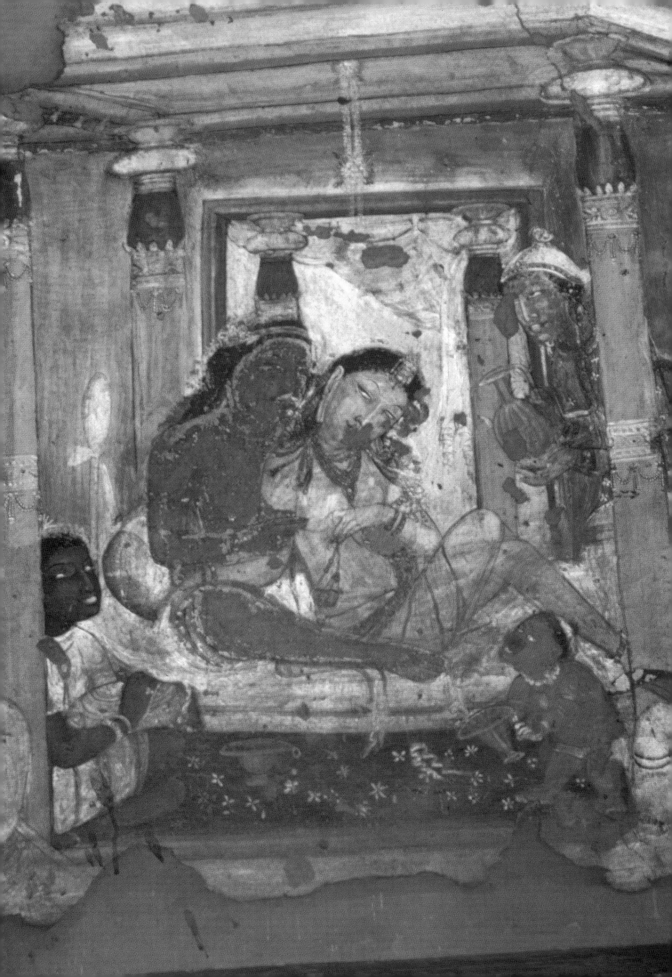

Oils for health
and beauty

Since the earliest civilizations, plants and plant extracts have been valued for their medicinal and cosmetic qualities. Ancient healing systems, such as Ayurveda, recognized the power of plants to promote health and well-being, and the earliest cave drawings confirm that primitive dwellers used natural colours to paint and dye their hair. Over thousands of years, it was discovered that the nuts and seeds of plants also yielded oils that provide the ideal lubricating medium for massage and can be combined with pure essential oils to have specific health-giving effects on mind and body. The long tradition of using natural vegetable oils to enhance the benefits of massage continues to the present day.

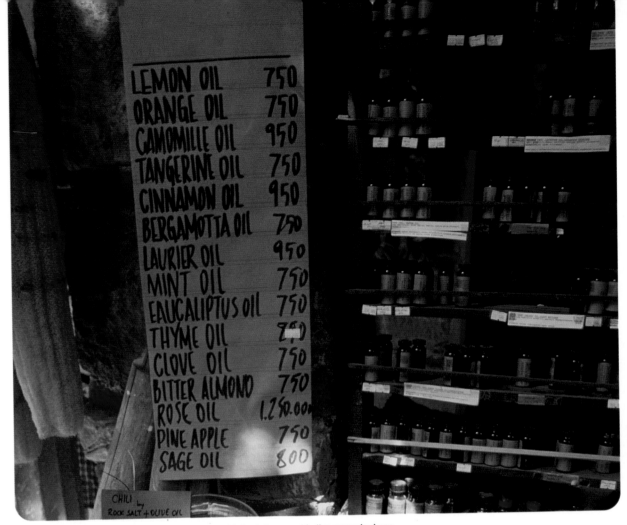

LEMON OIL	750
ORANGE OIL	750
CAMOMILLE OIL	950
TANGERINE OIL	750
CINNAMON OIL	950
BERGAMOTTA OIL	750
LAURIER OIL	950
MINT OIL	750
EAUCALIPTUS OIL	750
THYME OIL	800
CLOVE OIL	750
BITTER ALMOND	750
ROSE OIL	1.250.000
PINE APPLE	750
SAGE OIL	800

CHILI by ROCK SALT + OLIVE OIL

ABOVE **A wonderful array of oils can be found in health food stores and Indian grocer's shops.**

Why use oils?

Warm vegetable oils, often mixed with different aromatic herbs and spices, are an essential part of a massage in India. These oils, which have become known as 'carrier' oils in the West, act as a lubricant and make the massage a smoother and more pleasant experience for both the giver and the recipient. They also complement the circulation-boosting effects of head massage by cleansing the scalp and nourishing, moisturizing and strengthening the skin and hair.

In the West, it is fair to say that most people would shy away from being seen in public with greasy-looking hair; in India, however, it is extremely common for men, women and children to go about their daily lives with an oil-drenched head. Indeed, it is this tradition of regular head massage with vegetable carrier oils that helps protect their hair from the drying effect of the harsh sun and accounts for the beautifully lustrous locks so prized in Indian society.

Choosing vegetable carrier oils

The main vegetable carrier oils used in Indian head massage are almond, coconut, mustard, olive, sesame and sunflower. You can obtain a selection of natural vegetable carrier oils from many health food stores, Indian grocer's shops, aromatherapy mail order suppliers and some supermarkets – but do choose the highest quality products. Check with a shop assistant before you buy, or ask a qualified aromatherapist to recommend some reputable suppliers. Look for oils that are unrefined, extracted mechanically by cold or warm pressing and are free from additives. Most vegetable carrier oils sold for cooking are highly refined and are extracted using extremely high temperatures, which destroys much of the nutritional content. Although these oils will not cause you any harm, they will not offer the same benefits either, and you may well end up smelling something like a wok or frying pan! If possible, always select organic oils, as these have been produced without the use of chemical fertilizers or pesticides. Choose these more nutritious oils for dressing salads, too.

- If you or your massage partner have an allergy to nuts, avoid using nut oils as small quantities may be absorbed into the bloodstream.

Oriental blends

There is a wide selection of ready blended scalp and hair oils, available in chemist's shops and department stores, that are suitable for Indian head massage. These blends are often formulated for different hair and skin types or mixed with herbs and essential oils to aid relaxation, increase energy levels or add an erotic note to the occasion. For an authentic touch, it is worth shopping around for blended oils imported directly from India and sold in Indian supermarkets and health stores. These oils are often blended with Eastern herbs, spices and fruits, such as brahmi and neem, which are not readily available in the West. Brahmi is a herb that is widely used in Ayurvedic medicine to balance all three doshas, stimulate the circulatory system and promote hair growth. Neem oil is extracted from the seeds of the neem tree, which is native to India and has cleansing and insecticide properties.

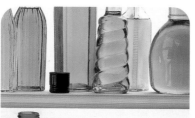
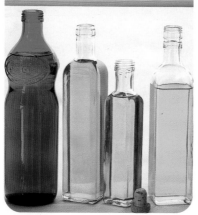

ABOVE **Take care when storing essential and blending oils.**

Commercial blended oils can provide a good starting point for using oils in head massage. They do vary greatly in texture and quality, however, so buy in small quantities and test a selection to identify the ones you prefer and find most enjoyable to use. Choose an oil that has a pleasant aroma and feels smooth on your hands. Some oils may have a rather unpleasant, synthetic aroma; others may leave a sticky residue on your hands and on the skin of your massage partner, or may be too watery to slide easily over the skin.

Pure essential oils

The vegetable oils used in Indian head massage can be applied on their own, mixed with another vegetable oil or blended with an appropriate pure essential oil. Pure essential oils are quite different from vegetable oils – and it is important not to confuse the two. Essential oils are non-greasy and extremely concentrated essences extracted from the petals, leaves, fruits and bark of aromatic plants. When used safely and correctly they can have a therapeutic effect on the mind, body and emotions. The oils enter the bloodstream in two ways: inhalation via the lungs and absorption through the skin.

Essential oils each have their own distinctive aromas that can have a profound influence on moods. The nasal passages contain large numbers of olfactory nerve receptors. These are closely linked to the part of the brain associated with emotions, arousal, feelings and memories. Certain smells can calm you down, wake you up or help you to concentrate. When blended with a vegetable carrier oil, tiny molecules of pure essential oils are absorbed through the skin and transported around the body to fulfil specific healing functions.

Choosing essential oils

A pure essential oil can enter the body within twenty minutes and may stay in the bloodstream for over 24 hours, so the purity of the product is crucial. Look for oils sold in dark glass bottles with a screw cap. They should be labelled 'essential oil', which ensures that they contain 100 per cent concentrated plant oil. A good guide is to check that the labels show the common name as well as the botanical Latin name and have specific instructions for use, including safety guidelines. Look for a batch number and expiry date. Essential oils are sold in health food stores, chemist's shops and through mail-order outlets. They should be stored in a cabinet in a cool dark room and not on a shelf, where they may be exposed to light and heat. A qualified aromatherapist will be able to suggest a suitable supplier.

Blending oils

Pure essential oils should be treated with great respect. They are highly potent and can be toxic if misused. Do not make the mistake of thinking that the more oil you apply, the greater the benefits. This is not the case, so use only tiny quantities. Adding that extra drop could cause skin irritation and other harmful reactions.

USING ESSENTIAL OILS SAFELY

The essential oils recommended on the following pages are safe for use in Indian head massage at home. However, you should always remember that all essential oils are very powerful and should be treated with caution.

- Never apply to the skin neat – always dilute with a carrier oil first. Wash off any spills immediately.

- Do not take internally.

- Keep bottles out of reach of children and pets.

- Avoid using any pure essential oils during pregnancy, when breastfeeding or on babies, children, or elderly people unless you are a fully qualified aromatherapist. Do not use in epilepsy, high blood pressure, asthma, hay fever or other allergic conditions, or any other contraindications (see page 257).

- Seek professional advice if you are taking homeopathic medicines, as some essential oils may adversely affect the treatment.

- Keep oils away from eyes. In case of accident, wash with plenty of water and seek medical advice.

- Do not use perfume or diffuse essential oils into the atmosphere while using essential oils for massage.

- Always obtain oils from a reputable source, make sure they are clearly labelled and always follow the instructions.

Before using essential oils, it is advisable to perform a skin test to check for sensitivity. Make up your chosen blend of oils. Rub a little of the blended oil on the inside of the wrist or behind the ears. Leave uncovered for 24 hours. Do not wash this area. Reactions often occur within a few hours. If you notice any signs of a rash, reddening or itchiness then you should not use the oil. Rinse off immediately with cold water.

Initially, it is best to err on the side of caution and use just one drop of a single pure essential oil for every 10 ml (2 teaspoons) of vegetable carrier oil. In the case of some oils such as rose, jasmine and Roman chamomile, you should add one drop to 30 ml (6 teaspoons). As you gain knowledge and experience of using pure essential oils, you can experiment by using a wider selection and different quantities, or mixing oils to give a synergistic (multiple) effect – but always follow the instructions and adhere strictly to the safety precautions.

When blending oils, ensure that your hands and all utensils are clean and dry. Measure the required amount of carrier oil (10 ml or 30 ml) into a small bowl or a measuring bottle. It may be advisable to use a 5 ml medicine spoon to ensure you use the right amount, as the size of teaspoons can vary enormously. Now add one drop of your chosen pure essential oil to the carrier oil – always buy essential oils in bottles with a special nozzle that allows you to measure one drop at a time accurately. Mix the oils in the bowl or shake the bottle, if it has a stopper. If you accidentally add more than one drop of essential oil, mix in the appropriate amount of extra carrier oil to restore the balance. Remember, essential oils are very concentrated. Wash your hands after blending.

Storing oils

Most kinds of carrier oil last for about six months before becoming unsuitable for massage. Once blended with a pure essential oil, they should be used within a month. Keep your carrier and essential oils in dark glass bottles with screw lids and store in a cool place, out of direct sunlight. Undiluted essential oils should be kept in a locked medicine cupboard. Keep the lid firmly closed, as they evaporate when exposed to the air. Most essential oils last from six months to a year.

BELOW **Essential and carrier oils should be kept in dark bottles.**

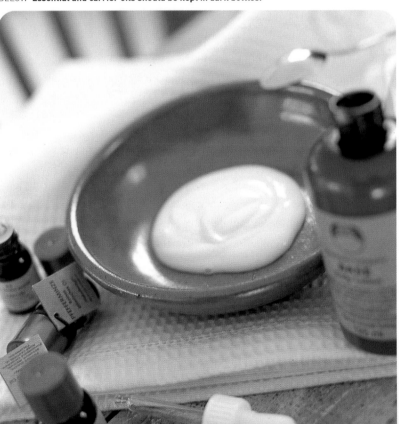

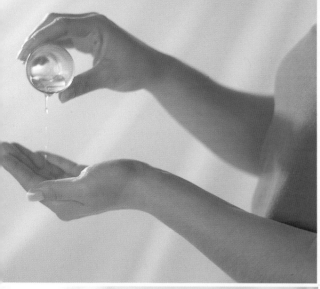

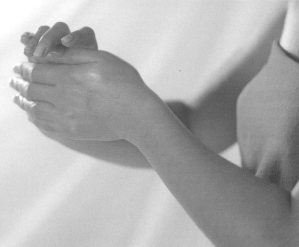

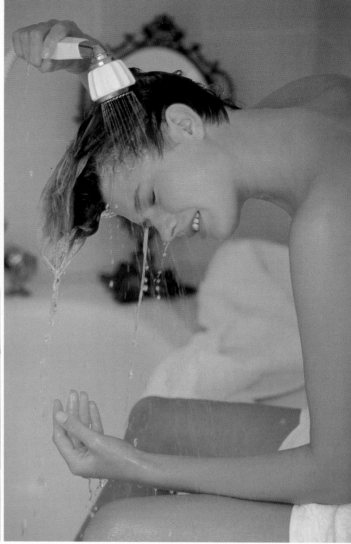

ABOVE **When removing oil after a head massage use shampoo first before rinsing.**

Applying oil

It is best to use around 10 ml (2 teaspoons) of oil for a head and shoulder massage. This may seem like a generous quantity but the hair does tend to absorb a lot of oil. The amount of oil you use will depend on your massage partner's hair length, skin texture and preference – and this can be adjusted on subsequent occasions. You need enough oil to allow your hands to 'slip' over the skin in a smooth and comfortable way and to prevent the hair roots being unduly stressed by the massage, but not so much that your hands slide and you are unable to feel the underlying tissues.

Pour the oil into a small plastic bowl or plastic bottle. Glass is best avoided as it can easily slip through greasy hands. Place the container on a paper towel on a nearby surface. If you are using a bottle, choose one with an easy-to-use dispenser so that you can replenish the oil easily. With a small bowl, you can easily dip in one or two fingers if you need more. If there is any oil left in the bowl at the end of the massage, throw it away immediately. Do not use it again, as it might spread infection.

Oil is best applied warm, as this provides a far more pleasant sensation and encourages absorption of the natural healing chemicals in the oils. Skin temperature, or a little warmer, is ideal. Warm the blended oil by placing the receptacle near a heat source or pour some oil into one hand and rub your hands together briskly.

• When washing out oil from your hair, put a small amount of shampoo directly on to your hair. The shampoo emulsifies the oil and can then be rinsed off more easily with warm water. Do not wet your hair first as the water will prevent the oil from combining with the shampoo and even after several washes, a film of oil will remain on the hair.

Oils for hair types

Different types of hair have their own unique properties – and often problems – and so, when planning to give an Indian head massage, for the best results choose the most appropriate carrier and essential oils.

Normal hair

Normal hair is glossy and strong with plenty of body and bounce. It is an indication of good health and well-being.

CARRIER OILS TO CHOOSE coconut, jojoba, sunflower.
ESSENTIAL OILS TO CHOOSE lavender, patchouli, rose, rosemary.

Dry hair

This type of hair tends to be coarse, brittle and lacklustre. It tangles easily and may be fly-away and hard to control. Dryness is often caused by over-exposure to the dehydrating rays of the sun, or the use of strong shampoos, heated hair appliances, chemical treatments and colourants.

CARRIER OILS TO CHOOSE coconut, jojoba, olive, sunflower, sweet almond.
ESSENTIAL OILS TO CHOOSE frankincense, jasmine, rose, sandalwood.

Greasy hair

Greasy hair tends to be rather dull and lank. It sticks to the scalp and is difficult to style. Oiliness tends to be due to a fatty diet, stress or hormonal changes, which can lead to over-active sebaceous glands (oil glands in the skin). Oily hair is common during puberty and around menstruation.

CARRIER OILS TO CHOOSE jojoba, sesame, sweet almond.
ESSENTIAL OILS TO CHOOSE geranium, lavender, rosemary, sandalwood.

Dandruff

A common scalp complaint – dandruff is often itchy and can be embarrassing, but it is not contagious. Dandruff is thought to be due to an excessive buildup of dead skin cells that are not removed by washing. The underlying cause has not been positively identified, but stress, fatigue, cold weather and a poor diet can all play a part. There are two types – dry and oily. Dry dandruff is characterized by dry, white flakes; oily dandruff by yellow, sticky flakes.

CARRIER OILS TO CHOOSE coconut, sweet almond.
ESSENTIAL OILS TO CHOOSE geranium, lavender, patchouli, rosemary, sandalwood.

Greying hair

This is associated with hereditary factors and the ageing process. Poor nutrition and prolonged stress can also contribute. A well-balanced diet and stress-relieving measures, including Indian head massage, are useful preventative steps to take.

CARRIER OILS TO CHOOSE olive, sesame.
ESSENTIAL OILS TO CHOOSE Roman chamomile.

Hair loss

To a certain degree, hair loss is perfectly natural. We can shed as many as 100 hairs every day, under normal circumstances. Excessive hair loss, however, can often indicate a problem, such as hormonal imbalance, high stress levels, extreme dieting, or muscular tension that hinders the blood circulation to the scalp. Chemical treatments often exacerbate the problem. Indian head massage can help reduce hair loss by encouraging mental and physical relaxation and stimulating the circulation. Avoid using vigorous massage movements if the hair is very thin, and do not tug on the hair.

CARRIER OILS TO CHOOSE mustard, sesame.
ESSENTIAL OILS TO CHOOSE geranium, lavender, Roman chamomile, rosemary.

- If you are seriously concerned about the condition of your scalp or hair, consult your doctor who may suggest a referral to a trichologist – a specialist in treating hair problems.

Nice or nasty?

Carrier and essential oils each have their own specific properties that should obviously be taken into account when choosing a lubricant for massage. However, the aroma is of particular importance. Give your massage partner the chance to 'follow his nose' by offering a selection of appropriate oils – he will know instinctively which is best for him.

If you or your massage partner strongly dislike a particular essential or carrier oil, then do not use it. If you get the opportunity, you might like to try a few different oils before you buy. Pat just a little amount on the inside of your wrist (as you would perfume) to get the best effect.

- The healing properties of essential oils have been known for many centuries. Hieroglyphics show that the ancient Egyptians used aromatic oils in their medicines. But the treatment system known as 'aromatherapy' dates back only to the 1930s. This system was devised by the French cosmetic chemist Prof René Gattefosse who burnt his hand during an accident at his laboratory. He plunged his hand into the nearest bowl of liquid, which happened to be pure lavender oil, and the pain eased immediately. His hand healed quickly with minimal scarring and there was no sign of infection. He was so amazed by his discovery that he began a study of essential oils and called his findings 'aromatherapie'.

Carrier oils

There are many types of carrier oil. The most commonly used in Indian head massage are coconut, mustard, olive, sesame, sunflower, sweet almond and jojoba. The one to choose depends on special requirements, personal preference and whether the oil is tolerated by the skin type.

Coconut (Cocos nucifera)

A cream-coloured semi-solid 'oil' derived from the dried flesh of the coconut. It is popular in the southern regions of India and is recommended for Indian head massage. It is a light oil that can be used on its own, in combination with other carrier oils or blended with essential oils. It is virtually odourless and mixes well with fragranced oils. Coconut oil is highly refined, so many of its nutrients have been destroyed, but it has softening/moisturizing qualities.

A common ingredient in many hair and skin care preparations, coconut oil is suitable for all skin and hair types and gives hair a glossy shine. Solid coconut oil liquifies when warmed. Warm by placing the bottle near a radiator or in a jug of hot water for a few minutes. Pour as much as you need into a bowl and stir before use. The oil left in the bottle will set as it cools and can be re-used. Fractionated or light coconut oil, which remains liquid at a wider range of temperature, is also available.

CAUTION May irritate sensitive skin. Test before using by applying a little oil to the skin and waiting for any reaction. Do not use in cases of nut allergy.

CASE STUDY

SNEEZES AND SNUFFLES

Generally very fit and healthy, Tony, 74, started suffering from recurrent coughs and colds after the death of a good friend left him feeling rather low. It seemed that as soon as one infection cleared, he caught another. His skin looked dull and his hair lost its usual shine. 'When the sniffles prevented me from going to my grandson's birthday party, I decided to do something about my health,' he explained. 'I went straight to our local health food store and was advised that stress may be lowering my immune system and that I should take some positive steps toward better health. One of the suggestions was a course of six Indian head massages.

'I liked the therapist as soon as I met her. She asked me lots of questions about my past and present health and lifestyle. I was pleased that she didn't put my health complaints down to old age but said that she would try to help my body rebalance itself. After the second session I had another dreadful cold and didn't go for a couple of weeks, but as soon as I had recovered I went straight back. Within a couple of months I felt on great form. My skin looked better than ever and the oils gave my hair a lovely soft feel. I have a head massage about once a month now – it's a real treat and it seems to keep the coughs and colds at bay. I have only had one cold in the last three months and that only lasted a few days.'

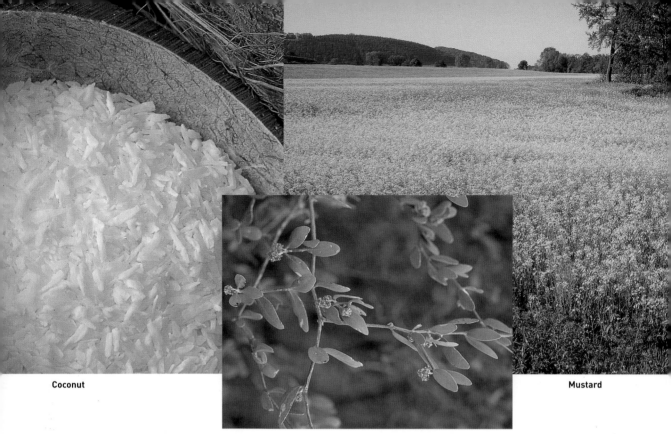

Coconut

Mustard

Jojoba

Jojoba *(Simmondsia chinensis)*

Jojoba (pronounced ho-ho-ba) oil comes from the fruit of an evergreen desert plant. It is extremely popular for skin and hair care and keeps well. It is an almost colourless, odourless liquid wax that is semi-solid at room temperature and solidifies when refrigerated. Excellent for all skin and hair types, jojoba oil contains vitamin E, protein and minerals, which are readily absorbed into the skin to give a moisturizing effect.

It has a similar structure to sebum and combines with it to remove the dirt, grease and grime that can block pores. It can also help reduce muscular aches and pains. As it is very expensive, it is best to use jojoba in very small quantities – dilute it in the ratio 10:90 with another carrier oil.

CAUTION Generally well tolerated.

Mustard *(Brassica nigra)*

Mustard oil is a highly viscous, deep-yellow liquid, with a very pungent odour. It should not be confused with the non-greasy mustard essential oil, which is not suitable for home use. Mustard oil is popular in India, especially in West Bengal. The oil is extracted from the seeds of the plant, which has long been prized for its medicinal uses. The crushed seeds are used in Ayurvedic medicine to help aid digestion and stomach disorders. Mustard oil is often used on its own as it has a powerful scent that does not mix well with essential oils. Mustard oil is very heavy and warming, a useful oil in the winter months. It helps stimulate the circulation of blood to the scalp and creates a warming, relaxing sensation that eases muscular tension, pain and stiffness. The best place to buy this oil is an Indian grocer's shop, where it is sold at a very reasonable price.

CAUTION May cause some irritation on sensitive skins. Test before using by applying a little oil to the skin and waiting for any reaction.

Olive *(Olea europea)*

Olive oil is a yellow-green, viscous liquid, derived from the fruits of the olive tree. It is readily available in most supermarkets and health food stores and is a useful oil for both massage and cooking. Look for products labelled 'virgin' and 'extra virgin', which contain high levels of unsaturated fatty acids and help moisturize dry skin and hair. Olive oil has similar properties to sesame oil and can help ease muscle pain and stiffness. It can be used on its own but, as it is rather thick and pungent, is best mixed 50:50 with another carrier oil, such as sweet almond.

CAUTION Generally well tolerated.

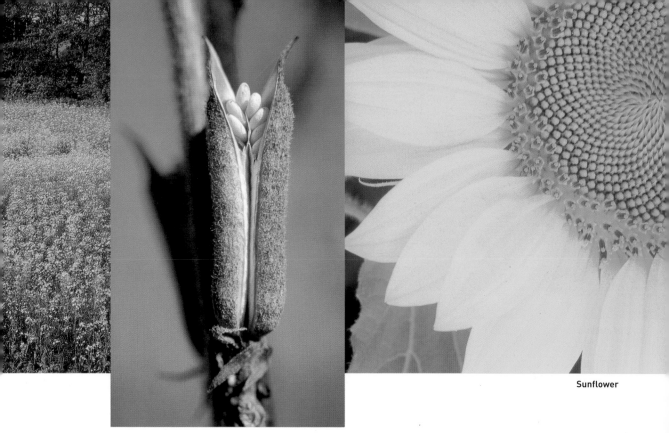

Sesame

Sunflower

Sesame (*Sesamum indicum*)

One of the most popular oils for massage in India, sesame oil is highly regarded in Ayurvedic medicine, both for internal and external use, and is reputed to prevent hair from turning grey. It is a golden-yellow, viscous liquid, derived from the untoasted seeds of the sesame plant, and has a light, slightly nutty aroma. Do not confuse it with the dark-brown sesame oil used in cooking. That oil is made from toasted sesame seeds and has a very strong smell.

Sesame oil is generally used on its own, but it can be mixed with other vegetable oils or blended with an essential oil such as sandalwood. Rich in vitamin E, iron and phosphorus, it is recommended for all skin and hair types and can help to ease muscular pains and stiffness. **CAUTION May irritate sensitive skin (olive oil is an alternative). Test before using by applying a little oil on to the skin and waiting for any reaction.**

Sunflower (*Helianthus annus*)

This produces a light, pleasant oil that is useful to keep at home for both massage and culinary purposes. Look for unrefined, organically produced sunflower seed oil, which is available in many health food stores. It is a viscous, golden-yellow liquid, with a sweet, nutty aroma, which is derived from the seeds of the sunflower plant. Organic, unrefined sunflower oil is often used in body massage. It can be used on its own or blended with other oils. It mixes especially well with many essential oils, including frankincense and lavender. The unrefined, organic oil contains high amounts of unsaturated fatty acids and vitamins A, B, D and E and is suitable for all skin types, especially dry skin. **CAUTION Generally well tolerated.**

Sweet almond (*Prunus amygdalus*)

Sweet almond oil is extracted from the kernels of the sweet almond tree. It is a pale yellow, viscous liquid with a mild fragrance. The oil is light and can be used on its own or as a blend. It is widely available, highly versatile and mixes well with most carrier and pure essential oils, especially Roman chamomile. Popular as a body massage oil, it is rich in unsaturated fatty acids and protein. It also contains vitamin A, some B vitamins and small amounts of vitamins E and D. Almond oil is often added to hair conditioners as it helps soften and protect the hair. It is useful for easing muscular pain and stiffness. **CAUTION Well tolerated by most skin types. Do not use in cases of nut allergy. Do not confuse sweet almond oil with the oil made from bitter almonds, which has culinary applications but is never used in massage.**

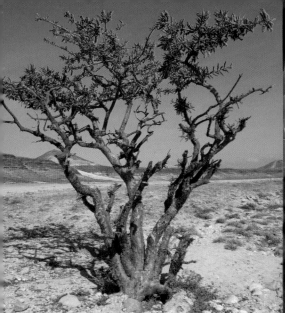
Frankincense

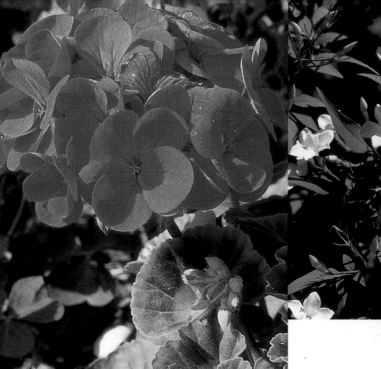
Geranium

Recommended essential oils

These oils are safe to use as long as you dilute them with a carrier oil in the correct proportions and follow safety guidelines. Ask a qualified aromatherapist.about other essential oils to use.

Frankincense (Boswellia carteri)

This is pale yellow or green with a warm, sweet, spicy aroma. Frankincense was one of the three gifts presented to baby Jesus by the three Wise Kings. It was so highly regarded at the time that it was almost as precious as gold. It is a balancing oil often used in meditation to aid concentration and focus thought. It is said to promote spiritual growth and help break links with the past. Throughout history, frankincense has been burnt on altars and in temples during religious rituals and applied to the sick to disperse evil spirits.

Frankincense can aid relaxation and lift mental and physical lethargy. It helps induce deep, slow breathing, especially when used in an aromatherapy burner or sprinkled on a handkerchief, and so can help clear sinus congestion. Suitable for all skin and hair types, it moisturizes dull, mature skin, acts as an astringent for oily skin and hair, and may also improve skin tone.

CAUTION Generally well tolerated. Not to be used in pregnancy or for babies and children.

Geranium (Pelargonium graveolens)

This is clear or pale-green with a fairly powerful sweet, refreshing, floral scent. It is a calming, strengthening and balancing oil that has a normalizing effect on the sebaceous glands, so making it useful for all skin conditions. Geranium is especially beneficial for improving the condition of very dry or very oily hair and skin. It is mildly astringent, a good skin cleanser and helpful for treating dandruff and head lice. Geranium oil is reputed to stimulate the blood circulation and boost the lymphatic system for speedy disposal of toxins and excess fluids from the body. It is often used to ease menstrual and menopausal tension and can help alleviate tension headaches.

Geranium is a versatile oil with a lovely scent. In Victorian England, geranium blooms were left at the sides of stairs so that the women's long skirts would brush against them and release the delightful perfume. The oil can be used to both soothe and uplift as it is a tonic for depression and has a calming influence on an over-active mind. Geraniums were traditionally grown in gardens and homes to keep evil spirits away. Try diffusing geranium oil into the atmosphere to create a harmonious mood in your home.

CAUTION May irritate very sensitive skin. Test by applying a little diluted oil to the skin and waiting for any reaction. Not to be used in pregnancy or for babies and children.

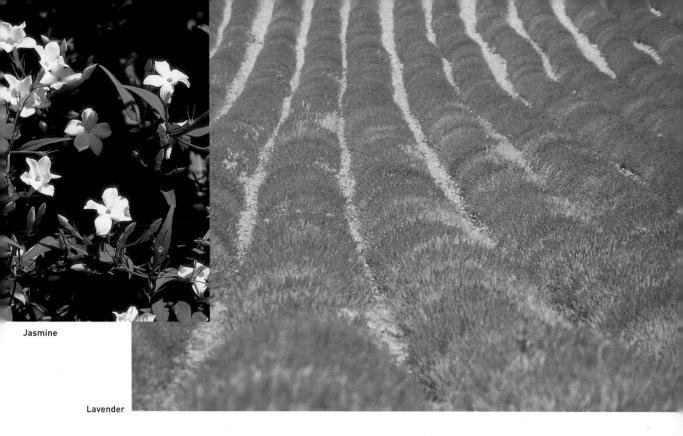

Jasmine

Lavender

Jasmine *(Jasminum officinalis)*

This is dark orange-brown with a rich, warm, heady, oriental aroma that tends to linger. Jasmine is known in India as 'queen of the night' or 'moonlight of the grove' because the scent of the delicate flowers is most intense at night. It is also called 'king of perfumes' because of its exotic fragrance, which is popularly used in soaps, toiletries, cosmetics and perfumes. Jasmine is a very common ingredient in hair oils in India and is beneficial for all skin types, especially dry, sensitive skin. It also has an ancient reputation as an aphrodisiac – Cleopatra is said to have bathed in jasmine oil to help make her seem more desirable to her beloved Anthony.

Jasmine is a balancing oil that can be uplifting and relaxing, revitalizing and restorative. It helps create feelings of optimism, emotional warmth and self-confidence. It is often used to deepen and regulate breathing, and is useful in massage for relieving pain and relaxing tense muscles. Jasmine essential oil is costly and should be used sparingly. You can use a pre-blended massage oil to experience the benefits of jasmine.
CAUTION Use very sparingly – the aroma can be quite intoxicating – one drop in 30 ml. It may cause irritation on very sensitive skins. Test before using by applying a little diluted oil to the skin and waiting for any reaction. Not to be used in pregnancy or for babies and children.

Lavender *(Lavendula angustifolio)*

This is clear or faintly yellow with a light, fresh, floral aroma. Lavender is a balancing, normalizing oil with cleansing properties. The name derives from the Latin word lavare meaning 'to wash'. In Tudor times, women scattered lavender over their floors to cleanse and deodorize the rooms. Lavender oil can help regulate sebum production, so it is suitable for all skin and hair types. It is also useful for clearing dandruff, stimulating hair growth and repelling head lice.

On an emotional level, lavender helps induce feelings of composure, peace, contentment and tranquillity. It can be used to lift anxiety and depression, harmonize mood swings and ease tension headaches. A natural sedative, lavender oil is often used to prevent insomnia and aid restful sleep. Sprinkle two drops on a handkerchief and place inside your pillow at night. Lavender oil is also helpful in first aid for burns, stings, bites, bruises and wounds, as it has painkilling and antiseptic qualities that aid the healing process.
CAUTION May not be tolerated well by people with hay fever, asthma or other allergic conditions. Not to be used in pregnancy or for babies and children.

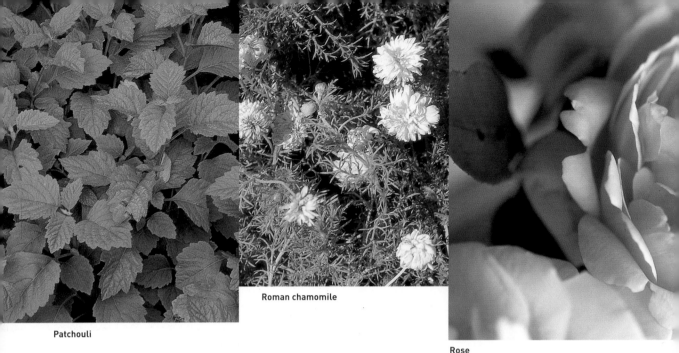

Roman chamomile

Patchouli

Rose

Patchouli *(Pogostemon cablin)*

This is dark-amber or reddish-brown with a rich, heavy, earthy, musky, sensuous aroma that people tend either to strongly like or dislike. Patchouli oil is often added to carrier oils for its exotic scent. It is highly evocative of the 1960s as it was the principal ingredient in many of the body perfumes of that era. In the East, dried patchouli leaves are used to perfume linen and fabrics, as the strong scent helps mask unpleasant odours and is thought to prevent the spread of disease and infection and to repel moths. Patchouli become popular in Britain during Victorian times, when cashmere shawls imported from India were a fashionable accessory. These shawls retained the lingering scent of the patchouli that was used for their transportation.

Patchouli is a balancing oil that is used for many stress-related disorders. It can promote relaxation and help calm a troubled mind. It moisturizes dry, mature skin and aids the shedding of dead skin cells. Patchouli can help ease scalp problems such as dandruff and improve the condition of oily hair and skin. It is also reputed to be an aphrodisiac.
CAUTION The aroma is not to everyone's liking. Always use very sparingly. Not to be used in pregnancy or for babies and children.

Roman chamomile *(Chamaemelum nobile)*

Pale yellow in colour, Roman chamomile has a mild, sweet, slightly fruity aroma. The ancient Egyptians held chamomile in such high regard that the plant was declared sacred and dedicated to Ra, the sun god. It is a gentle, calming oil with a pleasant aroma that helps relax mind and body. A wonderful oil to use at the end of a long, tiring, stressful day, it can lift anxiety, doubts and worries. Roman chamomile is beneficial for any stress-related disorder including tension headaches and insomnia. Commonly used in hair rinses, Roman chamomile has a lightening effect on fair hair and adds lustre and colour to grey hair. It is a good oil to choose for dry skin and hair conditions. It should be used very sparingly, however – one drop to 30 ml (6 teaspoons).
CAUTION It may cause irritation on sensitive skins. Test before using by applying a little diluted oil to the skin and waiting for any reaction. Not to be used in pregnancy or for babies and children.

Rose *(Rosa centifolia; Rosa damascena)*

So pale-yellow as to be almost colourless, rose has a deep, sweet floral smell. It is traditionally considered a 'female' oil and associated with Venus, the Roman goddess of love and beauty. The Romans crowned their brides and bridegrooms with roses. Rose petals are collected at sunrise, when their scent is strongest, and processed within 24 hours. It takes around thirty roses to make a single drop of oil, which accounts for the high price. However, it is a very versatile and pleasant oil to use. It suits all skin and hair types and is a very effective moisturizer for dry, mature and sensitive skins. Rose-water is a mild, soothing, lightly perfumed tonic that can be used in massage if your partner has a greasy scalp.

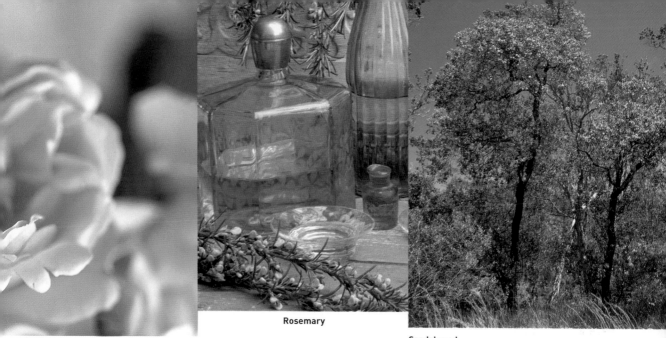

Rosemary

Sandalwood

Rose aids meditation and relaxation and encourages mental alertness and optimism. It may help ease the symptoms of some menstrual disorders and is believed to stimulate the lymphatic system. Like jasmine, rose essential oil is expensive and should be used in small qualities. It is often sold ready diluted in a base oil, but do follow the instructions on the label very carefully to ensure that you use the correct amount.

CAUTION Generally well tolerated but may cause a reaction in some very sensitive people. Use one drop per 30 ml of carrier oil. Test by applying a little diluted oil to the skin. Not to be used in pregnancy or for babies and children.

Rosemary (Rosmarinus officinalis)

This is clear or very pale yellow with a strong, fresh aroma. Rosemary has long been associated with improving brain power and mental alertness. The Greeks used to put twigs of rosemary in their hair to help boost concentration, while Ophelia in Shakespeare's *Hamlet* refers to its memory-enhancing powers: 'There's rosemary, that's for remembrance.' It is an excellent oil to diffuse in an aromatherapy burner while studying or meditating.

Rosemary is an invigorating, energizing oil that can help stimulate the blood circulation to the scalp and so improve the condition of the hair and promote its growth. It is said to enhance the colour of dark hair. It has an astringent action that helps tighten skin and harmonize greasy hair and skin. Rosemary is a useful oil to treat dandruff and protect against head lice.

CAUTION May irritate very sensitive skin. Test before using by applying a little diluted oil to the skin and waiting for any reaction. Do not use if the person suffers from epilepsy or high blood pressure. Not to be used in pregnancy or for babies and children.

Sandalwood (Santalum album)

This is clear or pale-green with a sweet, woody, sensual, distinctly oriental aroma that lingers for a long time. Sandalwood is included in the ancient Ayurvedic texts as an important therapeutic plant. In its powdered form, sandalwood is a popular incense and has been used as an aid to meditation for at least 4,000 years. The wood was used in India for sacred carvings and in the building of ancient temples. Sandalwood trees are now protected in India and regarded as the property of the Indian government. One of the oldest known scented materials, the aroma of sandalwood eases nervous tension and anxiety, making it a useful aid to relaxation and self-healing. It is also reputed to boost the immune system and induce restful sleep.

The diluted essential oil can help soothe and soften dry, mature skin and acts as a mild astringent for oily skin and hair. It is known to help relieve itching and so may ease the irritation caused by dandruff.

CAUTION May not be well-tolerated by people with very sensitive skins. Look for the highest quality oil, which comes from the Mysore region of India. Test before using by applying a little diluted oil to the skin and waiting for any reaction. Not to be used in pregnancy or for babies and children.

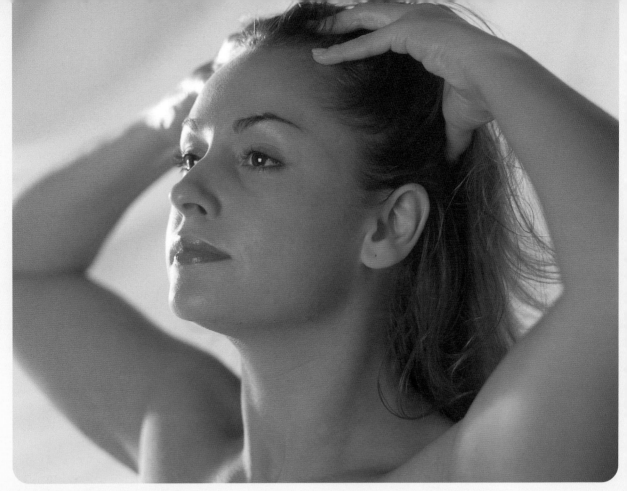

ABOVE **Treat yourself to a head massage.**

Self-massage

Follow the tradition of Indian women and give yourself
an oily scalp massage once a week to encourage your
locks to grow strong, shiny and more manageable.
Massage stimulates the flow of blood and lymph through
the scalp, bringing fresh supplies of oxygen and
nutrients to the hair follicles and removing any toxins
and waste products that could hinder healthy growth.
Natural vegetable oils can help cleanse, nourish and
improve the condition of your scalp and moisturize,
strengthen and protect your hair, helping to promote a
glossy sheen.

There is no need to shampoo your hair first unless it is
very dirty. If you wash your hair before massage, towel it dry
before you begin. Comb through with a wide-tooth comb.
• Scalp massage with oil is very beneficial for dry hair or
  hair that has been treated with chemicals. However,
  do wait a week after a perm or other treatment using
  chemicals to allow your hair to settle. If you have any
  doubts, ask your hairdresser.

Choose an oil or blend of oils to suit your hair type and
mood. Rub some oil into your hands and then, working
from the front of your head to the back, stroke it evenly
all over your scalp. Now place your hands in a claw-like
position on your head, fingers well spread-out, and
make small rotations with the pads of your fingers and
thumbs all over your scalp. The pressure should be firm
but comfortable. Feel your scalp moving beneath your
fingers. Keep your fingers moving so you do not spend
too long working on the same area.

Self-massage can make your arms ache, so try resting
your elbows on a table. Continue for at least five minutes
until you have covered the whole of your head. Include the
hair line and temples where muscles tend to get very
tense, so restricting the flow of blood to the hair follicles.
You may also like to try some of the other movements
from the step-by-step suggestions in the following
chapters. Finish with some gentle stroking movements to
soothe and relax. Cover your head with a warm towel and
rest. It is best to keep the oil on your head for at least half
an hour before washing to gain maximum benefits.

Top-to-toe massage

A weekly full-body massage using organic vegetable oils is an integral part of Ayurvedic recommendations for a long and healthful life. It is obviously not as enjoyable as being massaged by someone else, but it is a very good way of keeping your skin and hair in good condition and also of giving you time to get in touch with your body. This routine is quick, simple and effective. Use an unrefined carrier oil or a special massage blend. Sesame oil is generally favoured for a full body massage in Ayurvedic medicine, but you may prefer to choose an oil with a more fragrant aroma.

- Undress and sit or stand on a towel you have spread out on the floor in a warm and comfortable place. Apply your chosen oil all over the body. Start with your head and massage your scalp with small, circular strokes.
- Now move downward, covering your entire body: face and arms first, then chest, legs and feet. Use the flat of your hand, not just your fingertips, to perform upward massage strokes, directing the venous blood flow back to the heart. Apply more vigorous strokes on your head, arms and legs and moderate pressure to the rest of your body. Be gentle over your face and abdomen. Use long strokes on the straight areas of your body, such as arms and legs, and large circular strokes over rounded areas and joints, such as elbows and hips.
- At the end of the massage, sit quietly for a few minutes and practise a relaxation technique (see page 252). If possible, leave the oil on your skin for at least twenty minutes before showering.
- If you do not have time for a full-body massage, just apply a lightly fragranced carrier oil to your face, neck and feet. This will only take a couple of minutes. Undress and wrap a warm towel around you. Sit on another towel. Apply the oil to your forehead, temples, ears and neck in gentle soothing strokes. Now massage oil into the soles of your feet. Sit quietly for a few minutes before washing your feet in warm water. This is a very relaxing massage to have just before bedtime.

Shirodhara

An Ayurvedic treatment session often concludes with a luxuriously relaxing technique known as Shirodhara, pictured below. After a head massage, warm sesame oil is dripped over the centre of the forehead in a slow, steady stream. In Ayurveda, the middle of the forehead marks the position of the 'third eye', an area of great spiritual significance. Shirodhara can continue for up to an hour and is reputed to help lift depression and relieve mental fatigue.

BELOW **Ayurvedic treatment in Sri Lanka.**

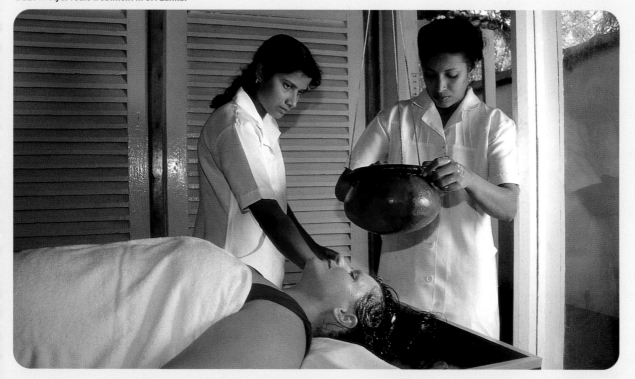

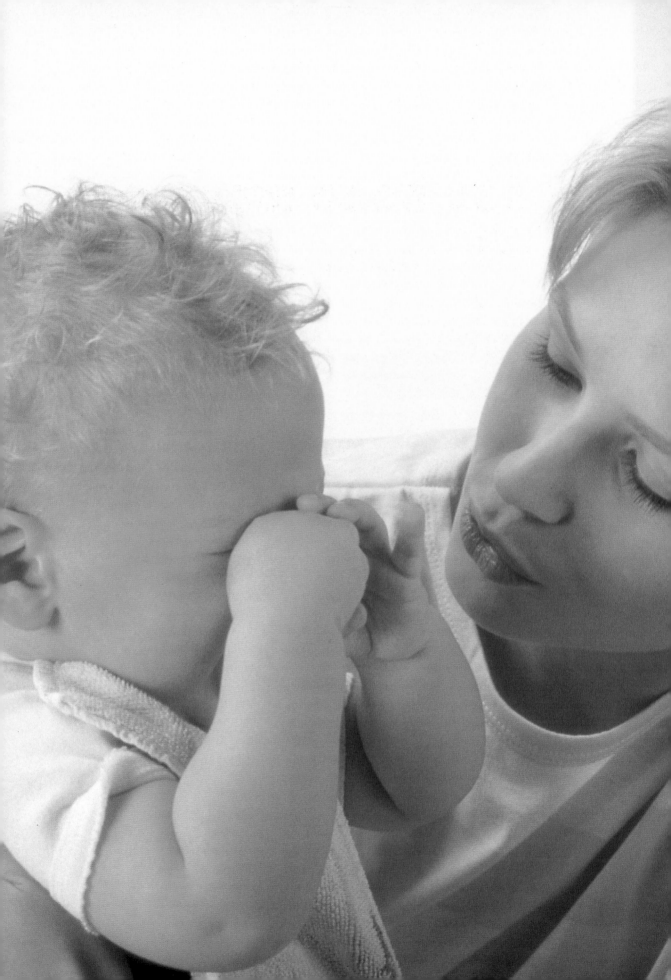

Indian head massage
techniques

Massage is a basic, nurturing instinct that we all share. We use our natural healing power of touch in our everyday lives, often without realizing it. Think how we instinctively rub a sore spot to ease the pain or offer comforting strokes to reassure an anxious child. These are all basic forms of massage that have been practised all over the world since ancient times. Indian head massage develops these intuitive skills into a flowing sequence of therapeutic movements. In India, the skills of massage are passed down through the generations. Children, who are massaged regularly from a very young age, instinctively pick up the techniques through their own experience. When they grow up and have children of their own they, in turn, share them with their offspring. Each person naturally acquires their own particular style. This can be readily adapted to suit the individual by including favourite movements or varying the speed and pressure of strokes in order to relax or stimulate.

Types of massage stroke

Massage of any kind can be classed as the manipulation of the body's soft tissues – the skin, fat and muscle and the connective tissue that holds the organs and underlying structures in place. It involves a series of movements using the hands. Each movement is applied in a particular way in order to have a specific effect on the area being massaged. Once you appreciate the essential differences between the actions and the benefits of the various manipulations, you can try other combinations of strokes and devise your own safe and effective routines to suit different occasions.

- With practice, you will learn to use your hands to detect factors that will influence your style of massage, such as the tightness of muscles, areas of tension, amount of fat and skin texture.

For ease of understanding, the different rubbing, squeezing, pressing, kneading, patting and tapping movements are classified by means of the widely recognized terminology of Swedish-style massage. This system was developed by physiologist Per Henrik Ling in the early 1800s and is now taught internationally to massage students. The main movements are stroking, effleurage, petrissage, frictions and tapotement. It is not easy to learn these movements from a book. Do remember, however, that the secret of a good massage is in applying each stroke with care and affection to make your partner feel nurtured and secure.

- Do not worry if you feel clumsy or awkward when you start to practise these different techniques. You will be pleasantly surprised at how quickly your movements begin to flow.

Stroking

Stroking is particularly effective on the face and scalp. These areas are well supplied with a mass of sensory nerve endings that quickly respond to touch and can strongly influence the way you feel, both mentally and physically. Soft stroking has an almost soporific effect on your mind and body, while faster, more energetic stroking will revitalize you, lifting lethargy and weariness. An Indian head massage often combines both gentle and brisk stroking to relax and refresh. A massage usually begins with gentle stroking in any direction to apply the oil to the scalp and help your partner get used to the sensation of touch. Gentle stroking is a slow, light and superficial gliding movement designed to soothe and relax the sensory nerves. It is the kind of smooth, rhythmical, repetitive action we naturally use to pacify a baby or stroke a pet. Your hands are open and supple so they mould to the shape of the part being massaged.

Brisk stroking or rubbing is widely used in Indian head massage. However, in the West, we tend to prefer a lighter touch rather than the more powerful approach adopted by Indian masseurs using traditional methods. Your hands work very briskly over the surface of the skin using short, invigorating movements back and forth in any direction – rather like rubbing out a mistake with an eraser. Wrists are flexible, with fingers held quite straight. Depending on the size of the area being massaged, you can use the palm, side or heel of the hand, or the pads of several fingers. Rubbing stimulates the blood supply to the local blood vessels and warms the area. This is, in fact, our natural response when we feel chilly – we rub the cold area briskly to generate warmth.

- You can give a very pleasurable massage by using stroking and effleurage movements alone. Change the overall effect by altering the pressure, speed, direction and length of stroke. Try it on yourself to feel how different variations have their own special impact.

BELOW **Stroking can be soft and gentle to promote a calming and soothing effect or brisk and energetic to revitalize.**

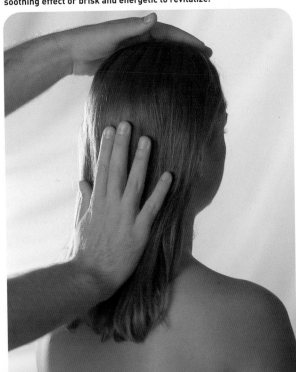

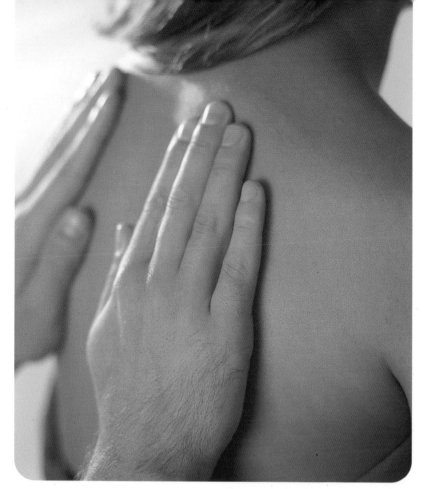

ABOVE **Effleurage is the use of pressure to create a light or firm stroke.**

Effleurage

This is a similar movement to stroking but is generally a firmer, smoothing action. It is like the relaxed hands of a sculptor moulding the contours of a piece of clay. Effleurage helps improve the superficial blood circulation – the stroke follows the direction of the venous flow back to the heart. If the stroke is directed toward the nearest set of lymph nodes, it also aids lymphatic drainage, so helping the body rid itself of toxins. Keep your wrists flexible and your hands supple. Your pressure should increase slightly toward the end of the stroke and then return with a light touch, maintaining some hand or finger contact at all times. On larger areas, like the upper back, use the palm of one or both hands. On smaller areas, use the soft pads of your thumbs or fingertips.

Slow effleurage, using moderate or light pressure, flows on naturally from gentle stroking and helps prepare the soft tissues for subsequent deeper massage movements. The underlying muscles are warmed and relaxed, thereby gradually easing any pain or soreness and allowing more freedom of movement. Once the muscles start to lose their tension, a faster effleurage action with deeper pressure can be uplifting and energizing.

- Practise whenever you get the opportunity. Hopefully, you should have no shortage of volunteers. The more you practise the movements, the more natural they become. Try massaging people of different builds, hair types and ages in order to broaden your range of experience.

Petrissage

This is a deeper movement than effleurage and so is mainly used on the muscles and fleshier areas. It is also called kneading because, as the name implies, the action is rather like kneading dough. The soft tissues are picked up and separated from the underlying structure and then compressed and released. Throughout this movement, your fingers or whole hands act like a pump, working on the deeper blood and lymph vessels to force blood and lymph back to the heart and squeeze out any toxins that have accumulated in the tissue spaces. The movement is slow and rhythmic with a deep but appropriate pressure. Be careful not to pinch and avoid working too long in one area, as this can cause discomfort and even bruising on sensitive skin.

- You may find it helpful to refer back to this chapter when you are reading the step-by-step instructions for different strokes and routines.

As with stroking and effleurage, your shoulders and wrists should be relaxed and your hands supple and moulded to the shape of the area being massaged. Your hands do not glide over the surface of the skin but press much deeper to move the skin against the soft tissues below. You will be able to feel the underlying tissues moving and feel any nodules of tension or tight adhesions as you roll the fleshy mass with your hands. Kneading is a circular movement with an increase in pressure on the upward half of the circle and a decrease on the downward half. Once the movement is complete, your hand moves smoothly to the next part so that the rhythm of the massage is not disturbed.

You can vary the kneading by using the palm and fingers of one or both hands, or the fleshy pads of fingers or thumbs. In an Indian head massage, most kneading movements are performed with the fingers or thumbs.

BELOW **Petrissage is a deeper, kneading movement made on the muscles.**

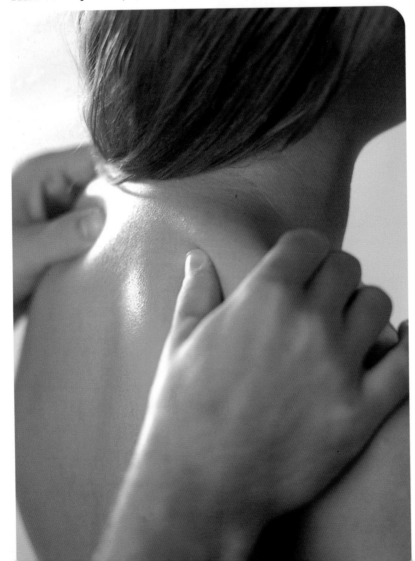

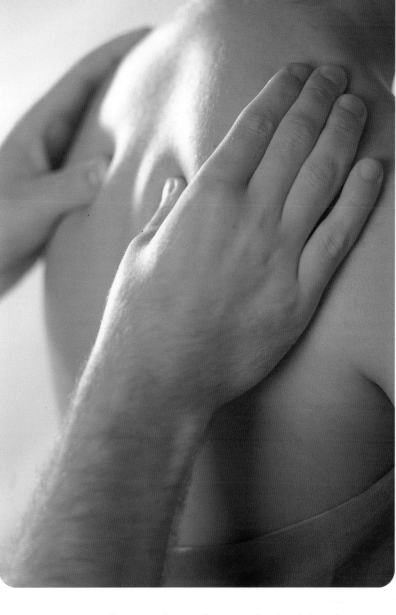

RIGHT **Frictions are deep, penetrating movements made with the pads of the fingers or thumbs.**

Frictions

Frictions are small, deep, penetrating movements that are generally carried out using the fleshy pads of the fingers or thumbs. The skin moves over the underlying structures so that one layer of tissue is pressed firmly against another. The frictions used in Indian head massage are circular, progressively increasing the pressure as you move deeper and deeper, or static, pressing on a single point. Circular frictions are an entirely different movement from finger and thumb kneading, where a mass of muscle tissue is massaged, with the pressure increasing on the upward half of the circle and decreasing on the downward half of the circle. Frictions are smaller, more specific movements that are localized on a particular spot and with a gradual increase in pressure.

Keep your fingers firm, pressing deeply by using your body weight. You can add more weight by placing one hand on top of the other or using two fingers or thumbs. Once you have completed the movement, usually after three seconds of static friction or after three complete circular movements, lift your fingers or thumbs and glide to an adjacent area.

Tense muscles can be very tender, so frictions should only be applied once the area has been warmed with more superficial movements. Start gently and increase the pressure. It may help to ask your partner to exhale as you apply the pressure and inhale as you relax the pressure. Do not work the same area for any length of time and stop at once if your partner experiences discomfort. Finish by soothing the area with stroking or effleurage.

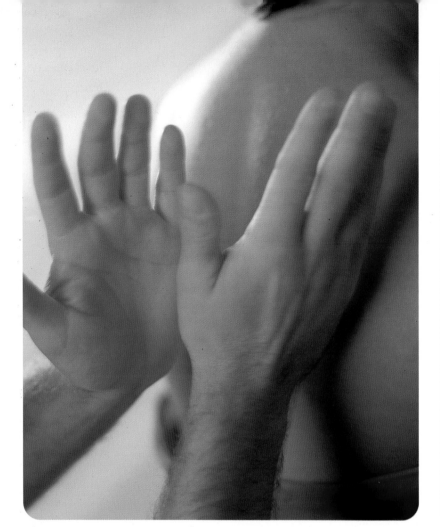

ABOVE **The rhythmical tapotement movements need to be practiced.**

CHECKLIST

BENEFITS OF TAPOTEMENT

- The tapping or striking action stimulates the sensory nerve endings in the skin and produces a feeling of exhilaration and 'get-up-and-go', especially if performed on either side of the spine.

- Tapotement, especially hacking, is very effective in increasing the flow of blood through the muscles and underlying tissues. This increased blood flow nourishes, warms and relaxes the tissues in the area.

- The alternate striking and releasing action can increase the tone in slack muscles as the fibres contract and relax in a reflex response. For this reason, it should not be performed on anyone with very tight, contracted muscles who would gain greater benefit from more relaxing movements.

- The brisk movement helps break up fatty deposits and softens areas of fatty tissue, so improving skin texture.

Tapotement

These movements, also known as percussion, involve striking or tapping the skin and then releasing in the same rapid, rhythmical way. Keep your wrists flexible and use your hands or fingers alternately to tap the skin with a light, springy movement. Your hands or fingers bounce back as soon as they land on the skin. It is best to start and finish each sequence with a lighter pressure to avoid an abrupt shock. When using these more vigorous movements, start and finish with stroking and effleurage to warm and prepare the area and then afterward to soothe the sensory nerve endings.

Tapotement movements for Indian head massage include tapping and hacking. Tapping is performed with the tips of fingers bouncing rhythmically up and down. Hacking is performed with the sides of the hands in a series of short, sharp taps. Begin hacking with your hands pushed together. Now take your elbows away from your sides and separate your hands. Keep your wrists flexible and move your forearms down and up so that the outer borders of your hands strike the area alternately. It is not a chopping action using both hands at the same time. Your hands move one after the other – strike, release, strike, release quickly and briefly in a brisk, rhythmical way. The movement comes from the elbows while your upper arms remain still. You should always work around any obviously bony areas and avoid using tapotement on a very thin person. Never hack on a very sensitive area such as the spine or face.

It takes practice to get the rhythm of hacking and if the rhythm is unbalanced it can be a very irritating. Before starting, practise hacking on different surfaces – a cushion, a kitchen work surface or a desk. Start slowly and increase speed without losing the rhythm.

- Practise these movements individually before you put them all together. Get constructive criticism from a willing partner or work on yourself to get a feel for the effect of the different manipulations.

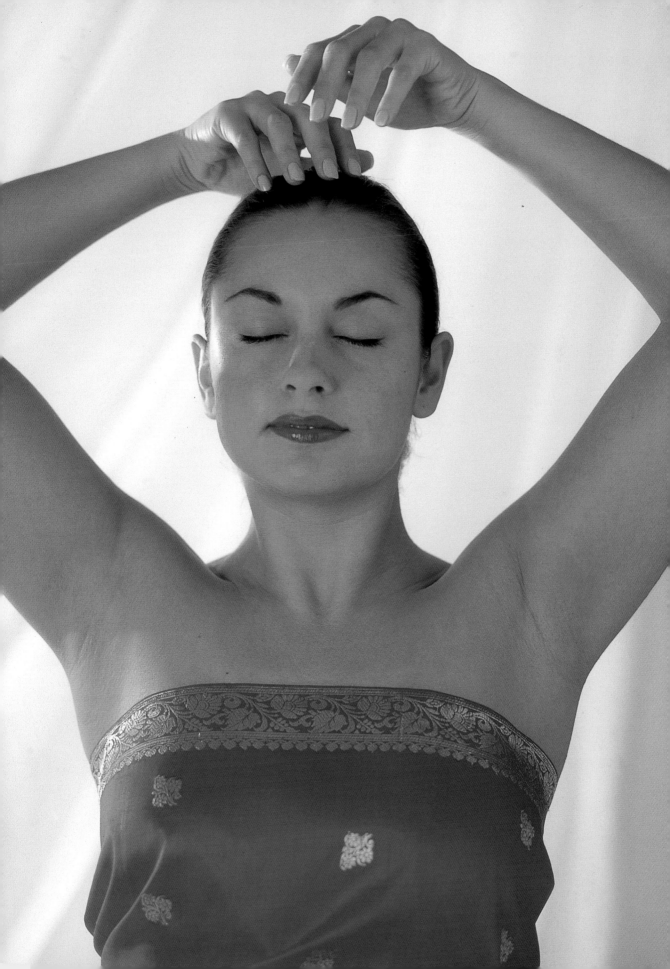

Massage guidelines

The following guidelines will help ensure a safe and effective massage.

- Always check that your partner is not suffering any conditions that may make massage inadvisable (see page 257).
- Massage should not cause severe sharp pain or discomfort. Stop if your partner feels dizzy, sick or nauseous. Ask your partner to tell you if she finds any strokes painful or in any way distressing so you can stop and quickly move on. Be guided by your partner. Never massage directly over the spine or any bony protrusions. Do not hack on the face.
- Make every effort to ensure your partner feels nurtured, cosseted and secure. Warm towels are a lovely extra. Spend time checking your partner's comfort and asking about any massage strokes that she particularly enjoys. Start with gentle, slow, caring strokes to relax and spread the oil. Slowly increase the pressure and speed.
- Be aware of your partner's body language. Around 70 per cent of all communication

RIGHT **Make sure your partner is comfortable and relaxed.**

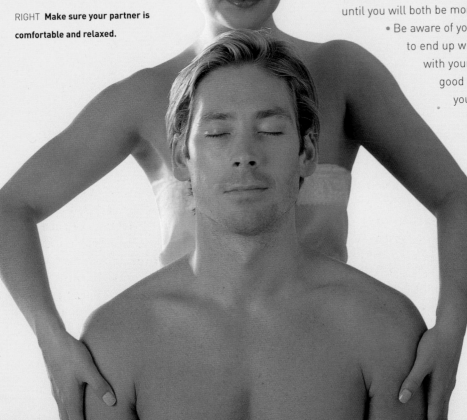

is by means of non-verbal messages and gestures. Take note of any flinching or stiffening that might indicate discomfort or unease. Similarly, look out for signs of evident enjoyment, such as relaxed breathing and a gentle purr of pleasure. Adapt your massage accordingly.

- Try not to chat too much. This will not only hinder your concentration but also upset the flow of the massage. Limit talking to a brief discussion of comfort, warmth and pressure. Background music can help discourage talk. At the start of the massage, advise your partner to let her mind empty. Discourage her from smoking, reading or looking around. Instead, encourage her to give herself totally to the massage. If her mind is still over-active, suggest that she focuses on the music, a favourite colour or the rhythm of your breathing.
- Do not massage for too long or too often. A massage of the scalp can be very powerful and stimulating – a weekly session lasting around half an hour is generally considered ideal. Be wary of being too rough, or working on the same area for too long a period, as this may lead to bruising of the skin or weakening of the hair roots.
- Choose a time when you are both in the mood for massage and there is little likelihood of being interrupted. Never try to coerce an unwilling partner, or rush a massage. If necessary, postpone the session until you will both be more receptive to the benefits.
- Be aware of your posture. You do not want to end up with aches and pains! Stand with your feet apart to maintain a good balance. You can then use your weight to increase the pressure. Keep your back straight and your shoulders comfortably relaxed.
- If you feel yourself slumping, make a conscious effort to lengthen your spine and neck. When you need to reduce your height, always bend your knees rather than your back, or kneel, if you find it more comfortable. Do not remain in one place, but

move around the chair so you do not need to strain to reach. Take deep, long and regular breaths to help calm and relax you both.

• Maintain continuity. An Indian head massage should be as fluid and rhythmical as possible, flowing smoothly between soothing, gentle movements and brisk, more vigorous movements. Try not to stop and start. If you forget a movement, improvise. Your massage partner will not notice. If you need more oil, keep one hand, or at least an elbow, in contact with your partner's skin for as long as you can. Never jerk both hands away at once as this can be surprisingly disconcerting.

• Judge the depth of the pressure. Most people prefer a fairly firm massage around their shoulders and scalp and a lighter pressure on the face, but everyone has different physical needs and a different pain threshold. Always check with your partner – if the pressure is too deep it can be painful. If your touch is too light it can be rather irritating. Either way, if the pressure is wrong the muscles will tense up in response. If an area is ticklish, try increasing the depth of the pressure or simply move on. Younger, fitter people tend to like firmer pressure, while older people and children tend to prefer a lighter massage. Decrease your pressure over sensitive or bony areas, to avoid causing pain. Be gentle over the face so you do not drag the skin. Increase pressure over larger muscles and fatty areas which may need extra work.

• Massage can be applied to relax and soothe, or to stimulate and invigorate. As a general rule, softer, slower strokes are calming, while faster, brisker movements are energizing.

• If you are using oils, always let your partner express a preference.

• Give your partner the chance to sit quietly at the end of the massage. This allows time to make a gentle transition back to the real world.

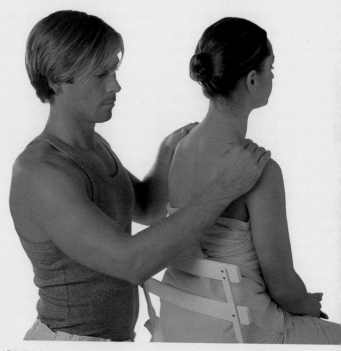

ABOVE **Use fluid and rhythmical movements for a successful massage.**

CASE STUDY

HARMONY AT HOME

Jessica, 15, says Indian head massage has helped improve her relationship with her mother. 'When my mother first started at college she kept asking to practise on me,' she explained. 'At first I wouldn't let her near my hair but I eventually gave in – as long as she didn't use any of her oils. I'm really glad that I did. It's hard to put into words the effect that it has – but it is amazing. I don't understand quite why or how you can feel so different in such a short time, but you do. 'I didn't really notice any change until after the third or fourth massage. It was quite nice to be massaged but that was it. Then I think I started relaxing, letting myself enjoy the massage. And I realized how much better I felt in myself afterward. Sort of happier and more confident. Mum has been giving me Indian head massages on and off for about six months now and we both notice that I don't get nearly so uptight as I used to – little things don't get me down so much. I feel much closer to Mum. I let her use oil now, and I'm sure my hair is less tangly and more bouncy.'

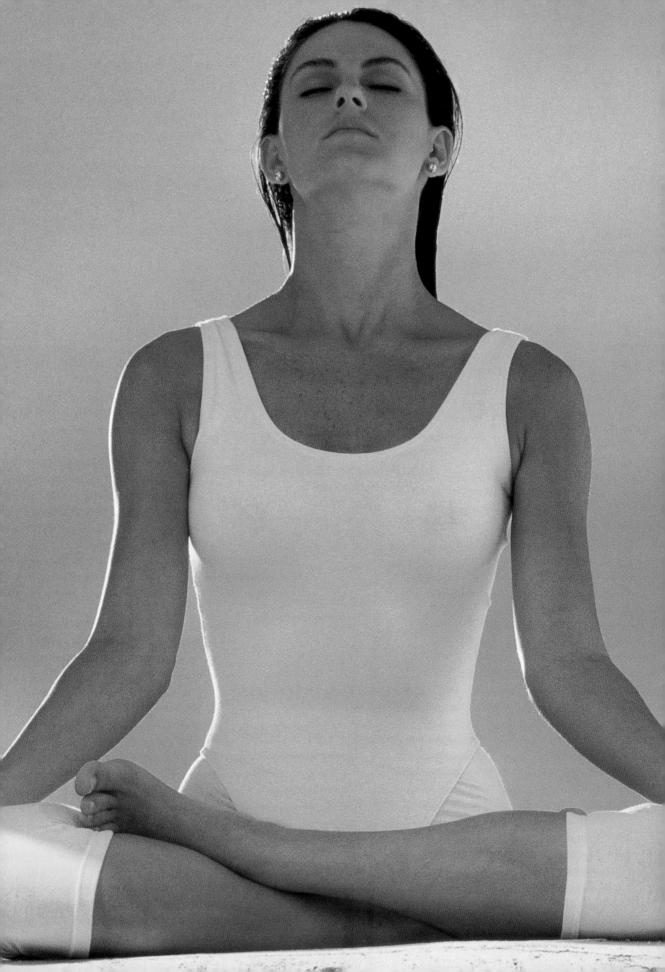

the art of
relaxation

Thorough preparation before an Indian head massage is very valuable. This includes making sure that both you and your massage partner are in a calm, relaxed state of mind, the atmosphere of the room is conducive to massage and everything you need is close at hand. It is also important to ensure that your partner is not suffering from a condition that might make massage inadvisable.

Relaxation techniques

Practising simple relaxation exercises before an Indian head massage can help your massage partner to enjoy a smooth transition from the hurly-burly of everyday life into a state of deep physical and mental ease. The chances are, however, that just telling him to 'relax' will only induce hunched shoulders and furrowed brows, so it may be helpful to offer some practical suggestions. The following relaxation techniques also offer useful strategies for managing stressful situations with inner peace, composure and serenity.

A breath of fresh air

When feeling stressed, your breathing tends to become shallow, uneven, rapid and noisy. This upsets the balance of carbon dioxide and oxygen within your body, which, in turn, leads to further physical and psychological tension. When relaxed, your breathing is deep, even, slow and quiet. The beautifully relaxed breathing of a child who is fast asleep in bed has an instantly calming effect. A good way of slowing your breathing is to focus on each breath as it enters and leaves your body – flowing smoothly and continuously in a balanced way.

1 Sit in a comfortable position, or lie on the floor, with your hands by your sides. Breathe in deeply through your nose, drawing the breath right down to your abdomen. Your abdomen should expand first, followed by your chest.
2 Rest for a moment, while still holding the breath, and then allow the breath to flow out, slowly and gently. At first, it may help you to rest your right hand on your abdomen until you get used to the feel of the movement.
3 Repeat this several times, concentrating on trying to empty the lungs. Practise this breathing technique for five minutes. If you sense that your breathing is becoming erratic, slow it down.

Step-by-step relaxation

Once you start to feel the difference between tense and relaxed muscles, you will recognize when you are holding tension and can then make a conscious effort to let go. Try the following full sequence, or a shortened version, wherever you are – watching television, while waiting for a train, or just before an important meeting. You will find that it eases aches and pains and gives you a greater sense of control and self-confidence. This progressive relaxation exercise involves tensing and relaxing the different muscles.

1 Sit or lie comfortably. Loosen any tight clothing. Breathe deeply and evenly, allowing the breath to flow to all parts of your body.
2 Tense the muscles in your forehead, hold for a count of five and then relax, releasing any tension.
3 Now concentrate on tensing the muscles of your eyes, cheeks and mouth, hold for a count of five and release.
4 Continue with your neck and shoulders, arms and fingers, first tensing and then releasing the muscles. Hunch your shoulders and then let them drop and relax – feel the tension easing. Grip your fingers tightly and then let go. It is a wonderful feeling.
5 Continue this movement working down your body, tensing, holding and relaxing the muscles.

▶ Visualizing paradise

Visualizations can help you to switch off from the stress of the daily grind and enter a more serene mental state.

1 Sit comfortably and quietly. Breathe in and out deeply and evenly. Close your eyes and imagine that you are in a pleasant location full of happy memories. You might be on a beach or in the country among the miracles of nature. Spend a few minutes in this place.
2 Use all your senses to re-create the feeling of being there, physically and emotionally. What can you see? What sounds can you hear? What can you smell or taste? Are you lying, sitting or standing? What can you feel against your skin?
3 Slowly open your eyes and gradually re-enter the real world.

Simple meditation

The following meditation is a useful aid to relaxation. Begin by meditating for a couple of minutes every day and gradually build up to twenty minutes once or twice a day. Before you start, make sure that you will not be disturbed. Set an alarm clock if you are concerned about the time.

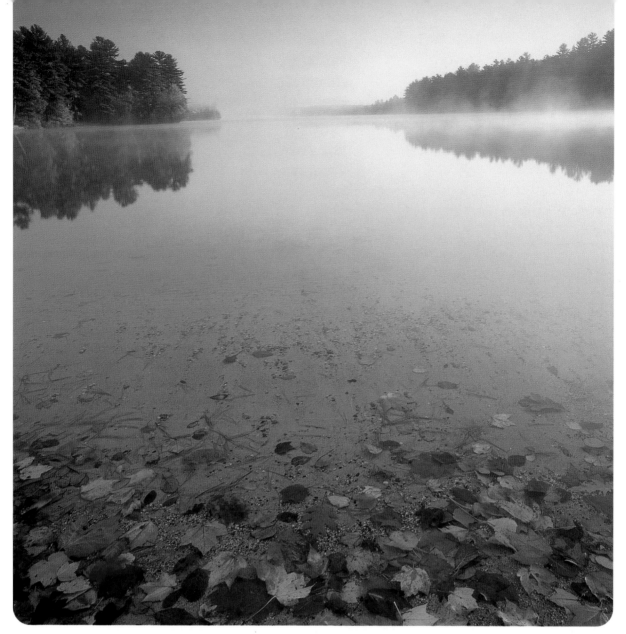

ABOVE **Visualize a scene that conjures up feelings of warmth, happiness, relaxation and serenity.**

1 Sit in a comfortable position. close your eyes and breathe in through your nose. Allow the breath to reach deep into your lungs. Exhale slowly through your mouth. Stay still and quiet for a few moments.

2 Feel your body relaxing completely. Start with the muscles of your scalp and face and slowly work down your body, releasing all the tension as you go.

3 Focus on a single word, such as 'one' or 'peace'. Keep repeating it aloud or to yourself. If you prefer, you can focus your attention on a favourite colour. Think of the colour in its lightest form. Picture it getting darker and richer, swirling around and forming exquisite patterns. Gradually, let the colour drain away so that it becomes paler and paler until it disappears altogether. At first,

all sorts of thoughts may keep coming into your head. Acknowledge them, but then go back to concentrating on your chosen word or colour.

4 It takes practice to empty the mind of stimulating thoughts or niggling problems – but it is worth the effort. A few minutes of inner silence on a regular basis is an exquisite experience with lasting benefits for physical and emotional health and well-being. Try to set aside a certain time each day to relax the tensions in your body and allow your mind to be free from daily pre-occupations. You will soon start to feel noticeably happier, calmer and more fulfilled. If you find it does not work at first, do not force yourself or try too hard. Wait a couple of days and then try again.

Feeling centred

Stress can affect your massage. Think how someone in a bad mood can alter the whole atmosphere at home or work. If you are tense and irritable, you can easily pass it on to others. If you are upset, worried or ill, your massage partner may well pick up on your negative mood. There is also a risk that you could take out your frustrations with excessively vigorous movements. And it works the other way, too. When you are feeling low or vulnerable, you are

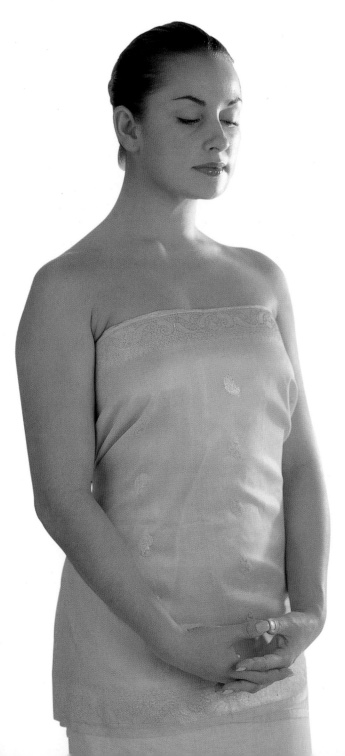

also more receptive to your massage partner's moods. To help make an Indian head massage a positive experience for the both of you, aim to get into a tranquil and confident frame of mind. This is often referred to as being 'centred' or 'grounded'. Try to create your own personal space so you can distance your emotions from those of your massage partner. The following sequence can help.

1 Take five deep breaths. As you breathe in, feel that you are absorbing calm and peace. Breathe out slowly, letting all your anxieties and tensions flow from you. Some people like to picture themselves surrounded by a strong bubble that protects them from any unpleasant or stressful thoughts or feelings.
2 Another way of detaching yourself and developing deep calm is to stand quietly for a few minutes with your feet firmly on the floor. Imagine that you are a tree with golden roots growing deep down. Picture the roots giving you strength and stability.

Helping hands

When giving a massage, you communicate with your massage partner mainly through your hands. They need to be warm, soft and supple to ensure a caring touch, yet well co-ordinated and flexible enough to perform the variety of massage movements so effectively used in Indian head massage. Aim to keep your nails clean, trimmed and filed to avoid scratching the skin. If possible, it is best not to wear nail polish when massaging as this could chip off, causing discomfort, and may even trigger an allergic reaction. Odours can linger on the hands, so make sure they do not smell of nicotine or the meal you have been preparing. Wear rubber gloves when chopping onions or garlic.

• When you are trying to relax and reassure your partner, the warmth of your hands matters more than you may realize. The touch of cold hands can give a nasty shock and may cause muscles to tense – think what it feels like to jump into an icy shower. So, before you begin, especially if your hands tend to get cold, rub them briskly together, or immerse them in warm water.

With practice, you will find that your hands become stronger and more flexible. Meanwhile, the following hand and finger exercises can help reduce muscle fatigue in your hands and improve your technique. Repeat them several times a day, whenever you get a free moment, and perform them as a warm-up routine just before giving a massage.

1 Hold your hands at chest level and shake them loosely and vigorously from your wrist for a count of ten.

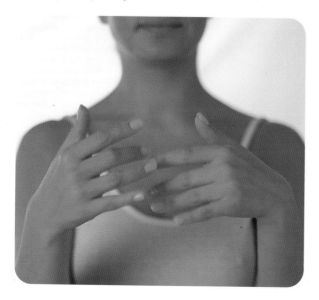

2 Make fists with both hands and rotate them from the wrist in a circular movement ten times. Repeat in the reverse direction.

3 Separate your fingers and thumbs and stretch them out. Hold for a count of ten. Repeat three times.

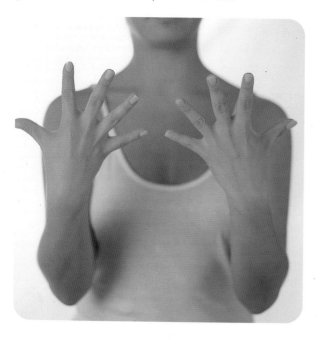

4 Put your hands on a flat surface with the palms facing downward. First, lift your thumbs, then each finger in turn, as though playing a piano. Return to the starting position by placing your little fingers on the surface, followed by each individual finger. Repeat three times.

5 Place your palms together and press one hand against the other for a couple seconds. Repeat ten times.

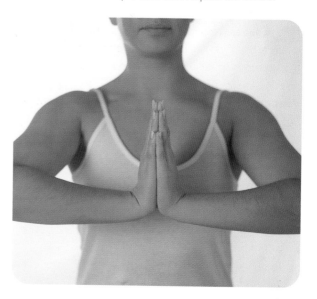

6 Hold a small rubber ball in your hand. Squeeze it as hard as you can, for a count of ten, and then release. Do this three times, then repeat, this time holding the ball in the other hand. This is also a great stress-busting exercise.

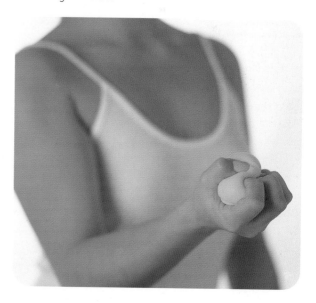

• The use of massage oils should keep your hands well moisturized. You may find that they are now in better condition than they have ever been before.

Creating a healing atmosphere

The art of relaxation is in creating a warm, comfortable and peaceful environment. It is worthwhile spending time and thought on getting the room fully prepared well in advance so you can both relax and enjoy the whole experience in tranquil surroundings.

Preparation

Get ready beforehand. For example, make sure you have plenty of towels and sufficient oil. Lay everything out ready so that, once you have started, you will not need to leave the room or search in drawers.

Check the room temperature. The room should be warm enough to encourage deep physical and mental relaxation without being too stifling. Even if you get pretty hot and sticky while massaging, your massage partner's body temperature can start to drop as tension is released. The benefits of massage will be spoilt if muscles tense and clench in response to the cold. Ideally, the room should be free from disturbing draughts, yet well-ventilated to allow a healthy circulation of air. Take note of the lighting. Avoid giving a massage in a room with harsh overhead or over-bright lighting. If possible, reduce the light level by turning down the dimmer switch or use only lamps or wall lighting. Shaded, natural light is preferable, or the gentle glow of a candle can add a special touch to the atmosphere.

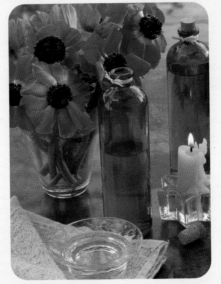

ABOVE **Create the right atmosphere in order to experience the ultimate head massage.**

Choose a suitable chair

The type of chair you use is very important to achieve the most effective massage. You will need one that is fairly upright, preferably without arms. Most kitchen chairs are ideal for the purpose, so long as they do not creak, squeak or wobble. The back of the chair should be low enough to allow you to reach your partner's upper back and shoulders. You must be able to massage without tensing, twisting or straining your back. Your partner should be able to sit comfortably with his or her feet resting firmly on the ground. It is a good idea to experiment with different chairs, using cushions if necessary, to find one that is exactly the right height for you both.

Mood music

Select background music with care. People who spend most of the day in a noisy work or home environment may prefer silence – so always offer the option of quiet. If you decide to play soothing music, choose a piece that you both enjoy. Most good music shops have a selection of tapes and CDs specially composed for massage and relaxation, often featuring natural sounds.

On a warm day, offer your massage partner the treat of an alfresco massage under the shade of a tree. Take some specially blended oil on holiday and offer an outdoor head massage in a scenic location.

Comfortable clothes

Dress for comfort and practicality. You need to be able to move freely, so choose something loose-fitting, short-sleeved – and washable. Some oils can stain so drape a towel over your chest or wear an apron and wash it immediately afterward. Always wear freshly laundered clothes, as the stale odour of food or smoke can be most unpleasant. Fresh breath is important too – it is remarkable how the smell of foods and cigarette smoke can linger. Wear your hair tied back from your face, both for hygiene and practical purposes. Remove your wristwatch and any bracelets, dangling earrings, long necklaces or rings that could interfere with the smooth flow of the massage. Wear low-heeled shoes or go barefoot – if your feet feel comfortable you will be more relaxed.

Avoid distractions

Turn off the television or radio, shut out the sound of traffic or other people, switch on the answerphone and hang a 'do not disturb' notice on the door. Check that children and pets are settled for at least half an hour. A valuable feature of Indian head massage is that it allows space in a busy life for some complete 'me' time. It gives your massage partner the chance to enjoy the comforting, stress-relieving sensation of being nurtured. Also if you are worried about being disturbed, you will probably find it more difficult to concentrate on the massage.

When head massage is to be avoided

- Like all forms of massage, Indian head massage is generally considered a safe, non-invasive therapy. However, there are a few occasions when it can actually cause more harm than good, so do check that your massage partner is not suffering from any conditions, known as contraindications, that could be aggravated by massage.

If you have any doubts – do not give a massage. Trust your intuition and postpone the massage until you have taken professional advice or are certain the condition has cleared up completely.

Points to watch

Never give a massage if your massage partner has any of the following conditions.

- Any recent injuries involving the head, neck, shoulders or limbs, including sprains, strains, fractures and whiplash. Massage to the area could make the injury worse and would also be extremely painful. Wait until you are confident that the injury has healed.

CHECKLIST

CONTRAINDICATIONS

- Fever.
- Swellings or inflammation.
- Severe bruising in the massage area.
- High or low blood pressure.
- Skin disorders.
- Scalp infections.
- Arthritis of the upper spine.
- Osteoporosis.
- Diabetes.
- Severe asthma.
- Epilepsy.
- Disorders of the nervous system.
- Protruding veins.
- Recent haemorrhage (bleeding).
- History of thrombosis or embolism.
- Recent head or neck injury.
- Recent surgery involving the head or neck.
- Any potentially fatal condition, such as cancer.

- A history of thrombosis (blood clots in an artery or vein) or embolism (blockage in an artery). Massage may encourage a clot or fragment to break away and enter the bloodstream, where it may become lodged and block the flow of blood to a vital organ.
- Any skin disorders or scalp infections, including weeping eczema, acne, psoriasis and head lice, as massage could irritate and/or spread the condition.
- Recent surgery. Massage might delay the healing of recently formed scar tissue.
- Any potentially fatal condition such as cancer. Although a trained masseur can often help relieve pain and induce relaxation in someone who has contracted cancer, there is a risk of making the condition worse. Try gentle stroking instead.
- Disorders of the nervous system, such as multiple sclerosis, which could be exacerbated by the stimulating effect of massage.
- Osteoporosis. This is a condition, usually associated with the ageing process, in which bones lose their density and become weak and brittle. Strong pressure on fragile bones could cause a fracture.
- A migraine attack. Although Indian head massage can help relieve recurrent migraines, massage during an attack could make the symptoms worse.
- Do not massage anyone who is under the influence of alcohol or drugs. It is impossible to know what reaction to expect in these circumstances, so do not take the risk.

Doctor's advice

Seek advice and consent from an appropriate medical practitioner if any of the following situations apply to your massage partner.

- Being prescribed medication, especially strong or long-term drugs, being under medical supervision, or receiving complementary therapies.
- A chronic (on-going) medical condition, such as diabetes, epilepsy, severe asthma, serious heart problems, oedema (fluid retention leading to tissue swelling) or acute back pain.
- High or low blood pressure, as massage can cause fluctuations in blood pressure levels.
- Pregnancy. Take particular care during the first three months, when the risk of foetal disorders and miscarriage are greatest. Keep strokes light and gentle. Check that your massage partner has not developed a medical condition such as high blood

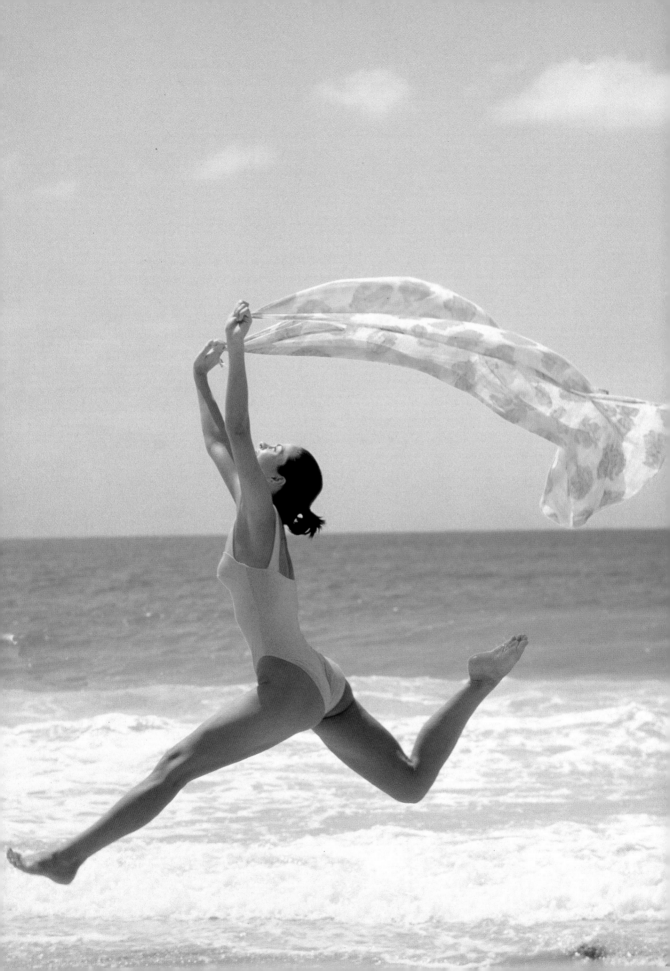

pressure or gestational diabetes, which are relatively common in pregnancy. Do not use pure essential oils during pregnancy and breastfeeding.

Look out for:

- Fever. Massage is not usually recommended for anyone with a temperature over 37.5°C (99.4°F). A high temperature generally indicates that the body is bringing its defence mechanisms into action to deal with an infection of some kind. Massage increases the body temperature and so might interfere with this natural healing process.
- Swollen, inflamed, bruised, tender or sore muscles, joints or areas of skin. Never massage over swollen lymph nodes. Avoid the affected part or postpone the massage, especially if the cause of the problem is not known, as you may cause further damage.
- Warts, skin tags, moles, boils, bruises, cuts and abrasions, broken skin, blisters, sensitive or protruding veins, areas of sunburn, bites or stings and unexplained lumps. In some cases, you may be able to cover the site with a small plaster. Work very carefully to avoid massaging directly over the area.

Look after your own health

When giving an Indian head massage, you are in such close contact with your massage partner that infectious or contagious conditions could easily be passed on. Be wary of massaging anyone who has a skin and scalp infection or is feeling generally unwell or nauseous. Cover any cuts or abrasions on your own hands to reduce the risk of cross-infection. Postpone the massage if you are feeling below par. You need to reserve your energy for the sake of your own health.

Pre-massage advice

- Ask your massage partner to wait at least an hour after eating a meal or exercising before having the massage, and advise him to avoid stimulants such as tea and coffee immediately before the massage.
- Check any possible adverse reactions or allergies to individual carrier or essential oils. Read all safety guidelines carefully. You must be completely confident that the oils you use have no potentially harmful effects.
- Do not use essential oils on babies, children or elderly people.

CASE STUDY

A GOOD NIGHT'S SLEEP

Peter, 60, was persuaded to try Indian head massage by his wife, Moira, because he was sleeping badly and felt permanently tired. 'I didn't want to take sleeping tablets,' he explained, 'but I was becoming desperate – and so was Moira. I was getting forgetful and irritable in the day, then at night I would toss and turn and keep her awake. I was prepared to try anything. Much to my embarrassment, I fell fast asleep during the first head massage. I don't really remember much. I felt quite weird when I woke up – not with it at all. I kept muddling up my words. But I sat still for a little while and soon came round. I almost floated

home, I felt so light and relaxed. 'I slept really well that night. It was a lovely surprise to wake up, look at the clock and realize that it was morning. I didn't sleep quite so well on the following nights, but then after my second massage, I had another good night's sleep.

Over a few months of regular Indian head massage and full body massage my sleep patterns have gradually changed for the better. I still get the odd night of wakefulness but generally I get about six or seven hours. I have far more energy in the day – and I'm sure my memory has got better.'

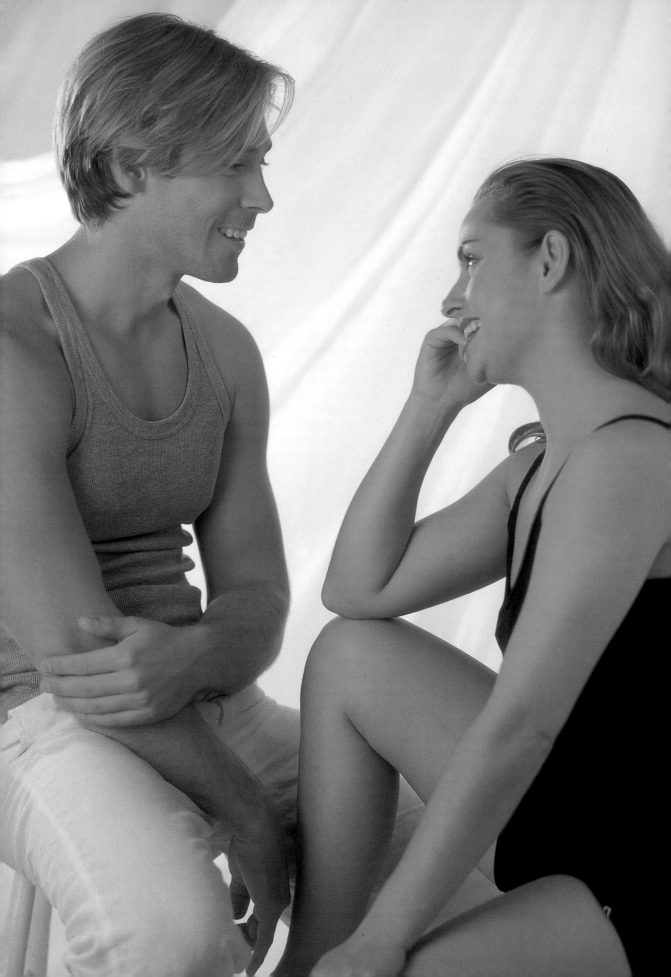

The full
works

An Indian head massage involves varying combinations of gentle,

soothing and brisk, stimulating movements to suit the mood, needs

and preferences of the recipient. The following routine takes around

20–30 minutes from start to finish but can be readily adapted by

spending longer on favourite strokes, omitting others, or adding

some of the movements featured in the other step-by-step

sequences throughout pages 276–99. A natural vegetable carrier

oil – with the addition of a pure essential oil if you wish – acts as

a wonderfully nourishing lubricant, but it is possible to perform the

massage without oil by doing it through light clothing.

THINGS YOU WILL NEED

- Upright chair with a low back.
- 10 ml of suitable oil in a small bowl (see pages 224–39).
- Large towel.
- Small towel draped over a chair back.
- Paper towels to wipe your hands and absorb any spillage.
- Soft background music (optional).
- Clock (helpful to keep an eye on the time).
- Apron (optional).

THINGS TO DO

- Dress in comfortable, washable clothes.
- Reduce the lighting.
- Check that the room is warm and free from draughts.
- Switch on the answerphone or unplug the phone. Make sure that you are not likely to be disturbed for the next half an hour or so.
- Remove any jewellery that may interfere with the massage.
- Wash your hands. Ensure your nails are short, smooth, clean and free from nail polish. Cover any cuts or abrasions with a plaster.
- Warm your hands; shake them from the wrists to release any tension.
- Breathe slowly and deeply, concentrating your thoughts on the massage you are about to give. Rehearse the different moves in your mind.
- Adopt a calm, centred approach (see page 254).

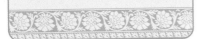

Before you begin

Never give a massage without first having a preliminary discussion with your massage partner. Most importantly, check that there are no contraindications that would make it inadvisable to continue (see page 257). Ask about past or current medical problems – particularly accidents, injuries or serious illnesses. Look at the condition of your partner's hair and skin and pick up clues about her general health and well-being. This is also an opportunity to ask questions that will help you to adapt the massage to suit your partner's needs and wishes. Find out if there are any areas that require special attention and ask how she hopes to feel afterward. Has she had an Indian head massage before? If so, ask if she experienced any adverse reactions (see page 302), were there any movements she liked or disliked and does she have any suggestions of her own.

- It might seem tempting to launch straight into a massage, but it is worthwhile spending some time reading through the preliminary steps described in this chapter until you are familiar with them, so you do not have to keep stopping to refer to them. You can rehearse the moves quite easily while sitting in a chair by practising on your own thigh and bended knee.

Let your partner know what to expect

The thought of having your head touched in such an intimate way can seem rather daunting. Give your partner the chance to ask questions. Explain the sequence of movements. Give a brief summary of the benefits and possible reactions (page 302). These are different for everyone and can vary every time.

Explain that comfort is an integral part of the relaxation process. Make it perfectly clear to your massage partner that she should tell you at once if anything about the massage feels painful or unpleasant. You can easily stop and then continue with another movement. Above all, explain that this is her time to relax, shut off from the outside world and thoroughly enjoy being pampered.

ADVICE FOR YOUR PARTNER

- Remove any make-up, if possible, to ensure optimum benefits from the oil.
- Remove earrings and necklace.
- Remove spectacles or contact lenses.
- Brush through her hair to avoid pulling and tangling.
- Tie up long hair with a clip, head-band or similar accessory.
- Adjust clothing. Your massage partner need not disrobe for a dry massage – a T-shirt or similar light clothing is suitable. For an oily massage, your massage partner should take off her upper clothing and adjust her bra straps to leave her shoulders bare. Wrap a large towel around her chest – warm it on a radiator first for extra comfort.

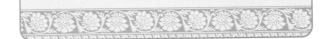

Massage sequence

- Try not to rush any of these movements. A gentle, unhurried pace will contribute greatly to the efficacy of the massage.

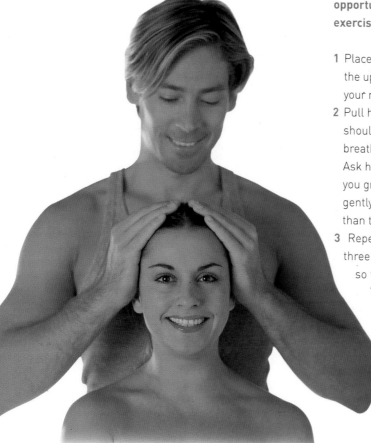

▶ ▲ Making contact

Resting your hands on your massage partner's head provides a reassuring, comforting moment of contact. It helps make your partner feel secure and creates an awareness of the touch of your hands on his head. This preliminary hold is a very important part of the massage as it helps to establish a bond that allows you both to relax, centre and focus on the massage. Your partner will appreciate the lovely sense of calm that it brings. With your partner seated in a chair, legs uncrossed and feet flat on the floor, gently rest your hands on either side of his head, your fingers facing toward the crown. Stay still. Hold for a minute and release gradually.

CAUTION Be careful not to press down too firmly on the head as too much pressure can hurt the neck.

▼ Deep breathing

During this deep breathing sequence, you may like to suggest that your partner imagines breathing in peace and tranquillity and expelling any doubts, fears or frustrations. You can do the same. This is also an ideal opportunity to guide your partner through a relaxation exercise (see page 252) if you feel it is appropriate.

1 Place a hand on each shoulder, with fingers resting on the upper arm facing downward. Turn your body so that your right hip is pushed into your partner's back.
2 Pull her shoulders gently back toward you. As her shoulders move, ask your partner to take a deep breath through her nose. Hold for a couple of seconds. Ask her to breathe out slowly through her mouth as you gradually release the shoulders, pushing them gently back into place. Take longer on the out-breath than the in-breath.
3 Repeat the move very slowly and deliberately at least three times. It helps to talk through the movement so that your partner knows what is expected. 'As I take your shoulders back, breathe in deeply and slowly... hold... now, as I release your shoulders, breathe out, long and slow...'

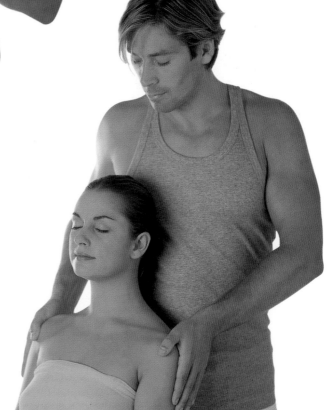

▼ Restful darkness

This helps relax the muscles at the back of the eyes, which can often get strained as a result of long periods spent reading or driving, especially in poor visibility.

1 Ask your partner to close her eyes. Hold the palms of your hands over her eyes with the fingers of one hand slightly overlapping those on the other, thumbs upward.
2 Press very gently so that she is in darkness but does not feel restricted. Hold for 30 seconds.

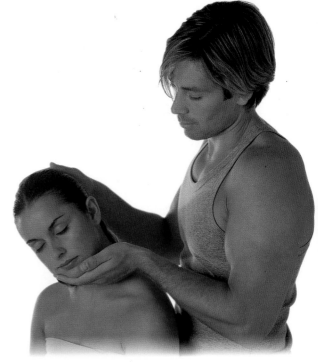

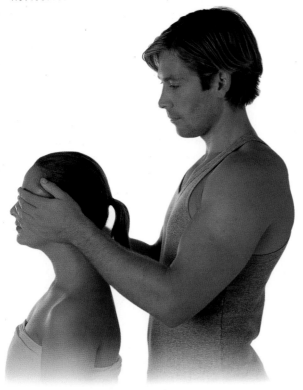

CAUTION Do check that your partner is not claustrophobic or fearful of darkness before applying this action.

• Apply each stroke with care and love to make your partner feel comforted, reassured and secure.

▶ ▲ Head roll

In this sequence, your partner may find it difficult to let go at first. If your partner appears very tense, you may like to spend a little longer on this move – but there is a risk of feeling rather like a nodding dog after a while! The movement should come from your partner's neck so that only the head moves, not the whole body.

1 Place one hand under your partner's chin for support. Place the other at the back of her head, just below the crown. Gently roll her head in a semi-circle, first to one side, then to the front and around to the other. Do not roll the head backward as this places stress on the neck muscles. Ask your partner to let you support the weight of her head so that you are directing the action.
2 Retrace the line of the arc going in the other direction. Do this at least three times, concentrating on detecting stiffness and tightness. Gently return the head to the upright position and take your hands away slowly.
CAUTION Keep the head well-supported throughout. Do not press on the throat, as this may restrict breathing.

▶ ▲ Stroking on the oil

This sequence uses long, confident movements that help soothe and relax your partner.

1 Pour warm oil into the palm of one hand. Some people love to have their hair saturated in oil; others prefer just a little. You can easily top it up during the massage if you find your partner has dry skin or long hair.
2 Rub your hands together so that your palms and fingers are warm and covered in oil. Explain to your partner that you are now going to stroke the oil into her scalp.
3 Place both hands on your partner's head, with fingers pointing forward and just touching the start of the

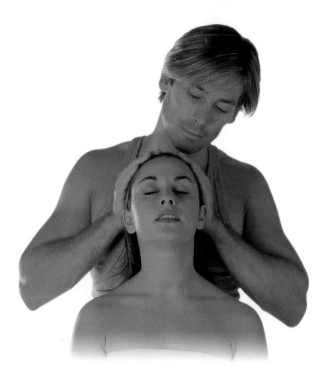

flowing movements as before to cover your partner's upper back and upper arms. Use the whole of the palms of both hands and the fleshy pads of the fingers. Start with a very light pressure and gradually make it a little firmer.

CAUTION Long hair should be tied up or pushed to one side.

- Keep breathing slowly and deeply. You will need a good supply of oxygen to help maintain your energy levels. Giving an Indian head massage can be more tiring than you might think. If you find yourself losing concentration, make an effort to think about the strokes.

▼ Thumb fans

This movement works on the powerful kite-shaped trapezius muscle, where many people store a great deal of tension. As you move your thumbs, you will start to feel some movement of the muscle fibres beneath and sense any tightness starting to ease. Your partner may feel some tenderness.

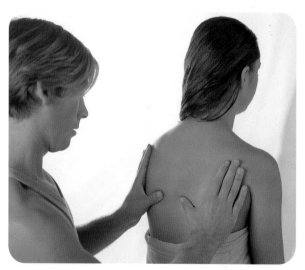

hairline. Stroke over the top of the head, using the flat of both hands and the pads of the fingers, and continue along the top of the shoulders. Repeat until you have applied oil to the whole of the scalp.
- Maintain as much contact as possible. It can be very disconcerting for your partner if you jerk your hands away suddenly at the end of a move.

▼ Warming up

These movements spread the oil and relax and soften the area ready for massage. Continue with the same

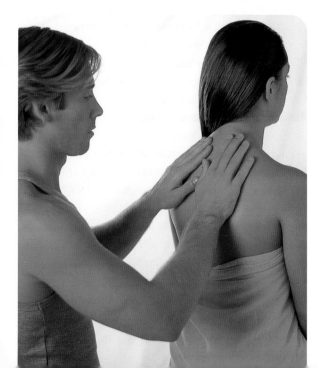

1 Place your hands flat on your partner's back, on either side of the spine, so that the heels of your hands rest just below the bottom of the shoulder-blades. Keep fingers slightly outstretched and resting on the skin.
2 Press fairly firmly with the sides of your thumb pads and, with one long sweeping fan-like movement, push them upward to the base of the neck and across the top of the shoulders. Your thumbs should stay in contact with the skin as you sweep them up to form a curved T-shape. Maintain a firm, even pressure throughout the stroke.

3 Continue until you have covered the whole of the trapezius. This is a deep effleurage movement that helps boost the blood flow to the area and warms and softens the underlying muscle tissues. Work this area for at least a couple of minutes.

CAUTION While working with your thumbs, keep your fingers relaxed so that you do not grasp your partner's shoulders too tightly.

• Never work directly over the spine, as this protects the spinal cord and contains a vast number of individual nerves linking the brain to all parts of the body.

▼ Thumb kneading

This sequence involves a petrissage movement that flattens and broadens the muscle tissues, helping to disperse any nodules of tension. It also helps squeeze out any excess lymph and encourages a healthy flow of nourishing blood to feed the muscle fibres and improve the condition of the tissues. Pay special attention to the upper trapezius (feel for the soft tissue that runs along the top of the shoulder) which tends to get very tight. You can also knead this area with the pads of your fingers or the palms of your hands.

1 With your hands held in the same position as before, make deep, circular movements with your thumb pads over the whole of the trapezius muscle. Keep your

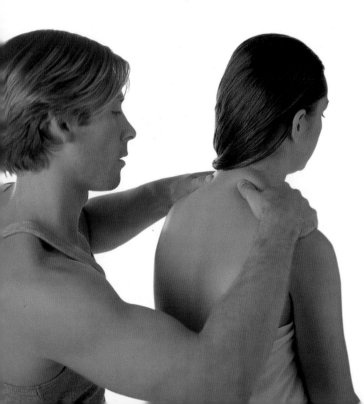

fingers relaxed as you work with the thumbs. Rotate the skin firmly against the underlying tissues so that you can feel the muscle fibres moving, stretching and loosening beneath your firm touch. Press, lift, squeeze and release the flesh in a rhythmic, kneading action. Stand firmly on two feet and lean into the movement, using your body weight to gradually increase the pressure on the upward move and decrease on the downward part of each circle.

2 Work upward with a continuous action so that your hands do not leave your partner's back and shoulders. Work the area for around five to seven minutes.

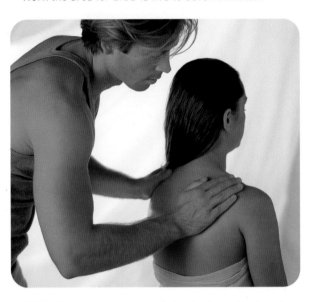

CAUTION Be careful not to press too hard or too suddenly and keep the movement flowing. Sudden, jerky actions will make your massage partner even more tense. Watch out for tell-tale body language or ask your partner if the level of pressure is bearable.

▲ Shoulder sweeping

This is a soothing, calming movement that is useful to include at any time during the massage. Deep massage to the trapezius may cause some discomfort but this is usually described as 'therapeutic' or 'positive' and can bring a great sense of relief. However, too much work on tight muscles can cause the fibres to contract even more and may cause bruising. If your partner is tense around her upper back and shoulders, take it in stages. Repeat the warming up, thumb fans, thumb kneading and shoulder sweeping movements two or three times a week until the tension has cleared.

1 Place your left hand on your massage partner's left shoulder for support. Place the palm of your right hand on the right shoulder-blade, fingers splayed and pointing toward the upper arms.

2 Push the whole of the flat of your hand upward in slow, generous, circular movements, sweeping across the top of the shoulder and tracing the outline of the shoulder-blade. Make sure the flat of your hand is in contact with the skin at all times. Keep your wrist flexible and mould your hand to the shape of your massage partner's back.

3 Use your body weight to increase the depth of pressure on the upward movement and decrease as you slide your hand downward. You can move your hand in a clockwise or anticlockwise direction, whichever feels most comfortable. Repeat at least four times. Now repeat the sequence on the other side, this time with your right hand on your massage partner's right shoulder.

▶ Ironing the shoulders

The sliding action of this movement helps lower hunched-up shoulders, relaxes the deltoid muscles at the top of the arms and drains toxins down to the lymph nodes in the elbow.

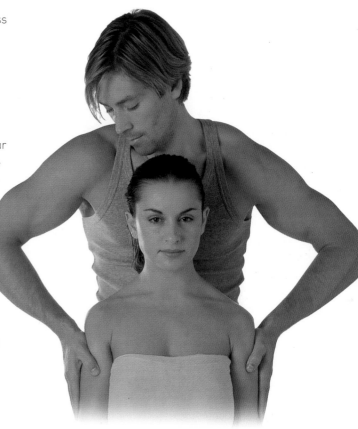

1 Place both hands near the base of your partner's neck. Using the outer edges of your hands, 'iron' along the top of the shoulders to the upper arm. Press firmly and evenly, keeping the hands in contact with the skin.

2 As you reach the top of the upper arms, change the position of your hands, without losing contact with the skin, so that the flat of the hands sweep downward in a firm, flowing effleurage movement toward the elbows. Do this at least three times.

• The benefits of Indian head massage are cumulative. A weekly session will help you look, feel and think better.

Easing a stiff neck

These movements help relax the tension that often builds up in the neck, so easing stiffness and pain and aiding neck mobility.

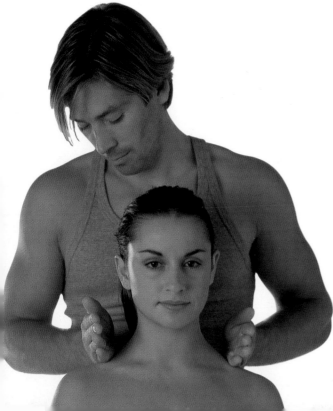

1 Place one hand on your partner's forehead. Ask her to drop her head forward so that you can support its weight and her neck is easily accessible for massage.

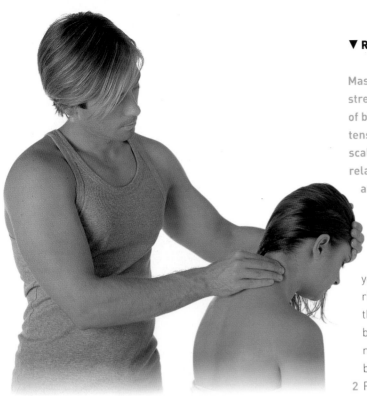

▼ **Relaxing scalp tension**

Massaging around the base of the skull can help stretch and soften constricted muscles, boost the flow of blood and release any build-up of toxins, so easing tension headaches. You may find that your partner's scalp is very tight, if she is under a lot of stress. As she relaxes, you should start to feel the scalp loosening and moving more easily.

1 With one hand supporting the head and your other hand in the same V shape position as in the previous sequence, make small static frictions with the pads of your thumbs and fingers along both sides of the bony ridge. Starting from the top of the spine, work out toward the ears. Press the scalp firmly along the ridge of the bone, hold for a couple of seconds, then release. Lift and repeat a little further along until the whole occiput has been covered.

2 Follow the same path, this time making small circular friction movements. Repeat on the same spot for three circles, then lift your hand and move to the next spot. Now do these two movements again, this time using the other hand to support the head.

CAUTION When working on the occiput you should massage the scalp against the bone and avoid pressing on the fleshy area beneath the bone, as this may cause nausea.

2 With the pads of your fingers or the palm of the other hand, make gentle, circular stroking movements with a very light pressure up the back of the neck to the base of the skull and along the bony ridge, known as the occiput, to the ears. Repeat three or four times.

3 Form a V between the thumb and first finger and lightly clasp the base of your massage partner's neck. Stand firmly on both feet, ensuring that her head is well supported with one hand at all times. Place your thumb on the fleshy area on one side of the bony cervical vertebrae and the pads of one or two fingers on the other side.

4 Starting at the base of the neck, work upward with a gentle kneading action. Lift, squeeze and release the muscles in a rhythmic, rotating movement.

5 Massage up to the bony ridge at the base of the skull, then give the muscles a slight stretch.

6 Repeat the movement, using the other hand over the same area – you will find that it feels completely different with each hand. It is best to work with your non-dominant hand first.

7 Finish with some soothing stroking up the neck.

CAUTION The neck area can be very tender, so ask your partner to tell you how much pressure feels comfortable.

• Never press hard on the neck. Stop if your partner experiences any pain, dizziness or discomfort.

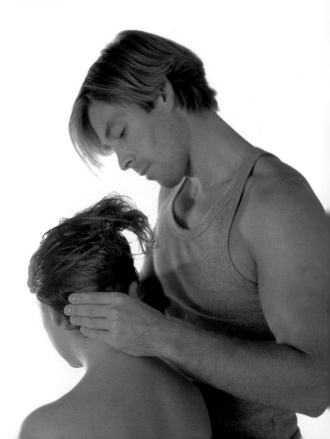

▼ Brisk rubbing

Brisk rubbing continues the benefits of the previous kneading technique by stimulating the blood and lymph circulation.

1 With the head still firmly supported in one hand, as before, use the fleshy pads of two or three fingers to rub along one side of the occiput from the top of the neck to behind the ear. Briskly rub along the bone backward and forward in a short, rapid sawing action. If you massage in a circular motion, hair tends to get matted.

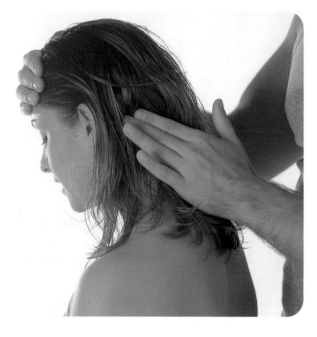

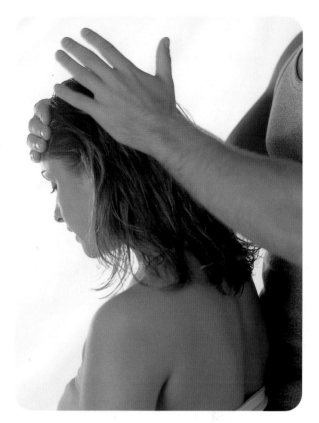

▲ Warming the scalp

The pressure should be firm so you are stimulating the local blood circulation and warming the area.

2 Change hands and repeat on the other side. Repeat three times. Try this rubbing movement with the heel or side of your hand.

CAUTION Keep your hand moving swiftly and do not stay in the same place for long.

• Be aware of your posture. Stand with your feet shoulder-width apart to maintain a good balance. Keep your back straight and your shoulders relaxed so you are in a comfortable position to give an effective massage without straining your back. Move around your partner's chair so that you do not need to strain to reach. Kneel on the floor or bend your knees if you need to lower yourself for a particular move.

1 Keep your partner's head well-supported with one hand, as before, and continue the brisk rubbing, moving up from the occiput to the crown. Keep your wrists fairly flexible and use the palm or heel of your hand in a rapid, waving action.

2 When you reach the crown, lift your hand and start again, a little further around the back of the head. Repeat several times so that the whole of the back of the head has been covered.

CAUTION Maintain a firm support for the head so that you can push against your supporting hand to increase the pressure without causing discomfort.

'Shampooing' the scalp

This movement usually comes quite naturally as most of us have experienced it at the hairdresser's. It is a friction movement that stimulates the blood and lymph circulation in the area and warms and loosens the scalp. As the scalp starts to move more freely, the tension is eased, bringing a great sense of well-being.

1 Place your hands on either side of the scalp, with fingers well spread out so that your little fingers are resting on your partner's temples and your thumbs are at the back of her head.

2 Place your fingers in a wide claw-like pose and use the fleshy pads of your fingers and thumbs to make small anticlockwise movements all over the scalp. Keep your fingers fairly rigid so that you can feel the scalp moving beneath them. Repeat three times.

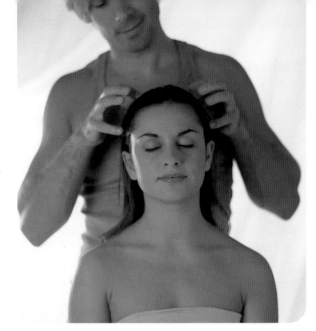

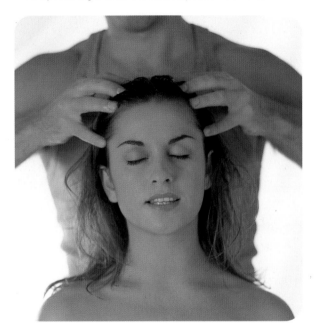

CAUTION Ensure that your partner's head is held firmly between your two hands and is well supported.

▶ Hair smoothing

This is a soothing, relaxing movement that contrasts well with the previous brisker strokes and helps drain any excess blood or lymph from the scalp. It provides an opportunity to put your partner's hair back in place.

1 Rest both hands lightly on your massage partner's head, with fingers facing forward. Using alternate hands, stroke from the top of your partner's head right down to her shoulders in a flowing, gently overlapping motion. As one hand finishes, the other hand starts so that continuity is maintained. Keep your fingers and hands soft and moulded to the contours of your partner's head, neck and shoulders.

▲ Finger tapping

The following action is rather like playing the piano or drumming your fingers on the table. It is an energizing, revitalizing action, a gentle form of tapotement that helps stimulate the blood circulation.

1 With the hands held in the same position as before, tap the pads of your fingers all over your partner's scalp and back of the neck. Keep your fingers flexible so you can tap the head quickly, energetically and firmly without being too heavy handed.

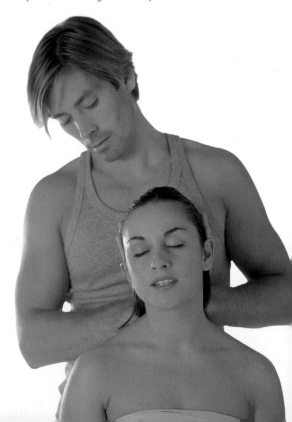

Facial massage

You are now going to massage your partner's face. But before you begin, there are some important points to consider. Firstly, check that your partner's neck is not strained. The head can become surprisingly floppy during a facial massage. If her head is allowed to fall back too far, it not only causes discomfort, but can also restrict breathing, leading to feelings of panic. Your partner's head should feel secure and supported throughout so that she can relax completely and gain maximum benefits from the massage.

Stand close to her back and use a rolled up towel to support her neck so that her head is resting firmly against your chest. Maintain this stance throughout. This position is also useful for a woman giving a massage who may feel slightly inhibited about having a man resting his head against her chest. Keep a rolled up towel ready so that you do not disturb the flow of the massage.

You should always keep your massage partner warm and cosy. Wrap a towel around her shoulders so that she does not get chilly while you are working on her face. Drape a towel over the back of the chair for this purpose. You can also use the towel to dab off any excess oil on your partner's back or shoulders.

Check the amount of oil on your hands and fingers. There should be just enough oil to provide light lubrication for a smooth massage without dragging the skin. Wipe off any excess. Look for any stray hairs that may be on your hands and remove them before you massage the delicate skin on the face.

▶ **Forehead stroking**

This is a very caring, soothing stroke that is wonderfully relaxing. Habitual frowning or worried expressions can cause these muscles to constrict, which leads to furrowed brows, tension headaches and eye strain. Gentle stroking helps to ease the tension away from these overworked muscles and smoothes away fine tension lines.

1 Place your hands on your partner's forehead so that your fingers overlap slightly, with the thumbs pointing upward. Using the flat of three fingers, stroke away from the centre of the forehead toward the area around the temples.

2 Start just above the eyebrows and repeat a little higher, gradually moving up to the hairline. Your hands work in alternate finger-over-finger strokes so that it feels like a single, continuous movement. Repeat around six times until the whole of the forehead has been covered. Keep the movement very slow, with a light, even pressure. Your hands should be soft and gently moulded to follow the shape of your massage partner's brow.

• Keep the pressure on the face very light. Do not drag the skin. If necessary, add a little more oil.

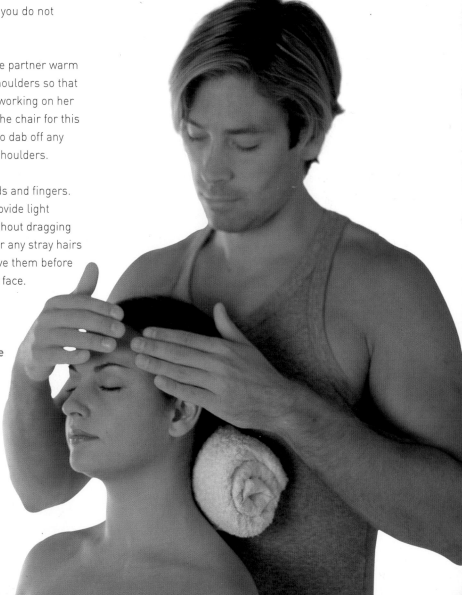

▼ Temple circles

The temples are another tension hot spot where constricted muscles are a common cause of headaches and eye strain. Massage helps boost the circulation of blood and lymph and relaxes the temporalis muscles. You can also try this movement using the heels of your hands. This is a very slow and controlled movement using a fairly firm pressure.

1 Place your hands over your massage partner's temples. Using the pads of two fingers, massage the temples with small, clockwise or anticlockwise

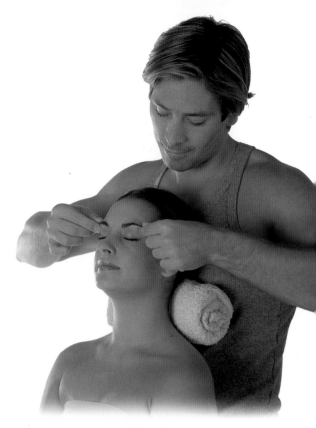

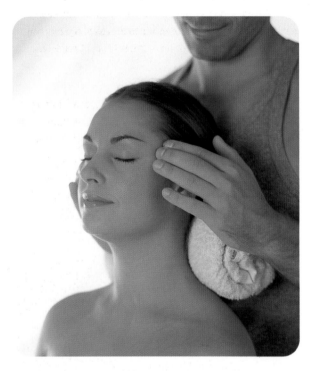

movements. Avoid digging in with your fingertips. Keep your fingers on the same spot – it is the skin that moves as you make the rotations. Make around twelve circles.

CAUTION It is important to find the right area of the temple. Feel for the shallow depression surrounded by a bony ridge at the corner of your partner's eyes. Work on this small area of soft tissue.

• Do not be concerned if you partner falls asleep – keep going. When someone has trouble getting to sleep, an Indian head massage in the late evening can work wonders.

▲ Eyebrow squeeze

This sequence helps relieve the tension that often builds up in the muscles and helps ease any congestion in the sinus passages around the eyes.

1 Gently hold your partner's eyebrows between your thumbs and index fingers. Gently squeeze, pressing fairly firmly against the bone. Hold for a couple of seconds. Start at the bridge of the nose and work out.
2 Lift and move to the next spot. Repeat until the whole of the eyebrows have been covered. Return to the starting position. Repeat three times. Finish with a few gliding strokes along the eyebrows.

CAUTION Do not apply pressure if your partner's sinuses are swollen or painful.

• When massaging near the eyes, be careful not to allow any oil to seep into your partner's eyes.

▶ Clearing sinus congestion

The compression action of your fingers helps draw out any lymph in the sinus passages. You may feel some slight puffiness in the area if your partner suffers from congested sinuses.

1 Place the index finger of each hand near the sides of your partner's nostrils. Following the line of the cheekbones (or zygomatic bones), apply small static frictions with the pad on one finger, pushing the flesh firmly up and under the ridge of the bones. Press, hold for a few seconds, release and move to the next spot. Work slowly and precisely along to the sides of the face, lessening the pressure as you reach the ears. Return to the starting position. Repeat three times.

2 Now make sweeping movements with one finger along the same paths to help direct the excess lymph to the lymph nodes near the ears, where it can be filtered and purified. Repeat these sinus sweeps three times.

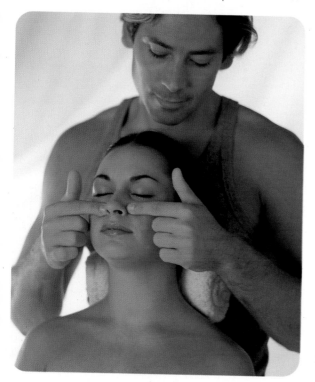

CAUTION Miss out this movement if your partner's sinuses are extremely congested or painful.

- Lightly rubbing and stroking the ears can have a very pleasurable and sensual effect – so save this for a romantic evening. Massage the insides of the ears too.

▶ **Releasing tension along the jaw line**

This is a similar movement to the back and forth waving type action performed on the occiput, but your pressure should be light. These movements help warm and soften the jaw muscles.

1 Place your fingers at each corner of your partner's mouth. Using the pads of your fingers, gently stroke, one hand after the other, outward across her cheeks toward her ears. As one stroke finishes so the other begins, in a flowing action. Repeat three times.

2 Using the pads of two fingers, rub lightly but briskly all around the sides of her mouth and outward to her ears. Always move upward to help tone and lift the muscles. You may also like to apply small, anticlockwise, circular movements around these areas. Finish by repeating the initial stroking action.

CAUTION Massaging around the jaw area can be extremely uncomfortable if your massage partner is wearing dentures. If possible, remove the dentures. If this is not possible, use a very gentle touch.

- Releasing tension in the facial muscles can have an almost instant effect. Your partner's face will look softer, more relaxed and refreshed.

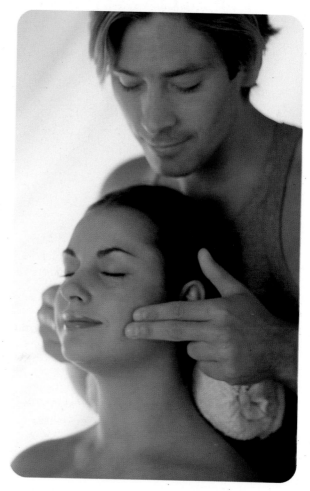

▼ Facial tapping

This is a soft tapotement movement that stimulates blood circulation and helps firm the facial muscles.

1 Tap the pads of your fingers very gently all over your partner's face and neck in a random, rhythmical fashion. The action is similar to 'Finger tapping' (see page 270) but your touch should be much lighter.

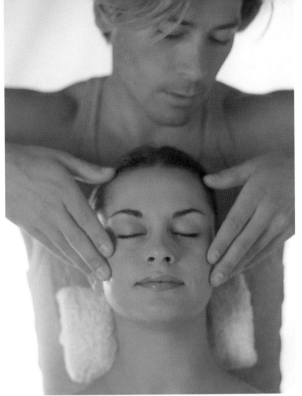

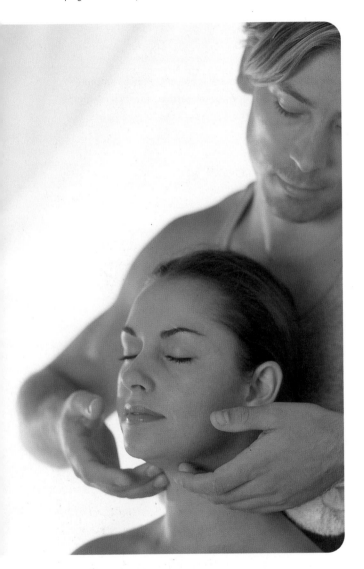

1 With the flat of four fingers, stroke from your partner's neck up the face to the hairline in long, gliding, strokes. Use alternate hands in a wave-like flowing motion so that as one stroke finishes the other begins. Keep your hands moulded to the natural shape of her face.
2 Finish each stroke with a soft, lifting action. Do at least ten strokes so that the whole of her face is covered. Do not miss out the upper lip area and sides of the face.

▼ Repeat restful darkness

By repeating the restful darkness sequence you allow your partner to enjoy the calming effect of total darkness.

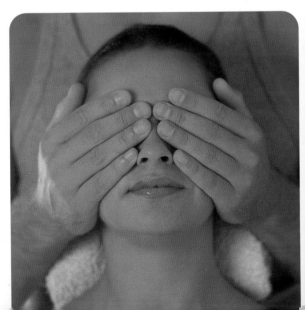

▶▲ Facial stroking

Follow on from the previous stimulating movements with gentle stroking, this soothes the many sensory nerve endings in the face and releases mood-enhancing endorphins to promote a sense of inner harmony and serenity.

▶ Final touch

Repeat the first sequence – 'Making contact' (see page 263). Maintain this reassuring hold for about half a minute and then gradually release your hands and step back. Stand silently by your massage partner's side for a couple of minutes to allow her to awaken slowly from a state of deep relaxation. She may feel very 'spaced out' and need time to gather her thoughts. Suggest that she stays seated while you wash your hands and bring her a glass of water. Advise her to put on a warm cardigan or sweater after the massage. If circumstances permit, wrap her hair in a warm towel and suggest that she rests for at least half an hour before washing off the oil.

• Oil will wash out of hair very easily afterward. The trick is to apply a little neat shampoo straight on to the hair. Do not wet the hair first. Rub in the shampoo, rinse in warm water and then wash as normal.

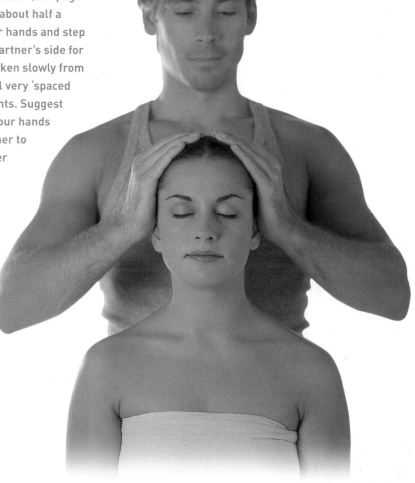

CASE STUDY

COMPUTER-AIDED TENSION

Steve, 38, works in a busy architectural practice as a computer-aided design technician. Deadlines tend to be so tight that he often spends all day working at the computer with very few breaks. 'When you're working you don't notice how tense your muscles have become,' he explained. 'It's only when you stop that your body feels stiff and painful. I often used to go home with aching eyes, a sore head and fuddled brain. But it wasn't really enough to bother about. Then, a couple of months ago, a local therapist wrote to the office offering his services in Indian head massage.

'I enjoyed the first session so much that I booked in for a weekly head massage. It only takes about 20 minutes from start to finish and it is all done at my desk. Afterward, I feel alert and focused. I seem to be able to get the work done much quicker with a more creative flare. I still spend long hours at the computer but I take more breaks. If I feel a headache brewing I massage my temples, which is very soothing. And now I enjoy the evenings far more because I don't have so many aches and pains to contend with. My children also tell me that I am far less grumpy!'

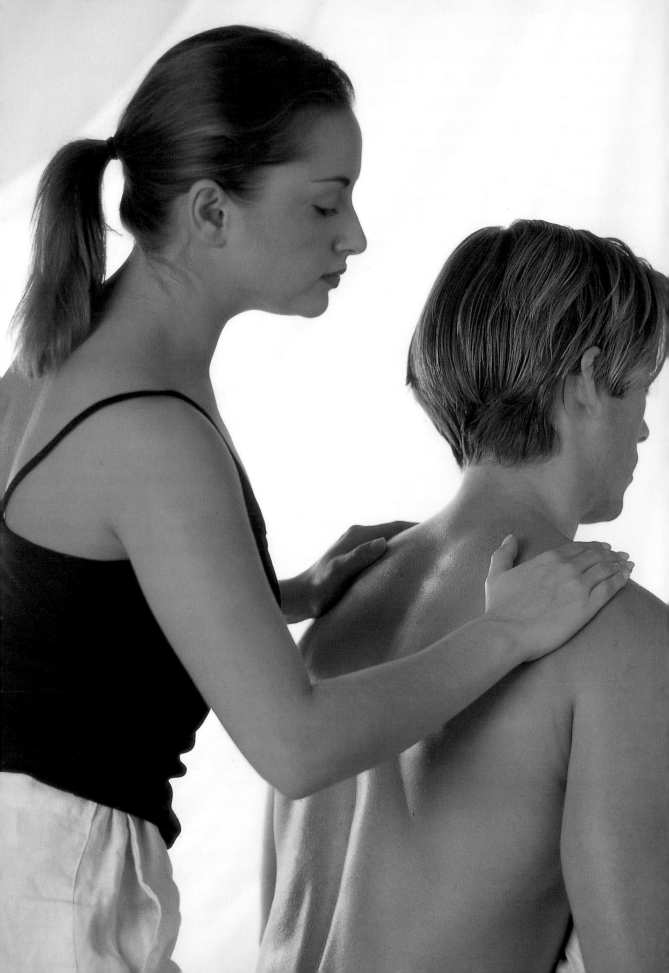

Instant
energy

A short, brisk Indian head massage can be amazingly revitalizing. Try this 5–10 minute sequence of stimulating movements to refresh and invigorate weary friends or family members. It is a perfect pick-me-up for those times when energy levels are low but the demands of living are high – such as during a mid-afternoon vitality slump, or in the evening when you have had an exhausting day at work or have spent hours travelling. Your massage partner may find it more comfortable to straddle a chair, preferably leaning against a large cushion or pillow covered with a towel. The use of oil is optional, depending on when and where you give the massage. The movements can be just as effective through light clothing.

Revitalizing breath

When you are tired, you naturally yawn to fill your body with reviving oxygen. Controlled breathing is a better way to combat lethargy. You and your partner can practise the following breathing technique together. It may help to imagine that you are breathing in energy, vitality and enthusiasm.

1 Start your routine by standing near an open window. Ask your partner to stand squarely, with his feet shoulder-width apart and arms hanging loosely by his sides. You should do the same. You should both feel as relaxed and comfortable as possible.

2 You both take in a long, slow breath through the nose. Hold it, while you count to four in your mind, then exhale slowly but strongly through your mouth, so you really empty your lungs. Take your time on the out-breath. This helps expel the stale air in your lungs and encourages you to take in more oxygen on the next in-breath. Repeat at least four times.

▼ Lowering the shoulders

This sequence helps to establish contact and encourages your massage partner to let go of any exhausting tension.

1 Your partner now sits down with his upper back easily accessible for massage. Place your hands on the top of his shoulders. Hold for a few seconds.

2 Gradually use your body weight to apply more pressure so that you are pushing down on his shoulders. Hold for twenty seconds then release. Ask him to exhale as you lean your weight down. Repeat three times.

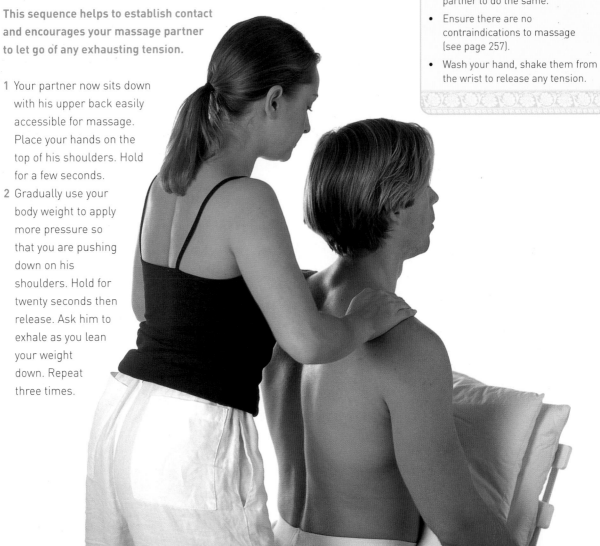

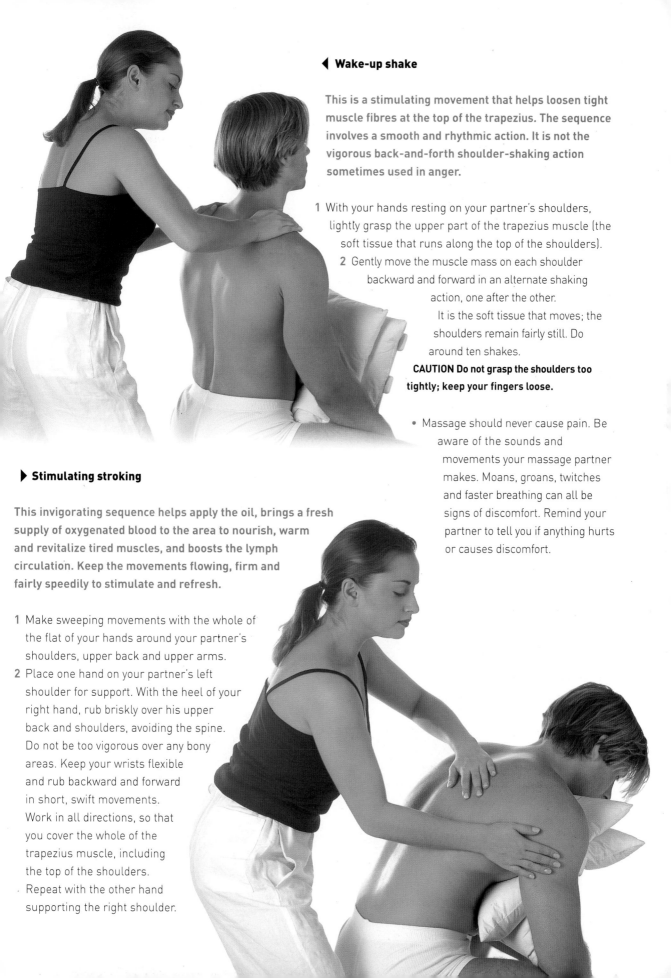

◀ Wake-up shake

This is a stimulating movement that helps loosen tight muscle fibres at the top of the trapezius. The sequence involves a smooth and rhythmic action. It is not the vigorous back-and-forth shoulder-shaking action sometimes used in anger.

1 With your hands resting on your partner's shoulders, lightly grasp the upper part of the trapezius muscle (the soft tissue that runs along the top of the shoulders).

2 Gently move the muscle mass on each shoulder backward and forward in an alternate shaking action, one after the other. It is the soft tissue that moves; the shoulders remain fairly still. Do around ten shakes.

CAUTION Do not grasp the shoulders too tightly; keep your fingers loose.

- Massage should never cause pain. Be aware of the sounds and movements your massage partner makes. Moans, groans, twitches and faster breathing can all be signs of discomfort. Remind your partner to tell you if anything hurts or causes discomfort.

▶ Stimulating stroking

This invigorating sequence helps apply the oil, brings a fresh supply of oxygenated blood to the area to nourish, warm and revitalize tired muscles, and boosts the lymph circulation. Keep the movements flowing, firm and fairly speedily to stimulate and refresh.

1 Make sweeping movements with the whole of the flat of your hands around your partner's shoulders, upper back and upper arms.

2 Place one hand on your partner's left shoulder for support. With the heel of your right hand, rub briskly over his upper back and shoulders, avoiding the spine. Do not be too vigorous over any bony areas. Keep your wrists flexible and rub backward and forward in short, swift movements. Work in all directions, so that you cover the whole of the trapezius muscle, including the top of the shoulders. Repeat with the other hand supporting the right shoulder.

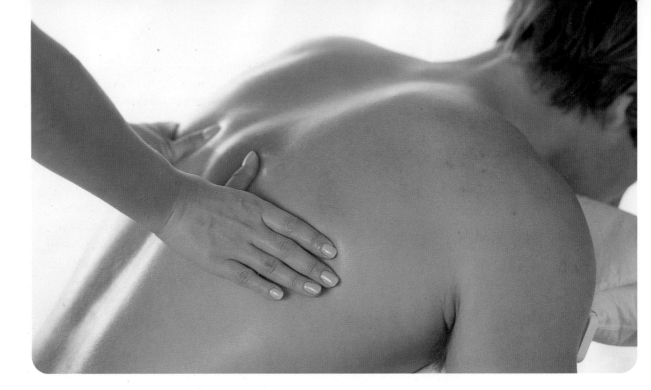

▲ Thumb pressures

This sequence uses a very deep, penetrating friction movement. It can be most effective in relieving muscular tension and stiffness around the shoulders.

1 With your fingers resting lightly on your partner's shoulder-blades, place your thumbs at the base of the shoulder-blades, on either side of the spine. Use the fleshy pads of your thumbs to press firmly in a state of friction. Hold for a couple of seconds and then release.

2 Lift your thumbs and glide up a little. Repeat step 1. Use your body weight to lean into the movement, gradually increasing the pressure. Ask your partner to exhale as you apply pressure and inhale as the pressure is released. Repeat until you have covered the whole of the large trapezius muscle. You may find that your partner's body moves forward as you press firmly.

CAUTION If your partner is very tense, these pressures can be painful if applied to a tender spot. If he shows any discomfort, use some gentle, soothing stroking.

• If you have any doubts about your partner's health, do not massage.

▼ Light hacking on the back

This is very effective for stimulating sensory nerve endings and can be most exhilarating. When you are doing this hacking technique correctly, you will hear a sound similar to the clip-clop of horse's hooves.

1 Hold your hands slightly apart, palms facing each other. Use the little finger side of your hands to work

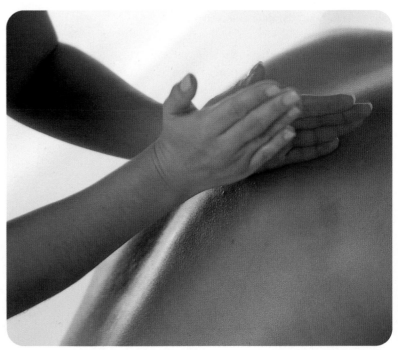

alternately in a hacking action (see page 246). Strike the upper back, then release, strike, then release. Keep your wrists flexible and fingers fairly relaxed as you move your forearms up and down. As soon as each hand touches the skin, it flicks back up again.

2 Hack across the whole area, including the upper trapezius. Keep moving your hands so as not to overwork any spot. Continue for around thirty seconds and then soothe and calm the area with some fairly speedy effleurage strokes.

CAUTION **Avoid massaging over the spine. Hacking over bony protrusions can be extremely painful for you and your partner.**

▼ Finger combing

This sequence uses a raking action that creates a completely different sensation to that of using the

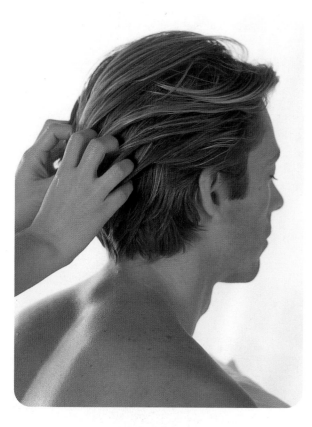

fleshy pads of your fingers and can often make your partner's scalp tingle. Try it on yourself. It is a useful energizing, circulation-boosting movement.

1 Place both hands in a claw-like position on the top of your massage partner's head, with your fingers facing forward, just touching the hairline. Keep your fingers fairly widely spread.

2 Use your fingertips to rake back firmly along the scalp, down to the base of the skull. Cover the entire scalp. Your hands can 'comb' the hair at the same time or with alternate strokes.

• Check that your pressure suits your massage partner. Everyone has their own preferences, so adapt to suit.

▼ Hair tousling

This action stimulates the circulation and helps loosen the muscles in the scalp. This can also be performed with one hand, using the other to support the head.

1 With your hands in the same claw-like position as in the previous sequence, use your fingertips to rub firmly and briskly in short random back-and-forth movements all over your partner's scalp. Keep your wrists very flexible and your touch light to medium. Start at the back of the ears and cover the whole head.

2 Keep your hands moving; do not stay in the same place for too long. You may start to feel a lovely, tingling sensation in your fingertips.

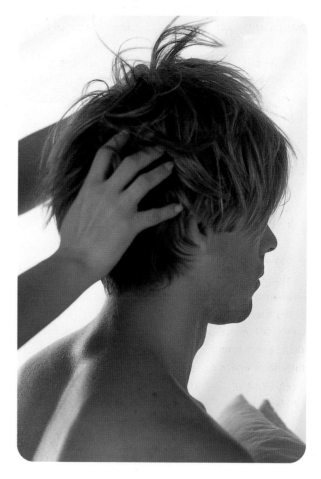

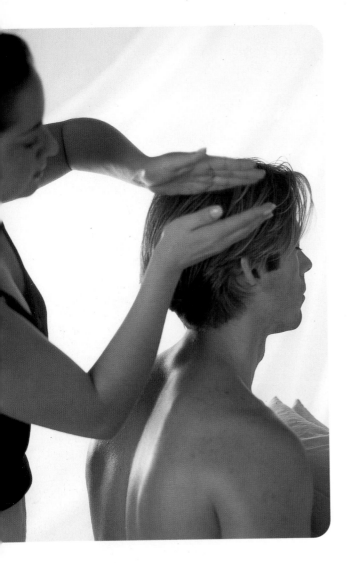

to flinch, use a lighter touch or move on to the next step. Keep your hands moving so you do not pull the same roots. Hold as much hair as you can.

1 Push your fingers up through your partner's hair and mould the flat of your hands to the shape of his head. Your fingers should be fairly widely spread with large bunches of hair between them. Press the palm of your hand firmly on his scalp around the occiput then grasp the hair roots between your fingers and give it a gentle tug to ease any tension and tiredness. Hold for a few seconds then release.

2 Reposition your hands and repeat the movement three times, until the back of the head has been completely covered. If your massage partner has very short hair, you can adapt the technique by clasping the hair roots between your fingers and thumbs, or in a clenched fist with the backs of your fingers against the scalp, and then gently tugging.

CAUTION Avoid this movement if your partner has very fine hair.

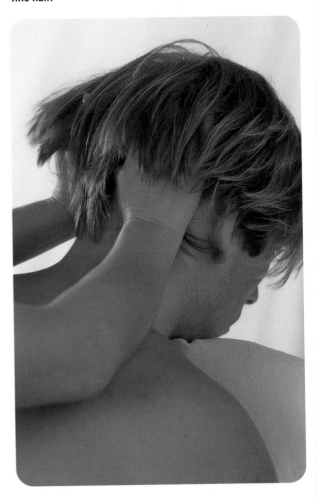

▲ **Gentle hacking on the head**

Using the same technique as in the 'Light hacking on the back' sequence (see page 280), hack very lightly and gently around the sides of your partner's head for about thirty seconds.

• Massage has a powerful influence on sensory nerve endings and can be used to relax or stimulate both mind and body. Energizing strokes are fast and brisk.

CAUTION Do not hack over your partner's crown as this can be a very sensitive area and should always be treated with extreme care.

▶ **Hair tugging**

This sequence is wonderfully revitalizing but be careful not to cause any pain. If your partner appears

▶ Final flourish

This finishing sequence will leave your partner relaxed and refreshed, ready to continue the day with renewed energy.

1 Repeat the 'Finger combing' sequence (see page 281) using first the fingertips and then the soft pads of your fingers to soothe and calm the scalp after the previous invigorating massage movements.

2 Complete the massage by using the flat of your hands to swiftly sweep down your partner's neck and over his shoulders and upper back several times.

3 Allow your massage partner to sit quietly for a few minutes while you wash your hands and bring him a glass of cool, fresh water. This is the ideal time for your partner to enjoy a refreshing shower.

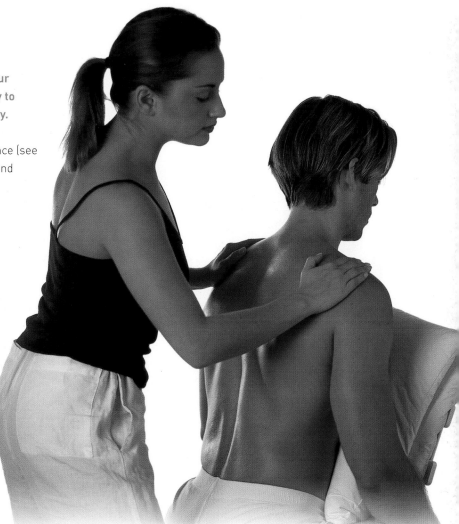

CASE STUDY

MANAGING A STRESSFUL LIFE

John, 46, runs his own painting and decorating business. He spends his spare time renovating an old barn where he plans to live with his wife and their two teenage children. With so many commitments and demands on his energy, life can be stressful at times. So when John heard that Indian head massage could aid relaxation and boost energy levels, he immediately booked in for a course of six sessions – and it has worked, but the results were not immediate. 'After the first massage, I felt so exhausted that I went to bed at eight in the evening. The next thing I knew, the alarm was going off. Even after such a good sleep, I felt tired all the next day. I also had a slight, niggling headache. Thankfully, I had

been warned that this may happen so I kept sipping water. I tried to view it as a positive sign that my body was being cleansed of all that alcohol and junk food.

'I am really glad that I booked six weeks of massages in advance – otherwise I might not have gone back. I must admit that I was bit disappointed at the time, I expected to be bursting with health and energy as soon as I walked out of the door. I felt a bit off-colour after my next two massages but it lasted only a few hours. Then after the fourth massage I had no ill effects, and felt full of energy. It was incredible. I feel much calmer and less hassled. I now realize that you have to listen to your body – you cannot keep soldiering on with only a few hours' sleep a night.'

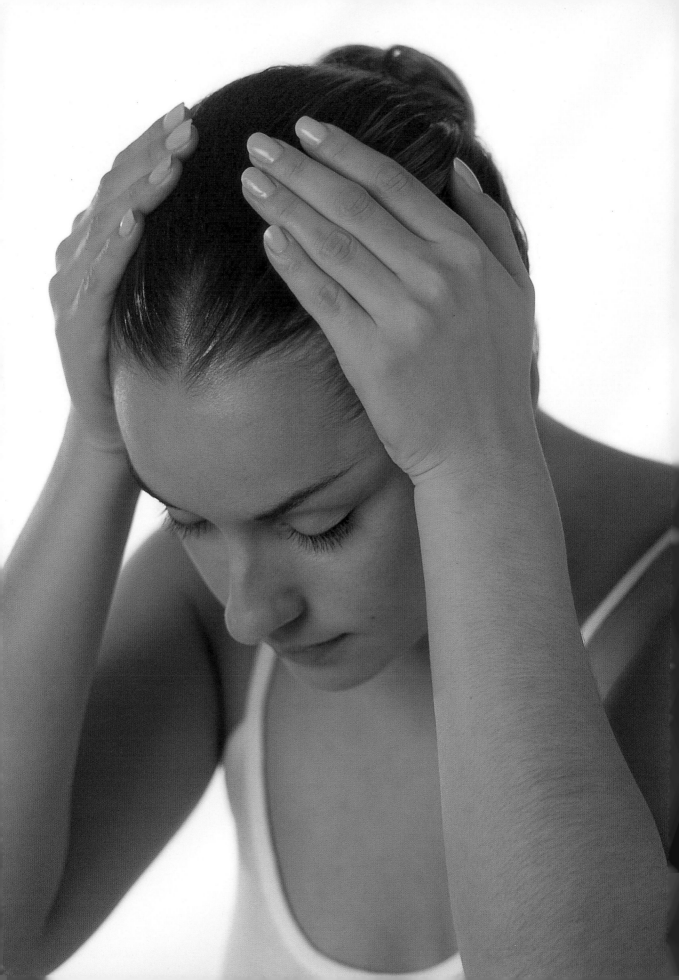

Ease your
headache

When a tension headache strikes you need instant relief. The following five-minute self-massage routine has been devised to ease the pain as soon as it starts, without having to resort to popping painkillers. There is no need to undress or use oil so you can easily perform it wherever you are – at home or at work.

Causes of tension headache

Headaches can cause different degrees of pain, ranging from a dull ache to very severe pain. They have a wide variety of causes, including lack of sleep, stuffy atmosphere, loud noise, changes in the weather, hormonal swings, food intolerances, dehydration, eye strain and poor posture. The most intense form of headache is migraine, which is often accompanied by nausea, dizziness and visual disturbances. However, the most common type is the tension headache, which can affect us all at some time or another. Indeed, it has been estimated that the stress-induced kind accounts for four out of every five headaches reported to family doctors.

Tension headaches are usually triggered by tightness in the muscles of the neck, shoulders, scalp and face. This restricts the normal flow of blood and lymph, leading to tenderness and pain, often in localized areas such as the base of the skull, temples, jaws, forehead or sides of the head. Muscular tension is often associated with stress, anxiety, tiredness and long periods spent working at a computer or driving a car. The pain is sometimes described as a 'tight band around the head' that gets worse as the day progresses.

It is hard to think straight when your head hurts. It is often tempting just to swallow a painkiller to clear the symptoms so you can carry on with your activities.

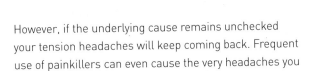

CHECKLIST

PREPARATION

- Turn off – or shut out – as much noise as possible.
- Allow fresh air to circulate around the room.
- Keep lighting to a minimum.

However, if the underlying cause remains unchecked your tension headaches will keep coming back. Frequent use of painkillers can even cause the very headaches you were trying to alleviate. The key is in relaxation.

- Most headaches are not a cause for concern. However, you should consult your doctor if the pain is very severe or persistent or the headache is accompanied by fever, vomiting, altered vision, stiff neck or a rash.

Self-massage for tension relief

A regular relaxation routine (see page 252) helps you cope better with the stressful situations that can lead to tension headaches. Massaging the neck, shoulders, scalp and face can also ease tension in taut muscles – thereby restoring the blood and lymph flow.

CASE STUDY

SOOTHING ROAD RAGE

Jane, 32, has been an insurance sales person for a year, and loves her work. However, it involves long hours and a great deal of time sitting in her car travelling between appointments. After a few months in the job she began to get shooting pains in her shoulders and had almost constant stiffness in her neck. 'I was getting really fed up and thinking of changing jobs,' she said. 'Then a friend recommended Indian head massage and after the first session I realized how tense I had become – both physically and mentally. I'm not a very relaxed person at the best of times, but I was getting very short-tempered – especially with other road-users.

'After just one Indian head massage my neck felt two inches longer and far more mobile, and the

constant nagging thud in my head had cleared. It recurred a few days later but my therapist said it would take a few sessions to clear the problem. She also advised me that Indian head massage doesn't work on its own. I needed to make some lifestyle changes too. She suggested that I take more exercise, correct my posture in the car and try to allow more time between appointments so I am not always rushing. I have learnt to recognize when I'm feeling anxious or certain muscles are beginning to tighten – and I make a real effort to relax. Now I feel happier and more tolerant than ever.'

▼ Breathing out tension

Start with a breathing exercise. Stop whatever you are doing. Sit down and close your eyes. Try to close your mind to outside disturbances. Focus on your breathing.

1 Breathe slowly and deeply in through your nose and out through your mouth. On the in-breath let the air flow right down to your abdomen.

2 On the out-breath make a long controlled sigh so that you slowly let out the breath as though exhaling all your tensions. The out-breath should take the same time as or longer than the in-breath. Repeat three times.

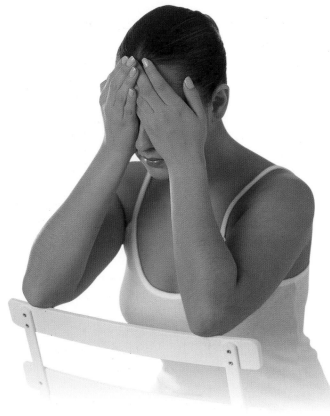

▲ Soothing darkness

Bathing in darkness has such as calming influence that it may be enough to lift a slight headache. Try to switch off from any circling thoughts, think of a colour or concentrate on your breathing.

1 Place your elbows, shoulder-width apart, on a table, chair back or desk in front of you. If you are in a stationary car, rest them on the steering wheel. Lean forward slightly so that your hands support the weight of your head, allowing the release of tension in your neck.

2 Place your hands over your eyes to create total darkness, enabling the muscles at the back of your eyes to relax. One of the most effective ways is to place the heels of your hands on your cheekbones, with your palms cupping your eyes, fingers pointing upward. Stay in this position for at least a minute, longer if possible.

• Headaches can sometimes be caused by dental problems and poor eyesight, so make an appointment with your optician or dentist if you suffer regular unexplained headaches.

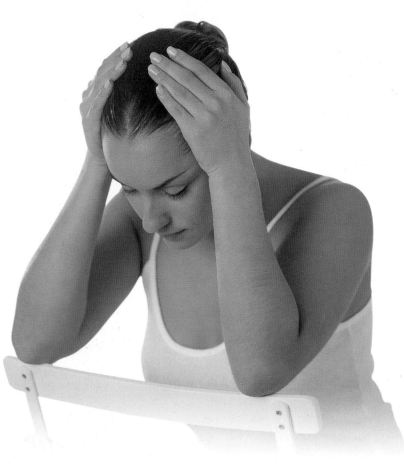

The comforting feeling of your hands against your head can help ease you into a state of relaxation.

1 Cradle your head securely between your hands so that the heels of your hands are resting on your temples and your fingers meet at the top of your head. Exert as much pressure with your hands as feels comfortable. Hold for a minute.
2 Move your hands a little further back and repeat this head hold.

▶ **Scalp lift**

This is a wonderful tension-busting movement that you can also use with your family and friends. It helps to ease away all the tension that can become trapped in the thin layer of muscle covering the head.

1 Interlock your fingers and slowly press the palms of your hands inward and upward against your scalp, so that the skin starts to move beneath your fingers.
2 Move to another position and repeat. You can repeat the move as often as you wish.
• Keep focusing on your breathing as you massage your scalp. Take deep calming breaths to help relieve any mental and physical tensions.

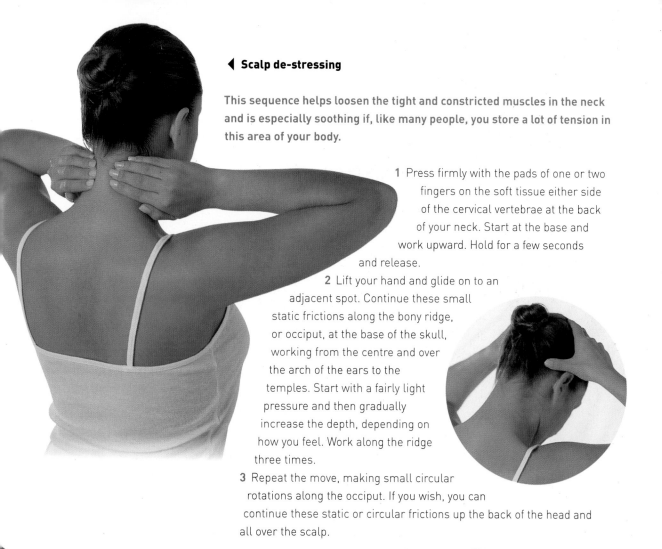

◀ Scalp de-stressing

This sequence helps loosen the tight and constricted muscles in the neck and is especially soothing if, like many people, you store a lot of tension in this area of your body.

1 Press firmly with the pads of one or two fingers on the soft tissue either side of the cervical vertebrae at the back of your neck. Start at the base and work upward. Hold for a few seconds and release.

2 Lift your hand and glide on to an adjacent spot. Continue these small static frictions along the bony ridge, or occiput, at the base of the skull, working from the centre and over the arch of the ears to the temples. Start with a fairly light pressure and then gradually increase the depth, depending on how you feel. Work along the ridge three times.

3 Repeat the move, making small circular rotations along the occiput. If you wish, you can continue these static or circular frictions up the back of the head and all over the scalp.

▶ Massaging the temples

You may instinctively rub your temples at the onset of a headache – it is a good pain-relieving movement. You will need to locate the soft indentation of both temples. This is often quite difficult to do on yourself, but you will know when you have found the right spot because it feels so good.

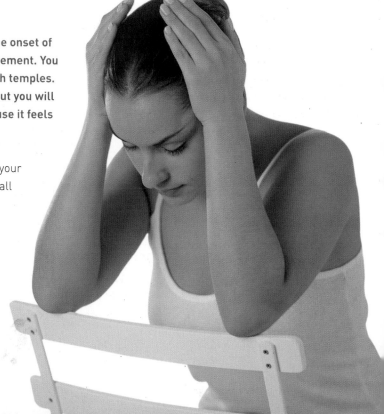

1 Place your hands on your temples. With the heel of your hands or pads of your fingers, make at least ten small circular movements, clockwise or anticlockwise, whichever feels best. Keep your fingers on the skin and move it against the underlying soft tissue to soften and relax the muscles.

• We all hold tension in different places around the head, neck and shoulders. Vary the routine and moves to suit your own personal needs. Massaging your own shoulders with gentle kneading can be very effective.

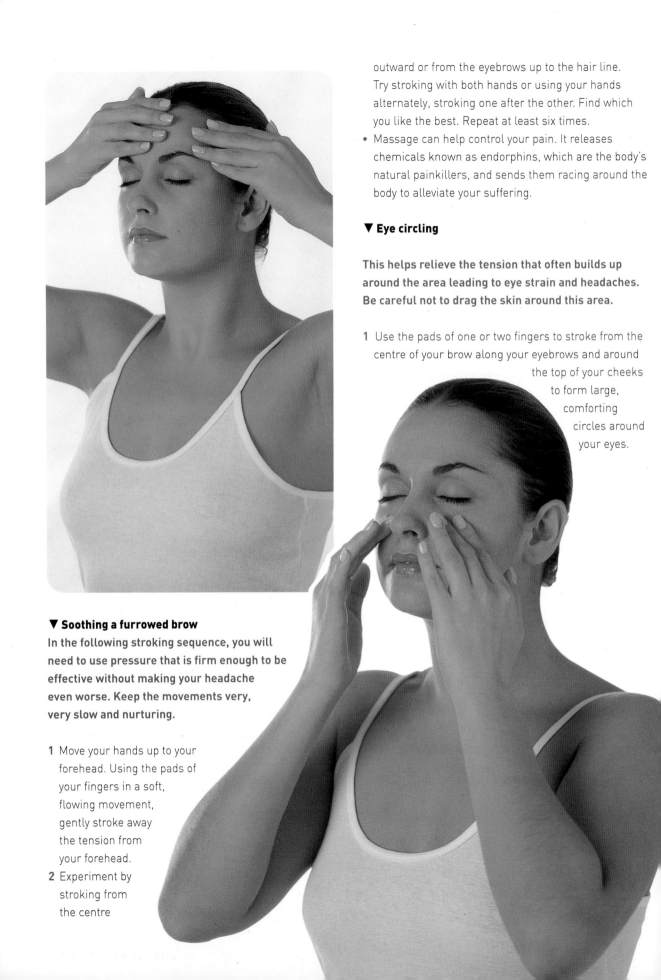

outward or from the eyebrows up to the hair line. Try stroking with both hands or using your hands alternately, stroking one after the other. Find which you like the best. Repeat at least six times.

- Massage can help control your pain. It releases chemicals known as endorphins, which are the body's natural painkillers, and sends them racing around the body to alleviate your suffering.

▼ Eye circling

This helps relieve the tension that often builds up around the area leading to eye strain and headaches. Be careful not to drag the skin around this area.

1 Use the pads of one or two fingers to stroke from the centre of your brow along your eyebrows and around the top of your cheeks to form large, comforting circles around your eyes.

▼ Soothing a furrowed brow

In the following stroking sequence, you will need to use pressure that is firm enough to be effective without making your headache even worse. Keep the movements very, very slow and nurturing.

1 Move your hands up to your forehead. Using the pads of your fingers in a soft, flowing movement, gently stroke away the tension from your forehead.

2 Experiment by stroking from the centre

▼ Loosening a tight jaw

If you tend to clench your teeth when under stress, this sequence will be especially beneficial.

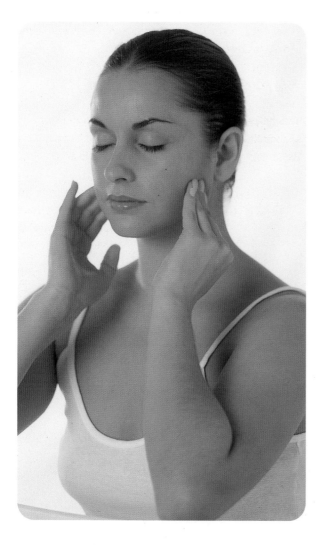

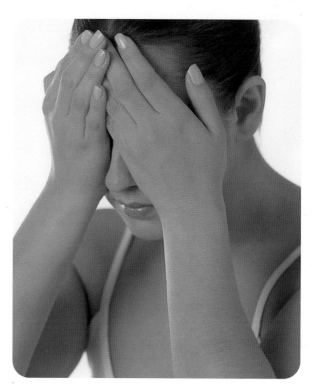

or does it seem glued to the bone? Regular scalp massage helps loosen and relax this layer of tissue, so helping to keep you free from tension headaches.

▲ Repeat final darkness

Complete your headache routine by repeating the first sequence. Stay in darkness for as long as you wish. If you have the opportunity, rest on a bed in a dimly lit or darkened room for half an hour or so after the massage. This enables your body to direct more energy toward relieving your headache.

Top up your fluid levels

Dehydration is a common cause of headaches. Drinking a glass of cool water regularly will restore the fluid you lose during the day and help flush the toxins from your body.

1 Place both your hands at the sides of your mouth and stroke the heels of your hands outward to the ears three or four times.
2 Now make small kneading rotations over the same area using the pads of your two middle fingers. Feel for any taut muscles. Move smoothly around the area to warm and soften the powerful jaw muscles. Finish by stroking the area again.
• A tight scalp is a sure sign of stress. When the facial muscles become taut with worry or anger, this causes a tightening in the layer of tissue covering the skull, leading to headaches and eye strain. You can feel the tension by trying to move your scalp. Does it move freely

• A cold compress can also help ease the pain of your headache. Fill a bowl with ice-cold water and add three to four drops of lavender oil. Place a folded face flannel on the water and let it absorb the oil floating on the surface. Wring out the flannel so that it is moist but not wet and apply it to the painful area for about fifteen minutes. Renew as necessary. Chilled eye masks are also wonderfully soothing.

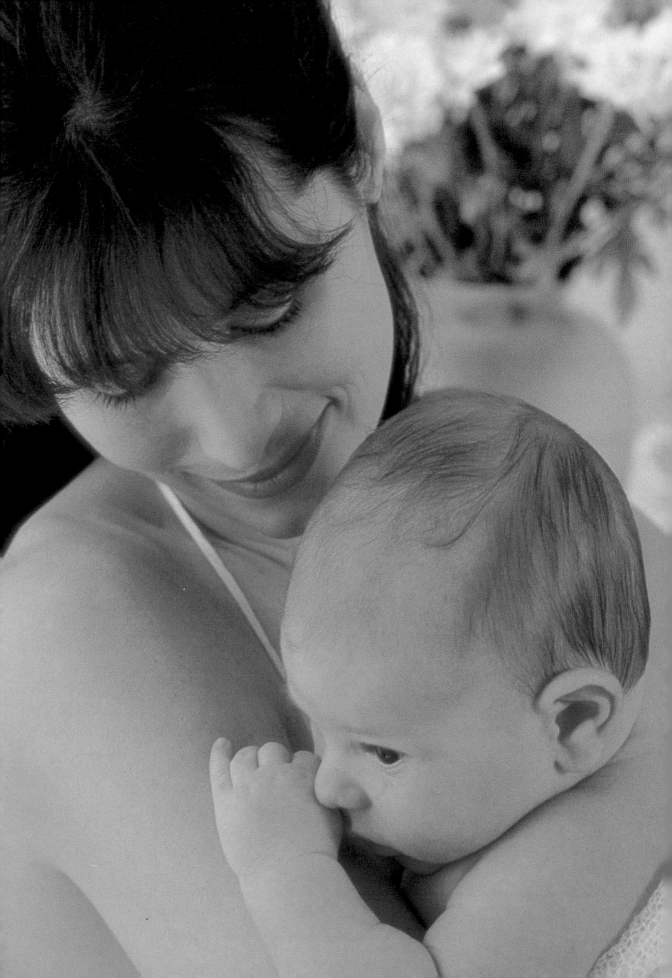

Family
focus

Everyone can benefit from Indian head massage – from the very young right through to the very old – not only physically, but also emotionally. Enjoying the pleasure of a caring touch brings tremendous comfort and a sense of security that helps establish a warm and loving atmosphere in the home.

The early days

The desire to nurture and be nurtured is innate. Babies and toddlers love to be cuddled, held and stroked and, as parents, we instinctively want to nurture and caress our offspring. Nature certainly knows best. Research in orphanages in Romania confirms that physical affection is crucial to a child's health and well-being. Lack of close physical contact in the first few years can hinder emotional, physiological and social development. By contrast, infants who are held, rocked and cuddled tend to be happier and more contented, throw fewer tantrums, suffer less colic, eat better and sleep more soundly.

The benefits of a loving touch can be extended still further by giving your baby a regular massage and continuing this practice throughout her childhood. Studies now show that massaging premature babies can help stimulate their growth and the development of their immune systems so that they gain more weight and thrive. The positive effects of massage, for both parents and children, are now so widely recognized in the West that most new mothers, and fathers too, are actively encouraged to share the soothing, loving experience.

The following sequence is for a quick and simple face, head, shoulder and arm massage. It is designed to introduce you to the pleasures of baby and infant massage. There is no need to make it a formal session, or to follow the steps rigidly. Aim to discover your child's likes and dislikes. You can massage your baby or toddler whenever you both feel like having some close contact with each other. Before or after bathing is a very popular time because this is such a lovely, cosy moment. She can be fully undressed or wearing a nappy, as you wish. But do make sure that she does not get cold. Stop as soon as your baby becomes fractious or seems to be no longer enjoying herself, and try again another time.

- If you would like to know more about sharing the many benefits of full-body massage with your baby, visit a class in your area. There, you will be able to massage your baby, with an expert on hand to guide and advise you.

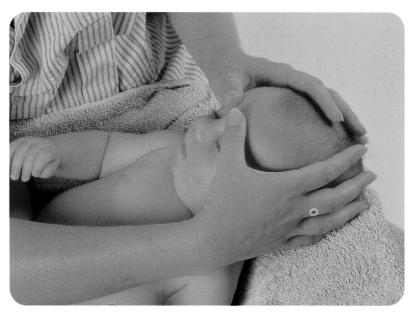

CHECKLIST

A FEW CAUTIONS

- Avoid nut oils and pure essential oils.
- Always get the go-ahead from your midwife or health visitor before massaging your baby. Some parents prefer to wait until after the six-week assessment.
- Do a skin test to check that she is not allergic to the oil. Apply a little oil to a small area of her arm or leg. Wait 24 hours. If you notice any red blotches, do not use the oil. If there is no change in the skin, try the test again to be completely sure.
- Wait at least an hour and a half after a feed.
- Do not massage if your baby is unwell, particularly if she has a fever or is being given any medication. If you are unsure, talk to your doctor.
- Work carefully around any areas of broken skin – but avoid massage if your baby has a rash or skin infection.
- Wait at least a week after an immunization.
- Do not apply oil to the face as it may get into your baby's eyes.

Until the age of about two or three, a baby's skull is very delicate and must be handled extremely carefully. Never press heavily on the skin or hair covering the soft areas on the top and sides of the head. These soft areas, called the fontanelles, are the spaces where the skull bones have not yet knitted. The fontanelles allow the bones of the skull to move during birth. The soft bones mould the skull to the shape of the mother's birth canal so that the head can pass down more freely. As your child grows, the skull bones start to fuse together to form a rigid structure.

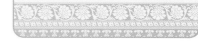

LEFT **Take immense care when massaging a baby's delicate head.**

Get comfortable

Try out several different positions to find out which one suits you best. Keep your baby facing you. Some options include:

- Sitting on the edge of a cushion with your legs stretched out in front of you in a V shape – with your baby lying on the floor between your legs.
- Sitting on a cushion, your back supported against a wall or heavy piece of furniture, with your baby lying on your lap. Your knees can be bent or straight.
- If you suffer from back pain, try resting your baby on a table or changing unit that is the right height for you. Never leave your baby unattended on a table or other high position.

Loving hold

Very gently, cradle your baby's head in your hands so that she feels secure and sure of your presence. Lightly rest the palms of your hands above her ears, with your fingertips touching at the top of her head. Keep the touch very, very gentle. Hold for a minute or so and establish eye contact.

CAUTION Do not exert any pressure on your baby's head.

Facial strokes

1 Support the side of your baby's head with one hand and very gently, slowly and rhythmically stroke the pads of one or two fingers across her forehead. Start at the centre and work out toward the temples.
2 Continue the feather-like strokes from the sides of her nose to her ears and under her chin. Trace a circular pattern over her face with the pad of your fingers, circling her nose, mouth and chin. Gently rub her ears.

Let your baby explore your face too. Encourage her to touch, feel and pat your face and head. If you wear glasses, take them off first.

Smoothing on the oil

1 Put a few drops of a suitable oil in the palm of one hand (half a teaspoon is plenty). Rub your hands together briskly so that they are warm and well lubricated with oil.
2 Gently stroke from the centre of her head down the sides and back of her head to her neck. Take special care to keep your touch very light, gliding over the surface of her skin and hair.

CAUTION Take extreme care to avoid pressing on the soft spot, or fontanelle, on the top of your baby's head.

Stroking the arms

1 Rest your hands lightly at the base of your baby's neck and gently stroke over her shoulders and arms with the palms of your hands.
2 Delicately trace small circular strokes with the pads of your fingers, spiralling up the arm. Cover the whole of the arm with soft, soothing strokes. Finish the massage in the starting position, with her head cupped between your hands.
- It is no coincidence that babies in India rarely cry – they are in almost constant close physical contact with their mothers. In many parts of India, babies are not taken outside for the first 40 days after birth. Instead, they stay close to their mothers in the warmth and peace of the home.

CHECKLIST

THINGS YOU WILL NEED

- A padded surface such as a changing mat for your baby to lie in comfort. Cover with a clean, soft, warm towel.
- Good-quality oil suitable for a baby's delicate skin. Unrefined, organic sunflower oil is ideal, or use an oil specially blended for babies.
- Spare towel or wipes to clear up any little accidents.

THINGS TO DO

- Ensure the room is warm and free from draughts.
- Check that your nails are short, clean and have no rough edges. Cover any cuts with a plaster.
- Remove any hand or wrist jewellery.
- Wash your hands in warm water.

Getting your toddler to sleep

Tempers can easily get frayed at bedtime. The following simple, impromptu massage movements may help your toddler get to sleep when she is over-tired and fractious. You do not need any oil, so your child can stay in bed in her pyjamas.

▼ Peace and quiet

Sit on the bed with your back resting against the bed-head or wall. Prop yourself up with pillows, if you will feel more comfortable. Your child sits between your outstretched legs with her head against your chest. You may like to support her back with a small cushion or rolled-up towel.

1 Ask your child to shut her eyes – often not as easy as it sounds. It may help to try sprinkling some imaginary sleepy dust on her eyes to close them but if she refuses to co-operate then she could just look at a book.

2 Rest the palms of your hands gently on her forehead, at the hairline, with your fingers slightly overlapping in the middle. Stay like this for a minute or so. It is very calming and allows you both to enjoy some stillness and peace. Breathe calmly and slowly. Listen as her breathing starts to follow yours.

• As you massage, smile, talk softly or sing quietly. Try to keep one hand in contact with her skin at all times. Focus on your breathing. Take deep, even breaths. Your child is very receptive to your moods, so try to stay as calm, confident and relaxed as possible.

▶ Sleepy stroking

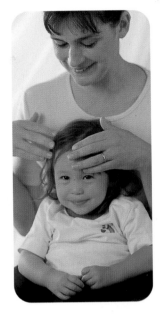

1 Place your hands on the top of her head and slowly and gently stroke down either side of her head to her ears. Repeat several times. Repetition is wonderfully reassuring. Sing or hum very softly.

2 Place the palms of your hands on her forehead and make some gentle circles in the centre above the eye-brows. Now stroke from the centre outward. You can use one hand – or two hands, alternating the strokes so that one stroke flows smoothly into the next. Keep the movements very slow and loving. Repeat as many times as you like. Continue these gentle, smoothing glides all over her face, working from the centre outward. Imagine that you are stroking her cares away.

3 Repeat the first step of 'Sleepy stroking' and finish by repeating step two of 'Peace and quiet'.

• If your baby or child seems to be continually upset and crying all the time, when she does not seem unwell and there is no obvious cause of her distress, you may want to consider consulting a cranial osteopath (see page 299), who may be able to help..

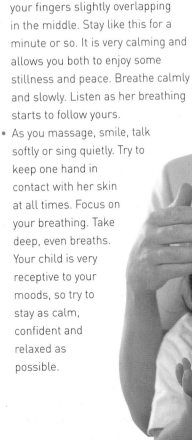

Growing up with Indian head massage

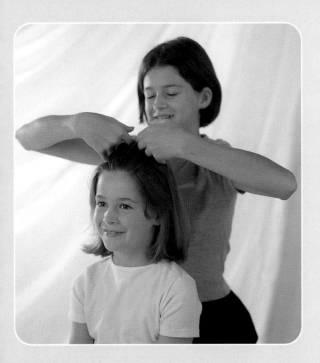 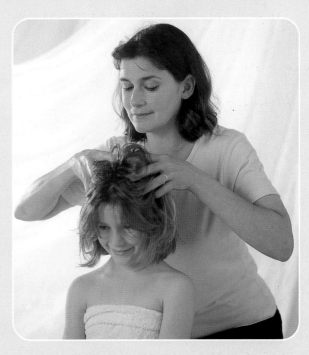

• Children are often more sensitive than we think and can get just as stressed as adults, sometimes even more so. Our modern world is full of pressures, choices and expectations. Young people are bombarded with the frenzy and noise of television, computers and video games. They may also have worries about friendships, homework, bullying and disturbing items on the news. Sometimes it can all get too much – leading to mental, physical and emotional overload. Frequent headaches, stomach upsets and muscle twitches are all signs of stress in children.

• Children over the age of about eight are often reluctant to be seen hugging or kissing their parents or siblings in public. However, when you are on your own together, they usually love the comfort of an arm around their shoulders and may well sit on your knee, especially when they are feeling tired or upset. Close physical contact with someone you love is a powerful way of soothing troubles and boosting confidence. The caring, relaxing sensation of an Indian head massage shared within the family may encourage the release of any feelings or concerns that are being bottled up.

• The massage movements on the previous pages can be adapted for children over about three years of age. If they fidget and wriggle, use a lighter pressure and reduce the length of the massage. Most children

generally do not like having oil in their hair, so it may be better to give a dry massage or use a very small amount of oil. It is virtually impossible to plan a session, so grab the opportunity when you are both in the mood for massage. This might be first thing in the morning, at bedtime, or any time during the day that your child seems to need some extra love and attention. Do not force your child; judge the right time.

Stormy times

It can be difficult being a teenager. This is a time of doubts, fears and turmoil. The change from childhood to adulthood can be very daunting, lonely and bewildering – with uncertainties about physical development, hormonal changes, relationship difficulties and the pressure of exams and career choices. A hectic lifestyle, fast-food diet and late nights only make matters worse. Although many parents and adolescents may seem to be at loggerheads most of the time, current studies show that they still usually hold a great affection for each other – they just do not always know how to show it.

Sharing an Indian head massage can be a way of helping you both to relax, unwind and look at your problems and disagreements from another point of view. It can help rekindle a bond between you and provide emotional

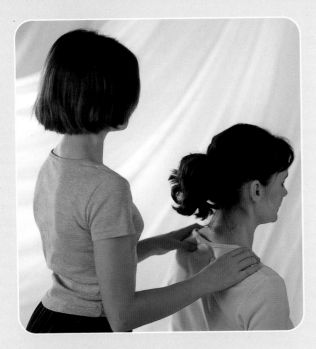

warmth and security to help you work through this difficult stage. Professional therapists are now being invited into some secondary schools to help boost the pupils' concentration and combat tiredness and exam stress. You can use some of the techniques from the previous pages to do the same in your own home – and ask your teenager to give you a massage, too!

Rubbing parents up the right way

Most children of around seven or eight years of age can give a very firm, relaxing and caring massage. Indeed, children often enjoy giving more than receiving. Think how they instinctively use their tactile senses to explore the world and how they love to rearrange your hair and softly stroke your face. They have few inhibitions about touch and find it perfectly natural to communicate love and affection through their hands. Most children enjoy experimenting with different moves and feel very proud of their achievements when you praise their efforts.

You will need to try out different positions for massaging, depending on your child's height. One of the most comfortable positions is sitting on a cushion on the floor, with your child sitting on a chair or kneeling on a cushion behind you. It is probably best that your child massages without oil, or uses only a tiny amount of oil, as you could both get rather messy. If you have already massaged your child, she may be able to copy your movements without any tuition. You may like to prompt her on occasion, however, so that you can enjoy your

favourite moves with the right depth of pressure. Do make it very clear that the spine must always be avoided. All you need to do then is rest and unwind as she kneads your shoulders, 'shampoos' your hair and rubs your back.

- Next time you are feeling uptight and stressed, ask your child or teenager for a massage – you will both feel a lot calmer and happier afterward.

Bridging the generation gap

In India, grandparents often ask their grandchildren for a massage to relieve their aches and pains. Massage can also be a way of forging a bond between family members of different generations – and a time to exchange news and stories. Many elderly people, especially those living on their own, have little physical contact with others. This can lead to feelings of isolation, depression and loss of self-esteem. A caring touch from a child can make all the difference. Although some children may be hesitant about cuddling their grandparents, they may find the more formal approach of touch through massage quite acceptable – even great fun. Your child can enjoy trying out the different massage techniques that he has already practised on you, although he may need to have a lighter and less vigorous approach if the grandparent is rather frail

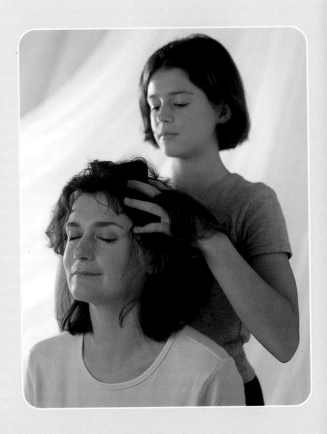

Cranial osteopathy

Many people ask if there is any similarity between Indian head massage and cranial osteopathy. In fact, the two are completely different therapies. Cranial osteopathy was developed in the 1930s by a US osteopath, Dr William Garner Sutherland. It is a highly specialized therapy that works by gentle manipulation of the bones in the cranium, the dome-shaped part of the skull that protects the brain. It is a common misconception that the cranium is one continuous bone. It is not. The cranium is made up of several bones that are connected by interlocking joints.

Therapists claim to be able to sense by touch the rhythm of the cerebrospinal fluid, which nourishes and protects the membranes that encase the brain and spinal cord. This fluid is said to pulsate at between 6–15 times per minute but can be disturbed by pressure on the head and injuries and tensions in the body. This cranial rhythmic impulse (CRI) is difficult to measure, but qualified practitioners have been trained to use delicate manipulation of the cranial and spinal bones to restore it to its correct rhythm. Blood circulation is also boosted and lymph and sinus fluids in the head are drained.

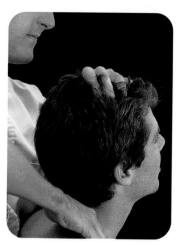

ABOVE **A cranial osteopath at work.**

Cranial osteopathy can be used on adults to help problems ranging from stress to physical pain. However, it is a particularly useful therapy for young children, when it is often known as paediatric osteopathy. It has been shown to relieve colic, glue ear and recurrent infections. It can even be used on babies to correct cranial bone distortions caused during a difficult birth. Early treatment, when a child's cranial bones are particularly flexible, can prevent problems later in life.

Craniosacral therapy grew out of cranial osteopathy but is more concerned with soft tissue than with bones. Founded in the 1970s by a Michigan State University osteopath, Dr John Upledger, it works on the principle that the CRI affects the whole body through the connective tissues that link all the organs, bones and muscles. Practitioners believe that it is the membranes that encase the brain and spinal cord that generate the CRI. Using subtle hand pressure on the body, usually around the head area or the base of the spine, they identify and relieve pain and tension and thereby re-establish an even, rhythmic flow of CRI. Unlike cranial osteopathy, the cranium is not manipulated. Craniosacral therapy can help nervous problems, pain and even paralysis. Patients also report feelings of deep relaxation and the release of tension.

CASE STUDY

BABY BLUES

Ruth, 30, was so exhausted after the birth of her baby, Joe, that she rarely had the energy to get dressed before midday. 'I had expected to be all excited and motherly but I missed my job and social life and spent most of my time in tears,' she explained. 'I looked a mess – my hair was all over the place and my skin was spotty. Then my mobile hairdresser said that she could give me an Indian head massage, which may help boost my morale and improve the condition of my hair and skin. It was the most wonderful feeling when she stroked my hair and face. I could almost feel the stress lifting. When I looked in the mirror afterward, it was a quite different person looking back.

'My hairdresser came back several times to give me a weekly head massage and always made time for a chat. Her caring touch and interest in my well-being helped me rebuild my confidence and I began to enjoy motherhood. She told me how to massage my own head using oils to help my hair regain strength after pregnancy and has really made a difference.

'She also suggested that I should try to massage baby Joe. Massage is now part of our bath-time ritual – he gurgles and smiles at me and we have a lot of fun. I still have my ups and downs but as soon as I start to feel low again I book in for a head massage to raise my spirits and put some colour in my cheeks.'

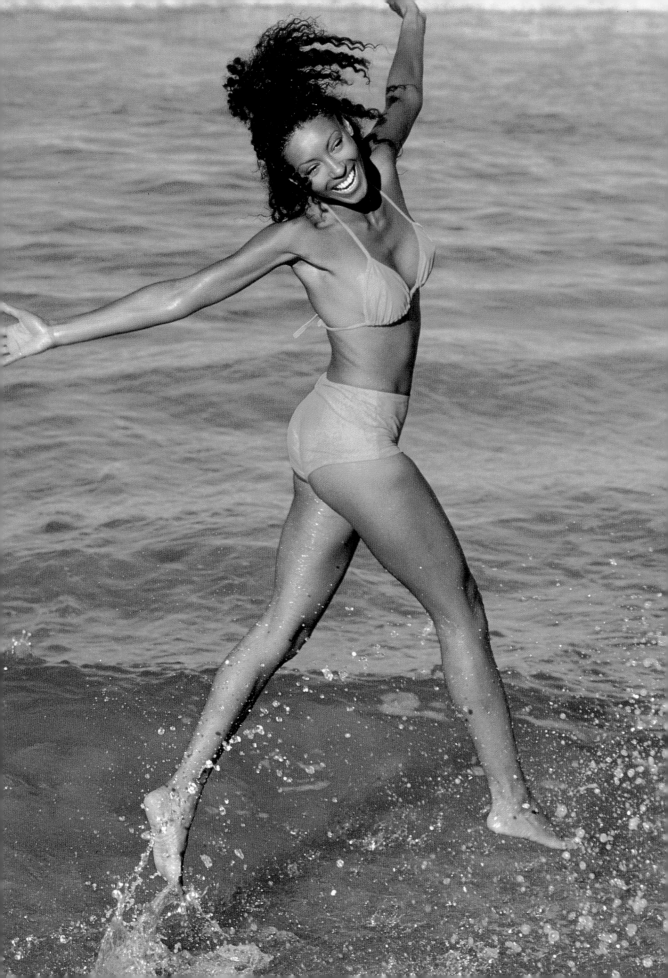

A healthy
lifestyle

Regular Indian head massage can often inspire a greater sense of self-awareness and enthusiasm for a healthier, less stressful lifestyle. As your friends and family start to appreciate the interaction of mind and body they may also show a positive interest in taking responsibility for their own health and well-being. It is useful to be able to offer some general tips and suggestions for a healthier way of life. Do not forget to follow your own advice.

Reactions to Indian head massage

Your massage partner may experience a range of mild reactions, known as contra-actions, during or immediately after an Indian head massage. These are different for each person and may vary on each occasion. Any transient reactions should be regarded as a positive indication that the body is rebalancing and cleansing itself – they are often a consequence of the body clearing out toxins that may have built up over a long period of time.

Common reactions during treatment

These contra-actions can be rather off-putting at first, so be aware of the most common ones and offer reassurance in advance. Once any initial mild ill-effects have passed, your massage partner should feel in much better health.

- Tell your massage partner not to fight sleep. His body needs it. Ensure that you are giving his head maximum support and continue the massage as usual. Gently awaken him at the end of the massage and allow time for him to 'come round'. He may feel quite disorientated for a while.
- It is not unusual for people to become quite tearful, angry or giggly during or after an Indian head massage. This is not a cause for embarrassment – laughing, shedding tears and shouting are wonderfully effective tension-busters and should be encouraged if your partner is feeling tense. Be open to sharing any problems, without being seen to interfere or judge. Be sensitive to the mood and ask if your massage partner would like you to continue or stop and talk. It may prove a perfect opportunity to discuss any concerns.
- Some people can suddenly feel hot and flushed or tingly as blood circulation is increased to the head and upper back. Others may feel cold and shivery as body temperature falls with general relaxation. Look out for body language and tune in to your massage partner's needs. Turn down the heat in the room or provide another towel for extra warmth. If your partner feels light-headed or dizzy, offer a glass of water and suggest that he rests awhile before getting up from the chair.
- Contra-actions are normal and should not last for more than two to three days. Encourage your partner to resist the temptation to suppress any aches, pains or other natural reactions to Indian head massage with over-the-counter medicines. Often conditions can get a little worse before they get better.

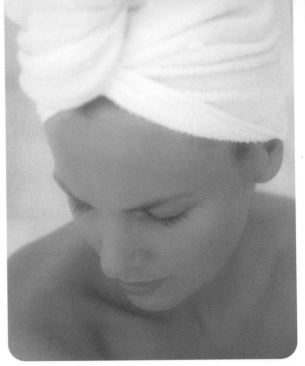

ABOVE **If oils are used during the massage wrap your partner's head in a warm towel for a while before washing.**

Common reactions after treatment

- Some people suffer varying degrees of tiredness. This is a signal that mind and body need rest to recuperate and recharge. Tell your partner not to ignore the signs. Suggest that he goes to bed for a few hours, if possible, rather than forcing himself to keep up a hectic pace of life. This post-massage tiredness usually lifts after the first few massages. Try to make the next massage in the early evening when there is more chance of resting afterward. Others feel a remarkable surge of energy after an Indian head massage – but do warn your partner not to over-do things or there is a risk of getting overtired.
- This contra-action passes, too, after a few massages. It is usually due to the release of toxins into the bloodstream or it may be a response to deep work on the muscle fibres. Occasionally, people may suffer some transient nausea or dizziness. Encourage your partner to drink plenty of water to help flush the toxins through the body.
- This can take several forms including more frequent bowel movements and urination (there may be some change in colour or odour). Your partner may also notice slightly increased perspiration, possibly a mild skin rash and an excess of mucus.

After massage

- If you used oils when you gave the massage, wrap your partner's head in a warm towel for at least half an hour before washing.
- Ask your massage partner to be still for a few minutes to enjoy the benefits of the massage. Suggest she takes it easy for the next twelve hours to ensure energy is directed toward helping the body to heal itself. She should rest as much as possible and avoid strenuous exercise.
- Advise her to drink plenty of still tap or mineral water and herbal teas to speed up the elimination of toxins from the body. She should also cut back on tea, coffee and colas, which act like a diuretic (increasing the flow of urine out of the body), and try not to smoke or drink alcohol for at least twelve hours to allow the body to detoxify itself.
- Heavy meals should also be avoided straight after a massage. The demands of digestion will divert energy away from the natural healing process. Light snacks, fresh fruit or raw vegetables are ideal.
- Your partner should take particular care when driving – deep relaxation may cause her reactions to be temporarily slower. If she feels light-headed, ask her to wait until she feels ready to drive and suggest that she keeps the window open.

Control your breathing

Breathing comes so naturally that most people do not give it a second thought. However, poor breathing can contribute to many health conditions ranging from dizzy spells and general lethargy to heart problems. Calm controlled breathing, on the other hand, increases your intake of oxygen, providing the energy you need for the proper functioning of every cell in the body, including the brain. The circulation of fully reoxygenated blood around the body boosts energy levels, relieves stress and helps you to think with greater clarity.

Bad breathing habits are often caused by a number of factors including poor posture, lack of exercise and a build-up of stress – which can all be corrected with a healthy lifestyle. Restrictive clothing can also hinder breathing, so avoid tight belts and waistlines. The most common fault is fast, shallow breathing, which means that the lungs are not being used to their full capacity. If breathing is not deep enough, inhaled air is not drawn down to the lower lungs where most of the blood circulates. Not only do you miss out on fresh oxygen, but carbon dioxide and other waste products are not being totally removed.

When you are breathing effectively, the movement comes from the diaphragm, not the chest. The diaphragm, the dome-like muscle that divides the chest and abdomen, pushes downward to allow more air to flow deep down into the lungs.

Exercise for energy

Our lifestyles have generally become increasingly sedentary over recent years. We tend to travel by car or bus, use labour-saving equipment and spend hours in front of the television or computer. So it is important to include regular physical activity in the daily routine. Regular exercise improves blood circulation, strengthens and tones muscles, encourages deep breathing, boosts the immune system and helps prevent a number of serious medical conditions including heart disease and osteoporosis. Exercise also releases tension and combats fatigue. Many people who exercise regularly find that they are far more alert and energetic.

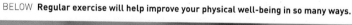

BELOW **Regular exercise will help improve your physical well-being in so many ways.**

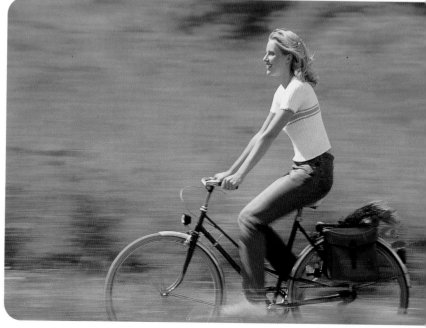

- Lie flat on the floor. Place one hand on your chest and the other on your abdomen. Your chest should be almost still and the hand on your abdomen should rise and fall in a rhythmic fashion. With slow, deep breathing the rate of breaths per minute usually falls from fifteen to about twelve.

Giving up smoking is possibly the single most important step you can take to improve your general health and prevent future illness. It is much easier said than done – but enjoying the benefits of regular Indian head massage may provide the perfect motivation to kick the habit – or at least to cut down. Keep reminding yourself of the benefits of giving up. Picture yourself feeling more energetic, positive and happy with glowing skin and shiny hair.

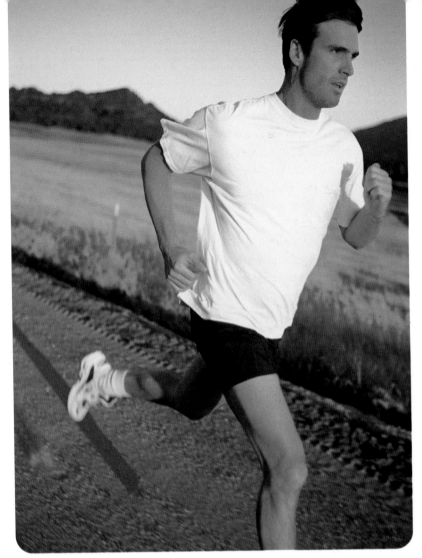

RIGHT **Keep yourself healthy by exercising on a regular basis.**

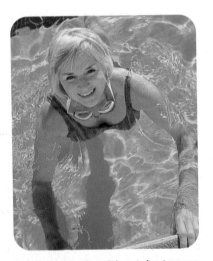

ABOVE **Exercise doesn't have to be strenuous – a gentler activity is just as beneficial.**

Be moderate

You do not need to sweat it out in the gym or on the squash court to reap the rewards of regular exercise. Around thirty minutes of moderate exercise carried out three to five times a week is the recommended prescription for good health. This can be any form of activity that you enjoy – swimming, brisk walking, dancing, housework and gardening are all ideal – so long as it raises your heartbeat and leaves you warm and slightly out of breath.

The suggested half an hour of activity can be taken in one session or accumulated during the day. Even small moves toward a more active lifestyle can bring significant health benefits: think twice about taking the car on short journeys, boycott the escalator, run up the stairs and put some extra elbow-grease into cleaning the windows.

Mind and body exercise

Many people enjoy significant benefits from taking part in an activity that exercises both mind and body – such as tai chi or hatha yoga. Regular practice will aid good posture, controlled breathing, self-awareness and relaxation to bring harmony and balance to your life. These activities also promote flexibility, increase strength and help maintain and restore good health and well-being. Some inverted yoga postures even complement Indian head massage by stimulating blood flow to the scalp.

Are you fit enough?

Walk up and down a flight of stairs three times – about fifteen steps is sufficient. At the end you should have enough breath to carry on a conversation. Stop if you feel dizzy, sick or uncomfortable during the test. While exercising, use the talk test to check you are working at the right level. You should still be able to chat. If you are gasping for breath then you are over-exerting yourself; if you can sing you are taking it too easy.

Get enough sleep

Everyone needs different amounts of sleep. The average is around seven to eight hours a night but we tend to need less as we get older. However, it is not necessarily the number of hours but the quality of your sleep that matters most. If you are getting too much sleep, you will feel sluggish. If you are getting too little, you will feel drained, tense and tetchy. A restful night's sleep repairs and restores the tissues of the body, rests and relaxes the mind and strengthens the immune system. You wake up feeling refreshed and ready to tackle the challenges of the day ahead. When you do not get enough sleep, however, you tend to feel irritable, lethargic and muzzy-headed. Your skin and hair become dry and lifeless and you may start to feel depressed and anxious.

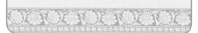

CHECKLIST

EXERCISE TIPS

- If you have any doubts at all about your general health, consult your doctor before starting any type of exercise programme.
- Warm up for five minutes before exercising to help reduce the risk of injury. Cool down afterward with slow, controlled stretches to prevent muscle stiffness.
- Start gently and gradually build up to your target. Vary your activities to stop boredom creeping in.
- Drink plenty of water during and after exercise to replace the fluids lost through perspiration.
- Stop immediately if you feel sick, dizzy or uncomfortable, or you get a pain in your chest or restricted breathing.

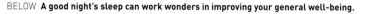
BELOW **A good night's sleep can work wonders in improving your general well-being.**

CHECKLIST

SLEEP TIPS

If you wake up feeling washed-out, the following tips may help.

- Check that your mattress is comfortable but firm enough to support your spine. A soft, sagging mattress can cause backache and tension.
- Avoid eating a heavy meal or drinking alcohol for three hours before bedtime. Alcohol may help you to nod off but it reduces the quality of your sleep. High-fat foods can also disturb sleep as they take a long time to digest.
- Do not go to sleep on an argument. Try to make up before bedtime.

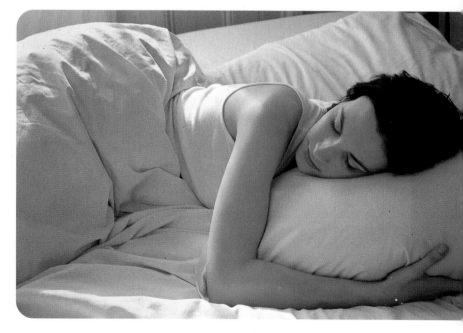

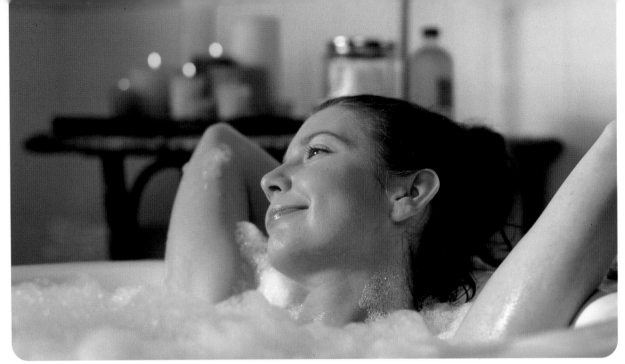

ABOVE **A soothing bath is one of the best ways to relax and relieve stress.**

Learn to handle stress

Stress is an inevitable part of life (see page 221). You cannot avoid it, but you can learn how to manage difficult situations in a calm and composed state of mind.

Try to identify and recognize the circumstances and people that make you feel frustrated, irritated and pressurized and work out strategies for avoiding them or limiting their negative effect on you.

Take five

Take a break during your lunch hour – anything to interrupt the routine and change the scene. If you feel that you are becoming stressed, try to go somewhere peaceful. Count to ten, have a good stretch, listen to some calming music or practise a relaxation exercise (see page 252). After work, take a few minutes alone to wind down so worries do not spoil your evening. Do not miss out on your annual holiday entitlement.

Manage your time

Stress is often caused by things that you know you ought to do, so do not put them off – tackle them now. Try to deal with paperwork and bills as soon as they arrive. However, be realistic about your targets. Plan your jobs and put them in order of priority. Try to allow plenty of time so that you do not need to rush. Learn to say 'no' to demands and delegate as much as possible.

Pamper yourself

Follow the guidelines over the previous pages. A good night's sleep, regular exercise and a well-balanced diet can help keep stress levels under control. Set time aside for yourself, away from responsibilities, to do something totally for yourself. Pamper yourself – book in for a facial, read a book, luxuriate in a warm bath or phone a friend for a long chat. A weekly Indian head massage is ideal.

ARE YOU STRESSED?

When you are finding it hard to cope with the stresses in your life, you may notice the following changes in your emotions and behaviour.

- Feelings of guilt when relaxing.
- Difficulty in getting to sleep or waking early.
- Impatience, irritability, intolerance of others, frequent arguments.
- Low self-esteem.
- Lack of appetite or over-eating.
- Excessive smoking and drinking.
- Nail-biting and teeth-grinding.
- Difficulty in concentrating and making decisions.
- Tension in the muscles of your neck, upper back and shoulders.
- Loss of interest in sex.
- Frequent headaches.

Simple enjoyment

Enjoy the simple pleasures in life – a child's smile, a butterfly floating through the sky or the sun rising at dawn. Smile and be pleasant to others. Surround yourself with friends or family whom you love and trust. Share any worries or troubles with those people you can rely on for positive support.

Have fun

A good laugh is brilliant therapy. A bout of laughing has been shown to relax tense muscles, soothe stress, deepen breathing, improve blood circulation, boost the immune system and encourage the release of 'happiness' hormones. It has even been referred to as 'internal aerobics' because it speeds up the metabolic rate and provides excellent exercise. Search out friends and situations that make you laugh. Re-read a funny article in a magazine or watch a comedy video. Try making yourself laugh out loud by remembering something amusing.

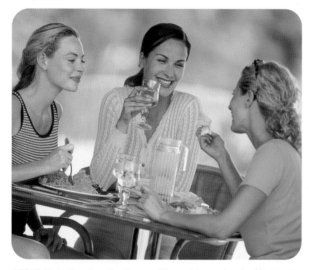

ABOVE **Make time to enjoy the sunshine and have a laugh with friends or family members.**

Enjoy some sunlight

The winter blues are often caused by lack of sunlight. A more serious problem, known as seasonal affective disorder (SAD); with symptoms including lethargy, anxiety and loss of self-esteem, is directly linked with the gloomy days of autumn and winter. Boost energy levels, lower stress levels and balance your levels of vitamin D by enjoying at least 30 minutes of natural daylight every day. It is surprising how much more alert and alive you feel afterward. But do wear adequate protection against the harmful rays of the sun.

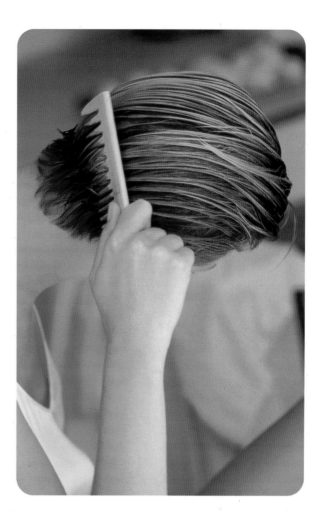

ABOVE **Use a wide-toothed comb on wet hair.**

Hair care tips

Some gentle care and attention with regular scalp massage using moisturizing vegetable carrier oils helps keep hair strong, shiny and easy to manage. Wash your hair frequently to keep the hair and scalp clean and free from debris. Use a small amount of gentle shampoo that has been formulated to suit your hair type. Rinse well afterward to ensure that your hair is free from residue.

Take care

Wet hair can easily be broken. Use a wide-toothed comb. Start with the ends and then work up to the roots. Limit blow drying as this can dry out and damage your hair. Allow your hair to dry naturally, away from direct sunlight, after wrapping it in a towel and squeezing out the excess water. If you are using a dryer, set it to medium heat and hold it a little distance away from your head.

HOW GOOD IS YOUR POSTURE?

Take a good look at yourself in a full-length mirror. Your weight should be evenly distributed, with your feet flat on the ground, knees pointing straight ahead. Your shoulders should be relaxed and at the same height. From the side there should be a straight line that runs from the top of your head, through your ears, arms, hip joints and knees to your feet. There should be a gentle curve in your lower back with your chin neither tucked in nor protruding forward.

POSTURE TIPS

WORKING AT A COMPUTER

- Have your chair – and desk, if possible – set to the correct height, your wrists level with or lower than your elbows.
- Sit with your feet flat on the ground, legs uncrossed.
- Sit square to the computer screen so you do not have to twist. Tilt the screen up a little to avoid squinting.
- Take regular breaks – get up and walk around for a few minutes every hour or so. Move your neck slowly from side to side or in gentle forward semi-circles to release tension.
- To avoid eye strain, try not to stare at the screen continuously. Allow your eye muscles to relax by focusing on distant objects.

DRIVING A CAR

- Check the height of the seat. You should be able to see clearly over the steering wheel without straining.
- Position the seat so you are not cramped and can reach the controls with ease.
- Sit with the base of your back fully against the seat back. Sit on your buttocks, not your spine.
- Hold the steering wheel fairly loosely, with your hands resting a little lower than your shoulders. Do not grip the wheel tightly, with your hands near the top of the wheel.

Brush regularly, using a brush with natural bristles, to distribute the natural oils and stimulate blood circulation to the scalp. Do not be too rough or you could cause breakage and damage, stress the roots and aggravate scalp conditions. Clean brushes and combs weekly to avoid spreading dirt and grime through the hair.

Protect your hair

Avoid using strong hair sprays and setting agents, which can dry out your hair and make it coarse, brittle and dull. Wear a sun hat or swimming hat or use a protective hair agent to protect your hair from the sun and when swimming in the sea or a chlorinated pool. Rinse your hair thoroughly in fresh water after swimming. Both salt and chlorine are dehydrating if left to dry on the hair. Avoid using curling tongs, heated rollers or chemical processes such as perming, crimping or tinting that can damage and dehydrate your hair. Get your hair trimmed regularly to reduce tangles and split ends. Above all, aim for a well-balanced diet, regular exercise and good-quality sleep.

Check your posture

Poor posture while sitting hunched over a computer or driving a car are common causes of shoulder and neck tension, leading to stiffness, poor circulation, headaches, eye strain and shallow breathing. Good posture can change the way you look and feel, giving you confidence and helping you move with comfort and grace. Correcting your posture does not mean adopting a rigid military pose, which can be just as harmful as slouching. Instead, you should lengthen and widen your spine, keeping your shoulders relaxed.

Think of lifting your breastbone to open up your rib cage. Picture your head balanced evenly and freely on top of your spine, with your limbs extending from the centre, allowing ease of movement. Try to be aware of any tensions in your muscles and learn to relax them and realign your body. If you are interested in improving your posture, consider taking lessons in the Alexander technique.

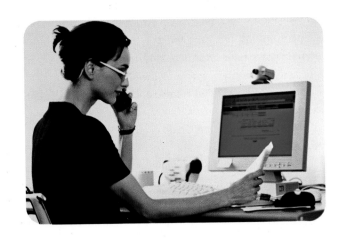

Alexander technique

The Alexander technique was developed by the Australian actor Frederick Alexander in the early 1830s. It is the perfect complement to Indian head massage and helps correct any misalignment between the head, neck and spine. Such misalignments often lead to a wide variety of problems ranging from headaches, migraine and chronic back pain to postural pain in pregnancy and even anxiety and depression.

Birth of a therapy

Alexander found that his voice often became strained and sometimes disappeared altogether during performances and so he began to look for the underlying cause. Studying himself in front of a mirror, he discovered the root of the problem – bad posture. Having taught himself to overcome such bad habits as arching his back before speaking, tensing his arms and legs and tightening his throat muscles, he went on to formalize the technique.

Re-learning good posture

We are all affected by years of sitting and standing badly, lifting and bending incorrectly and even walking tensely. Even turning a tap on and off can cause damaging twisting of the back. Small children have beautiful posture, moving with no apparent effort. However, with age we lose this natural posture. Shoulders stoop, spinal misalignment worsens, joints become distorted and bad habits become entrenched. There is also damage caused by repetitive movements, especially at work, and accidents. We can usually learn to live with minor twinges but for some people the pain of musculoskeletal problems can be severe and debilitating. The Alexander technique teaches you how to identify postural problems and rectify them by allowing the body to re-learn its natural posture. It is not a treatment session, but a course of lessons. The interaction is between teacher and pupil. This is not a massage therapy, and 'enjoyment' is not the aim. Nor is relaxation for relaxation's sake, although it might be the end result. It requires input from pupils, who are expected to practise the techniques in their daily lives.

Therapy lessons

With practice, there is a release of inappropriate muscle tension and a natural realignment of head, neck and spine. The result is a better balanced and more efficiently functioning body. Pain, even gastrointestinal

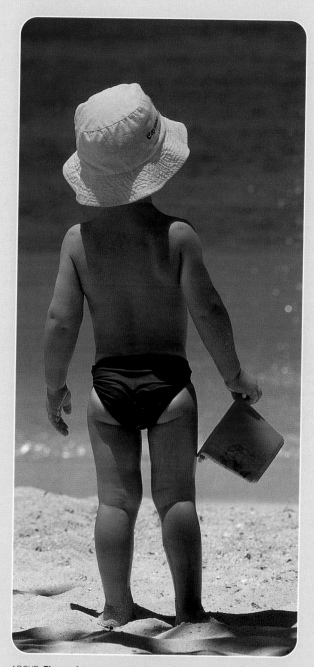

ABOVE **The perfect posture held by a child.**

disorders and breathing problems, can be alleviated. Lessons last between 30 and 45 minutes and a course can consist of anything from 15 to 30 lessons, depending on how quickly the pupil learns and adopts the appropriate techniques. Most doctors these days consider the Alexander technique to be helpful, and even some private medical insurance policies cover the costs of this therapy.

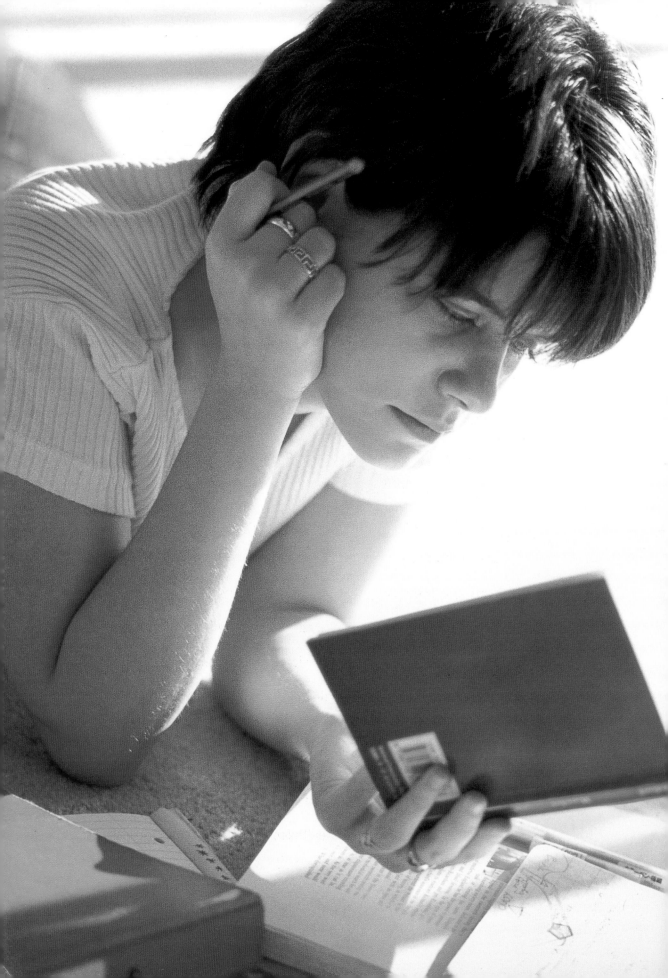

Taking it a
step further

If you have enjoyed practising Indian head massage on family and friends, you may be thinking about developing your massage techniques and knowledge or training to become a professional therapist. There are many short courses and workshops on the subject, run by colleges of further education or by private centres and tutors. Some are also run on a correspondence basis. Courses are structured either for those who simply wish to find out more about this fascinating therapy as a hobby, or those who would like to take Indian head massage more seriously. For many people, Indian head massage can be an extension of their existing qualifications in complementary health, hairdressing or beauty, and may even be a stepping stone to a new career. To find out more information about courses in your area, look in your local newspaper, search the Internet, telephone nearby colleges that have a health and beauty department or ask at your health food store or natural health centre.

Joining a massage course

A course on Indian head massage provides a great opportunity to meet other people who share a common interest in the health and well-being of others. Learning in a group situation, with the guidance and support of an expert tutor, can be an enlightening, inspiring and refreshing experience. You will find that everyone has something different to offer fellow students – new insights, varied backgrounds and a whole range of talents. It is usually good fun as well as being highly informative, and there is the added bonus that students practise on each other.

Choosing a course

It is important to select the right level of course for your experience and aspirations. Most colleges and private centres offer preliminary interviews that provide an opportunity to meet your tutor and ask questions – perhaps about the course curriculum, assessment procedure, facilities or pre-entry requirements. Most courses include practical work, often working on a range of clientele. You should also be taught human anatomy and physiology and the safe use of oils. Depending on the length and type of course, you may be expected to carry out case studies at home, complete homework and sit practical, oral and written tests or examinations.

Do not make any commitment or part with any money until you are happy with all the various elements of the course and feel able to establish a good rapport with your particular tutor. It is often a good idea to look at several centres, study different prospectuses and ask for feedback from past and present students before making your final choice. Do be sure that you have the time and energy to attend all the sessions and tackle the tasks within the course. It may be helpful to persuade a friend or your partner to join you. You will then be able to exchange massages, discuss the projects and boost each other's confidence.

BELOW **Looking the part is important if you are going to be taken seriously.**

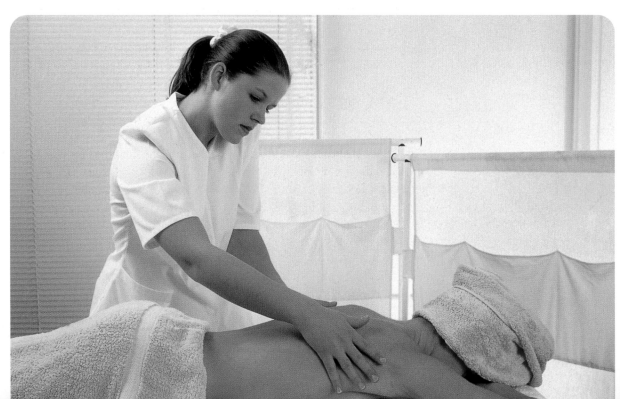

A professional approach

If you would like to set up in business, make sure the training and qualification you will receive are recognized within your industry. Once you have received a practitioner-level qualification, you will then be able to register with an appropriate professional body and obtain insurance. Associations lay down certain obligations including a strict code of ethics or practice and disciplinary procedures that act to reassure the public that you offer a high quality of service. Members of the public are always recommended to check that a practitioner carries the relevant professional qualification, which can be verified by their particular society or organization.

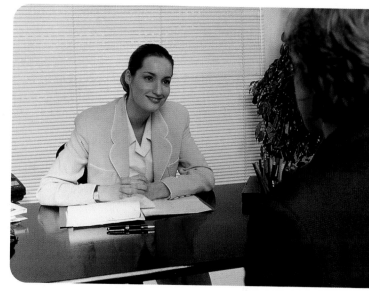

ABOVE **Ask your bank or local enterprise agency for guidance.**

Setting up in business

Many people choose to use their qualification in Indian head massage to set up their own small business. If this idea appeals to you, choose a course that has a business element and provides you with the necessary preliminary information to help ensure the success of the venture. You may be expected to draw up a business plan, which will consider issues such as: whether you will work at home, set up a salon or become a mobile therapist; how you will promote and advertise your business; designing brochures and setting charges; purchasing equipment; obtaining the necessary finance to meet initial and on-going expenses – and whether it is a viable financial proposition. If your course does not offer advice, ask your bank or a local enterprise agency for guidance in starting and running a small business.

Career opportunities

Indian head massage is becoming increasingly popular in the West as a health and beauty treatment, with a wide range of options for trained therapists. It is an ideal stress-relieving treatment to offer anyone who has little time to spare or feels inhibited by taking off their clothes for a full-body massage. Hairdressers learn the techniques so they can include a scalp massage in their regular services. Beauticians are now able to offer Indian head massage using a range of oils.

- Completing a course is just the beginning. One of the joys of taking an interest in a subject as varied as complementary medicine is that the learning process never ends. Keep reading books and magazines, practising your techniques, talking to others and attending courses, workshops and exhibitions to stay up-to-date with current ideas, techniques and products.

Combining therapies

Some complementary health practitioners combine Indian head massage with another therapy such as full body massage, aromatherapy or Reiki, or use some of the movements to relax clients before a treatment such as reflexology. Therapists working in clinics, hospitals and rehabilitation centres have found it an extremely beneficial part of a long-term treatment plan. Indian head massage has also been adapted so oils need not be used and clients do not disrobe. Many therapists make regular visits to offices and schools where they give shorter sessions to help relieve tension before an important meeting or exam, or simply to help people cope with the demands of hectic schedules. Indian head massage is also offered as a refreshing pick-me-up on long-haul flights and in VIP lounges at airports.

Finding a practitioner

If you would like to have a regular Indian head massage, it is a good idea to spend some time finding the right therapist for you. Look at adverts placed in local newspapers and on the Internet – or ask for recommendations from friends, family and work colleagues. Colleges sometimes give special discounts for treatments offered by students as part of their course work – and many clients continue to receive regular massage from these students after they qualify.

When booking an appointment with a therapist it is obviously important to check their level of competence – ask about their training and professional qualifications. Above all, it is essential to find someone whom you trust and respect. You need to feel comfortable and secure with them. A good practitioner will always spend time finding out about your medical history, current health and lifestyle. These details are used to check for contra-indications and work out a treatment plan for your approval. Avoid anyone who offers miracle cures or suggests changing your conventional medicine without consultation with your doctor. Your therapist should have a professional attitude and appearance and answer your questions thoroughly and accurately, giving information about the possible effects.

If you do not feel comfortable with the therapist, try someone else. Trust your judgement. Every practitioner has his or her own personal approach, which may suit some people but not others. Always offer feedback after a treatment so that you are getting exactly the kind of massage you desire – some like it firm and vigorous, others prefer a more gentle, soothing sensation. The choice is yours.

CASE STUDY

CHANGING CAREERS

When Jackie, 52, a primary school teacher, enrolled on a one-day workshop in Indian head massage, she had no idea that two years later she would be a mobile therapist. 'The title of the course captured my imagination,' she said. 'I wasn't sure what to expect but it sounded interesting – and it was something different to do on a Saturday. However, by the end of the morning session I was so inspired that I didn't want the day to end. I've always loved receiving massage but I never realized that giving massage could be so fulfilling. It was like a whole new world was opening up for me – I felt on a real high and couldn't stop talking about it.

Since that first workshop, I have done a series of weekend courses to gain professional qualifications in Indian head massage. I have also trained in full-body massage and reflexology and plan to study aromatherapy next year. The children have all left home now – so it is the perfect time to change career. At the moment, I'm building up my client base so I can combine teaching with evening and weekend appointments but I eventually hope to give up teaching altogether and set up my own salon at home. Being a complementary therapist may not be as financially rewarding as some occupations, but there is certainly a lot of job satisfaction.'

Acupressure, Tui na, Shiatsu

Many Indian head massage therapists incorporate other therapies into their treatments, such as acupressure. This therapy also works on the head, neck and shoulders – as well as other parts of the body – to relieve tension and create harmony of mind and body. Other therapies, such as Tui na and Shiatsu, are also based on acupressure. Each therapy takes a very different approach, however.

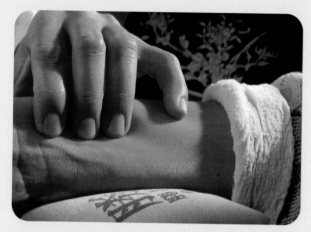

ABOVE **Acupressure is acupuncture without the needles.**

Acupressure

This is acupuncture without the needles. Like all traditional forms of Chinese medicine, it can trace its origins back to before 2000 BC and is based on the theory of 'qi', or life energy. The practitioner aims to stimulate the flow of qi throughout the body, so relieving ills and promoting health and harmony. Working on channels in the body known as 'meridians', the therapist, who is very often an acupuncturist as well, uses fingers and thumbs, and sometimes even feet and knees, to stimulate acupoints and boost qi.

Pressure is often applied in the direction that the meridian flows and acupoints on both sides of the body are massaged to maintain balance. You may feel a slight discomfort when an acupoint is pressed, but the therapy is excellent for relieving stress and can help with problems ranging from arthritis to insomnia and from fatigue to digestive disorders. With guidance from a therapist, or even a good book, you can practise on yourself.

Tui na

This is the name of the most common form of traditional acupressure practised in China and is gradually becoming known in the West. The name 'Tui na' literally means 'pushing and grabbing' and refers to the style of clinical massage practised by doctors in hospitals in China. Like acupressure, the guiding principle behind Tui na is that all pain, whether chronic or acute, is the result of an imbalance of qi life energy.

Exponents of Tui na use squeezing, kneading and stroking movements to focus deep pressure along the qi meridians. This is intended to re-energize, invigorate and release blocked energy and allow qi to flow unhindered. The result is relaxed muscles and pain relief. One of its main uses is to treat pain caused by problems of the musculo-skeletal system, such as a slipped disc. In the West, it is now being seen as a useful alternative to orthodox treatments such as anti-inflammatory drugs, prolonged bed rest and even surgery.

Shiatsu

This is also related to acupressure, although far more robust. Its roots are in traditional Chinese medicine and a belief in qi energy, but it was developed in Japan in the early twentieth century and has been greatly influenced by Western medicine. The name 'Shiatsu' literally means 'finger pressure' and was devised by a Japanese practitioner, Tamai Tempaku, who combined traditional Eastern techniques with an understanding of Western knowledge of physiology and anatomy.

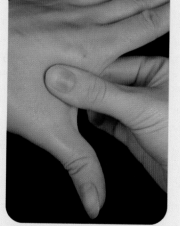

The practice is holistic – seeking to treat the entire body – with treatment usually beginning just below the navel, where it is believed that qi is stored. Practitioners use a wide range of techniques and the session can be extremely physical. Knees, elbows and even feet may be used to stimulate blood and qi flow, employing stretching and squeezing actions to disperse blocked qi and rocking movements to counteract agitated qi. Shiatsu can help with disorders ranging from headaches and migraines to asthma, stress and musculoskeletal pain.

LEFT **Shiatsu or finger pressure.**

Index

Resources

Reading

Cash, Mel, *Sport and Remedial Massage Therapy*, London, Ebury, 1996.
This is an excellent book for massage therapy students.

Cash, Mel, and Ylinen, Jan, *Sport's Massage*, London, Hutchinson, 1998.
This is a great reference for all aspects of sports massage techniques.

Norris, Chris, *Back Stability*, Human Kinetics, 2002.
Physiotherapist Chris Norris looks at posture and the muscles around the spine.

Sanderson, Mary, *Soft Tissue Release: A Practical Handbook for Physical Therapists*, Corpus Publishing, 2002.
An in-depth look at STR techniques.

Organizations

American Institute of Massage Therapy
1570 Brookhollow Drive, Suite 200, Santa Ana, California 92705, USA; tel: 714 432 7879; www.aimtinc.com; info@aimtinc.com.
A California-based school for accredited sports massage training.

American Massage Therapy Association
820 Davis Street, Suite 100, Evanston, Illinois 60201–4464, USA; tel: 847 864 0123; www.amtamassage.org.
Represents 46,000 massage therapists in 27 countries, and funds and reports on the latest research.

International Massage Association
www.imagroup.com
A database of massage therapists from all over the world with links to the healing arts. Please note that the IMA is not a regulatory body.

London School of Sports Massage
28 Station Parade, Willesden Green, London NW2 4NX, England; tel: 0208 452 8855; www.lssm.com.
Runs weekend courses at Regent's College, London.

Southern School of Massage Therapy
Founded by Paul Wills, this school, based in Kingston, Surrey, England, trains massage therapists. For more information tel: 07816 834 705 or search www.ssmt.net.

Sports Massage Association
PO Box 44347, London SW19 1WD, England; tel: 020 8545 0861; info@thesma.org; www.sportsmassageassociation.org.
A new body designed to promote and regulate sports massage in the UK. Contact to locate a practitioner.

Picture credits